To my wife, children and parents
— Floris

To Verony Manders — Hermans
— Tania

Dizzy Me

ISBN 978-90-6299-265-2

Photos: © Manly Callewaert, Pierre-Francois Migeotte, David Plas, Sportograf, Swoosh-e, Tania Stadsbader, Dian Thys, Matthias Van den Hoof, Leen Vandeweghe, VUB, Floris Wuyts

Illustrations: Pieter Rombaut, Luc Sanspoux, Charlotte Van den Hoof, Maxim and Charlotte Wuyts

Kugler Publications
P.O. Box 20538
1001 NM Amsterdam, The Netherlands
www.kuglerpublications.com

Kugler Publications is an imprint of SPB Academic Publishing bv, P.O. Box 20538, 1001 NM Amsterdam, The Netherlands

Cover design by Willem Driebergen, Rijnsburg, The Netherlands

The "VN08" on upper left of the photo on the back-cover is a reference to the eighth brain nerve; the "Vestibulo-cochlear Nerve".

Table of contents

I thought it might ruin my career. But nine years ago, something urged me to begin the online blog that ultimately became this book, hoping that it might help others in my position. I was thirty-eight, married, had three kids, was working in marketing, hyperactive and driven. From the outside, I seemed to be in good health, but for the last fifteen years I had been subject to attacks of dizziness. To look at me, you would *think* I was healthy – which meant my journey towards relief was lonely and difficult. Different doctors offered different diagnoses, all shots in the dark, none of them helpful. The medical profession didn't know what to do with me. Were they even taking me seriously?

I wanted to puncture the myths about my condition. We Dizzy Deans and Donnas are not drunk or crazy. We are not imagining things. It's not just 'all in our heads'. And that's why I wrote my book. I ripped off the mask I had been wearing for fifteen years, gave my disease a face and a name – and the result was *Dizzy Me*. The book sold out quickly, and its effect on my career was, all things considered, more positive than negative. Of course, when I apply for a job I get Googled, and it's easy for prospective employers to learn my history. Which makes them cautious.

Vertigo is a form of dizziness – though not the only form, as some doctors seem to think. It hits you at the most basic level imaginable. Sometimes it pops up out of nowhere, completely unexpected. Sometimes an attack drags on for what feels like an eternity. It robs you of your self-confidence, makes it impossible for you to stand, walk, work or live like a normal person. You are constantly afraid that the next attack is waiting to strike. Its causes are so complex that many sufferers can't get a conclusive diagnosis. And when your illness is invisible, it's hard for other people to understand what you're going through. No wonder that many of my fellow sufferers have been curious about the human being behind *Dizzy Me* and have reached out to me.

In return, my book has reached out to many of them. It has given them hope. But we have still got a long way to go. I want to tell my story to doctors, too, to nurses, caregivers, physical therapists. There is so much work still to be done. And that's why I have revised the book now, and why I have crowd-funded this English translation. Floris, my wonderful co-author, has stood by my side all along, and I remain ever grateful for his support. I hope that the audience we are trying to reach will carefully read his *Handbook for Doctors*, which consists of Chapters 5-7 of this volume.

Nine years have gone by since my surgery in 2008. Today, I feel nine years younger… and I am the proud mother of twins: the third Dutch edition and first English edition of this book I have titled *Dizzy Me. Shedding Light on balance.* And very proud to announce another little sister to be published soon: my first child book '*Wobbly Wilma*'.

— Tania Stadsbader

PS — What started out as a silly pseudonym has become a nickname I am proud of. I am not trying to be cute or inflate my self-importance, but, since it's now one of the ways people address me and refer to me, I capitalize both words when I use it to refer to myself in these pages.

Foreword

Just when I thought I can barely accept the level of incompleteness of this work, my eye drops on a new scientific article or a new insight of which I think it should be added to this book. The one that flabbergasted me today was that there is a significant correlation between the weather and Ménière's disease. The lower the atmospheric pressure and the higher the humidity, the higher the risk for a Ménière attack.

This example illustrates that science is about an emerging truth. Day after day, we try to understand nature, and by performing repeatable scientific experiments and clinical trials, we try to unravel the mechanisms behind certain observations and diseases. Old ideas and opinions have to be replaced with new findings and insight. In case of vertigo, I'm delighted to see that the past decade, many new discoveries have been made to better understand the dizzy patient. The first Flemish edition of Dizzy Me published in 2010, covered only half of the twelve vestibular disorders that I discuss in the current book. The newest scientific criteria of for example Ménière's Disease (2015), Vestibular Migraine (2012), Vestibular Paroxysmia (2016) and Persistent Postural Perceptual Dizziness (2017) are described.

This book also tries to build bridges and fill in gaps. This is one of the few books where the voices of the patients are put together with the voice of the clinicians and scientists. The science tries to explain the cause of the disorders, while the voice of the patients explains how the symptoms are experienced, from morning till evening. This provides a unique cocktail of stories of patients seeking help and trying to understand what is going on in their heads mixed with the pure science of explaining certain mechanisms behind these sensations of vertigo.

I hope this book will help many more dizzy patients to understand their complaints, and to guide clinicians in their search for a cure of the dizziness. It is certainly no rocket science.

— Prof. Dr. Floris Wuyts
University of Antwerp

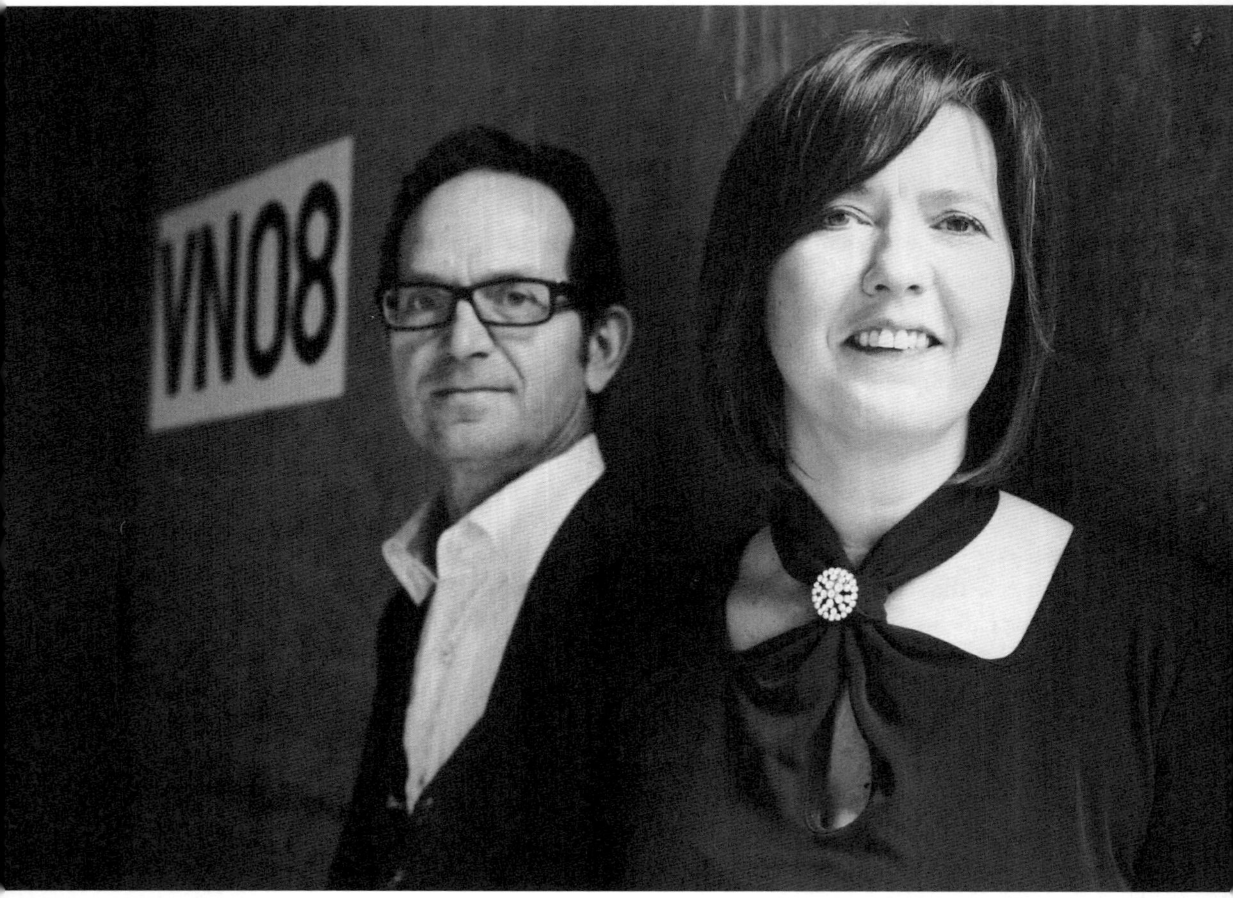
VN08

A party in my head...

... and I am not the only one!

Dizziness is a common complaint in our society, but it's hard to talk about. Why? As much as 30% of the population suffers from it - or has suffered from it at some time in the past. In some cases, the problem is one of balance: 11% of women aged 70 and above and 4% of men aged 70 and above have experienced dizziness which can be attributed to problems with their vestibular system, originating either in the inner ear or in the brain. So my case was far from unique. Dizziness afflicts many more people than you might imagine. The incidence of complaints increases with age - so, as the population ages, doctors will find themselves dealing with it more and more frequently. I didn't make the numbers up, by the way. They have been published by Neuhauser[1].

---

1 Neuhauser, H.K. et al. (2005). Epidemiology of vestibular vertigo. A neurotologic survey of the general population. *Neurology, 65*(6), 898-904.

If I win this lottery, I promise!
I will treat myself to a ride in a hot-air balloon.
I will go to every carnival I can find.
First I will gobble down an order of fries, with a big apple beignet for dessert.
My stomach full, I will ride the rides - they can bounce me up and down and spin me around as much as they want.
I will brave a haunted house and bungee jump from a bridge and loop the loop in a stunt plane.
From that day on, I will not just sit on the sidelines feeling sorry for myself!

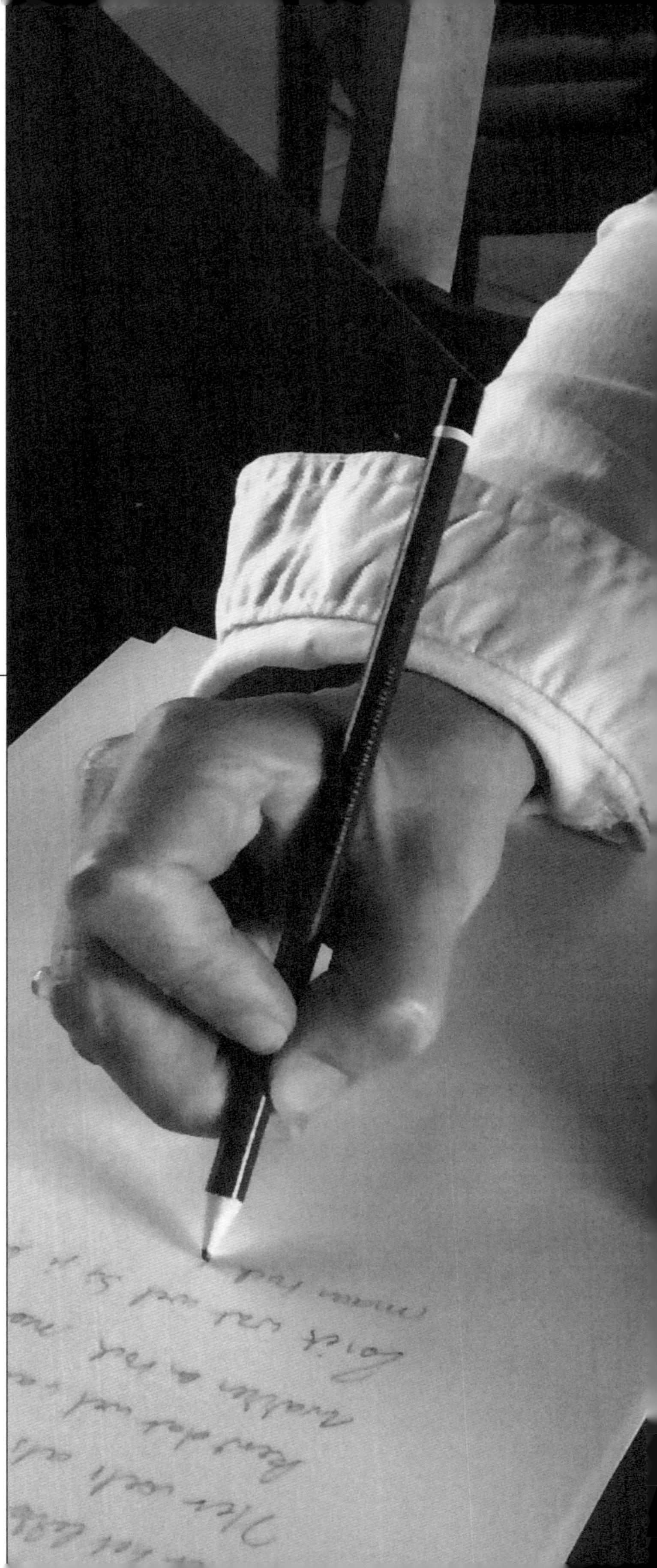

Chapter 1

A Party in my Head

Seven percent of the population is regularly troubled by dizziness. It's not a life-threatening condition, but it has a significant impact on the quality of life. Some types of dizziness show up without warning and are extremely intense, with attacks lasting several hours before fading away. When this happens, you don't dare drive a car, go shopping, or even leave your house. You can look this up, if you don't believe me. And dizziness has so many possible causes. I speak from personal experience: one by one, I have investigated them all.

Party in my head. We owe the fact that we can stand up and move around without dizziness to our amazing vestibular system, a gift from Mother Nature. Until relatively recently, though, in my case that system was far from amazing. And it took years before I was able to learn why. It wasn't until September 2007, after fourteen years of searching, that a vestibular researcher discovered the true cause of my trouble. All human beings, it turns out, have tiny calcium crystals (technically called 'otoconia') in their ears that enable us to stand erect without difficulty. But the crystals in *my* ears might as well have been snorting crystal meth, for all the good they were doing me.

From pillar to post. For years, I was offered incorrect diagnoses by a parade of specialists. Was the root cause of my problem hyperventilation? Did I have a brain tumor? After I underwent extensive brain-function testing, there was talk of Ménière's disease, of Ménière's syndrome, of 'lazy' vestibular organ and a 'deviation' and poor circulation in my vestibular system. Or maybe it was just a hormonal problem, or fatigue, or stress, or something wrong with my neck.

The first person to come up with a suggestion that made actual sense was my veterinarian. Because, believe it or not, it turned out my dog had the same condition! The vet had a good laugh when I told him about my original diagnosis of hyperventilation. Yes, I *did* hyperventilate, that one time, but surely that was just a panic reaction to my first bout of dizziness. That first doctor told me he saw photos of terrified patients, clinging desperately to a table leg, their only lifeline in the middle of a vertigo attack. He was the one who advised me to solicit other opinions.

After the scanner and the brain-function test, I wound up seeing an ear, nose and throat doctor (ENT) for a while. He never had a lot to say, just ran me through the usual battery of diagnostic tests and, every time, asked me if I could still hear okay. Over the next few years, I met a few more doctors cut from the same cloth. They would write me a prescription for Betaserc, apologize that they didn't really know how to treat me – and extend a friendly invitation to come back in a year for another check-up. They each had their own thoughts about what was wrong with me. Of course I also tried manual therapy – but none of it helped.

Full tilt boogie. Back then, I suppose I should have considered myself lucky to suffer an average of only one attack a year – but still, that one attack had to be endured. You do whatever you can to get through it. The people around you doubt that it's anything physiological. 'Must be psychosomatic,' they say, trying to be helpful. And, yes, from the outside it looked like I was in perfect health, fussing unnecessarily over nothing.

But there *were* those occasional crashes – and over time they began to strike with more frequency. The best way I can describe it is to say it felt like somebody grabbed the back of my head and stuffed me into a washing machine on spin cycle. Add severe nausea and vomiting to that, and you will begin to get the picture – and these episodes lasted anywhere from a full day to several days… and sometimes went on for weeks. The worst part of it, though, was the fear I lived with *between* episodes: when it hits me again, what will happen to me? You can imagine the impact this had on my everyday life.

Reaching into a kitchen cabinet for a jar of peanut butter wasn't just 'reaching into a kitchen cabinet for a jar of peanut butter', like it would be for a normal person. Something as simple as leaning back in a beach chair with a good book? Forget it. And imagine driving a car on a busy road and suddenly realizing you can't turn your head to the left or right. That's a pretty serious handicap, right? But my sickness wasn't even recognized as a real condition.

Hormonal ping pong? When I was pregnant with Charlotte, my youngest, the situation became unbearable: thirteen weeks of dizziness! Why? There wasn't anything visibly wrong with me, was there? Unfortunately not. My gynecologist was morally supportive, but there was nothing he could do for me physically without putting my baby at risk.

All I could do was retreat into manual therapy and homeopathy. My condition was given yet another name: 'disharmony in the neck'. Oh, plus poor circulation.

I saw a kinesthesiologist several times. Sometimes that was effective, but other times it left me feeling worse. Strange as it may seem, some of the manipulation was similar to treatments that would later truly help me, but I didn't know that at the time. My gynecologist thought the answer was obvious: 'Once upon a time, you had an ear infection. That's all there is to it.'

During the months of my pregnancy, I could often be found huddled at the foot of the stairs, unable to move - while my son Arthur, my second child, lay helpless and alone in his crib. I was scheduled for induced labor at thirty-seven weeks, in order to release me from my misery 'a little ahead of schedule'. Charlotte had a plan of her own, though, and at thirty-six weeks and five days my placenta ruptured and she was delivered in the nick of time. And guess what? The moment she was born, my dizziness disappeared. Maybe it had been hormones, after all.

Thanks, Google. The vertigo attacks continued to come and go, some of them worse than others. In July of 2007, my friend Linda Riondato died. She was such a sweet woman, full of life, beautiful, glowing with health. I liked her very much, and it was a terrible shock when the letter announcing her passing arrived. She wasn't even thirty, presented the same symptoms as I had. In her case, though, it actually was a tumor. Why her and not me, you wonder - and you comfort yourself with the thought that you are the lucky one…

So I did my best to live a normal life, to work, but the attacks were coming more frequently and, after an especially debilitating episode in late August of 2007, I felt like I had come to the end of my rope.

How long will this one last? How much of a break will I get before the next one? Maybe I should ask for another scan? 'Sweet dreams, honey,' my husband whispers, but how sweet can my dreams be when I am forced to lie in the same cramped position all night, trembling with fear? Will this torment ever end? Will I grow old like this? Thanks, but no thanks. I would rather die.

Well, not really. In many ways, I loved being alive - and I felt responsible for my three little ones. As soon as I was able to sit up straight again, I rolled up my sleeves and - since no one else seemed able to help me - dove into Google on a do-it-yourself research expedition, hunting for a plausible explanation of my illness.

The internet led me to several articles in Eos, a Dutch popular-science magazine, and those articles introduced me to Professor Floris Wuyts. A trained physicist - and a lecturer in physics at the University of Antwerp - he is also the research director of AUREA, the Antwerp University Research center for Equilibrium and Aerospace, a world-class facility specializing in the study of balance. I learned that his department had recently acquired a € 500,000 swivel chair, which was being used to study the vestibular systems of astronauts, who came to Belgium from around the world to consult with Professor Wuyts. Such detailed investigation into the causes of dizziness was only being done in a handful of hospitals around the world.

One unique feature of AUREA, I read, is that they have the ability to map out almost the entire vestibular system, while other labs have only been able to measure about twenty percent of it. Amazing - but no guarantee that the cause of vertigo could be determined in any one particular case.

Why had no one ever told me this place existed? To me, it seemed like my last chance at a resolution. I had nothing to lose. So I screwed my courage to the sticking-place and took action.

Naming the baby. Despite much skepticism, outright disbelief and advice to the contrary - from, amongst others, my doctor - I e-mailed Professor Wuyts a history of my forteen years of misery:

> Dear Professor Wuyts,
>
> For the last fourteen years, I have suffered from severe attacks of vertigo. They happen several times a year and last from two to four weeks. I have gone through various tests in the hospital (administered by three different ENT doctors). They all agree that something is wrong with me, but they haven't been able to pinpoint the cause or determine whether my problem is Ménière's syndrome or BPPV or something similar.
>
> Meanwhile, I have been seeing a kinesthesiologist for manual therapy on my neck, because the doctors agree

that I am dealing with a combination of two issues: a 'defect' in my inner ear and a misalignment of my cervical vertebrae, which constricts the blood flow to my vestibular system.

The kinesthesiologist helps a little, but the Betaserc I have been prescribed doesn't seem to do me any good at all. As I understand it, the pills are supposed to reduce the pressure caused by the overproduction of fluid in the ear, but if that's not the cause of my distress, I am taking medication that is in fact unnecessary and will not be of any value.

My current episode began on August 25, and the last few days I have experienced extreme dizziness, an inability to turn my head or my eyes, vomiting, hypersensitivity to light and sound - there has been no loss of hearing - a feeling of pressure in my head and behind my eyes, and a tension in my neck which makes everything else even worse. This morning I was able to sit up a little, and I spent some time online looking for information that could lead to a lasting solution. This is how I learned about you.

I hope that you may be able to help me to finally identify the cause of my illness and guide me towards proper treatment. Is there a long waiting list for an appointment with you? Would your testing even be possible if my symptoms suddenly disappear? I am guessing that such testing is performed on an outpatient basis - is that right? I eagerly look forward to your response.

With best wishes,
Tania

After that, things developed quickly. I was invited to AUREA for testing. And within fifteen minutes of putting on Professor Wuyts' video spectacles, my condition was finally given a name: Benign Paroxysmal Positional Vertigo (BPPV).

Harmless but treacherous. BPPV is a notoriously disruptive form of vertigo that strikes during certain head movements. 'Benign' means 'not life-threatening', and 'paroxysmal' means that the symptoms occur suddenly. So a diagnosis of BPPV indicates that the patient is afflicted with non-life-threatening dizziness that attacks without warning during certain types of head motion.

This is different from Ménière's disease, different from an infection in the vestibulo-cochlear nerve. It's not a matter of improper brain function or anything of that sort. No, the cause is simply the loosening of those tiny crystals in the utricle, which is one of the two otolith organs in the inner ear. Nothing could be simpler or more boring.

To give me more insight into my condition, I was handed a snow globe, just like we had on the mantel when I was a child. Shake it up, and the snowflakes drift. Pretty! But that pretty drifting is pretty debilitating when it happens inside the human ear.

You could look it up! BPPV has in its turn a cause, but that varies from patient to patient. In older people, it often results from the natural degeneration of the inner ear. But I was only twenty-three when the misery began. A second possibility is trauma to the head – and, yes, I remember a time when I fell flat on my face after a night of partying… but that happened when I was barely twenty-one, two years before my first attack. So let's figure that, in my case, the answer lies behind Door #3: a virus in my inner ear.

This diagnosis meant that I could toss my Betaserc in the trash and consider myself lucky to have been afflicted with the best possible type of vertigo. 'The best possible type of vertigo' might sound oxymoronic, but what I mean is that it's the easiest type to treat, requiring only a certain special physical manipulation that causes the wayward crystals to return to their original positions.

And more good news: BPPV is self-limiting. This means that the symptoms eventually disappear even without treatment. They have a tendency to crop up suddenly and vanish just as abruptly. Which is what makes the condition so treacherous.

Free at last! Professor Wuyts freed me from years of torment – or should I give the credit to Dr. John Epley? When I returned home, I found a physiotherapist trained to administer what is known as the Epley maneuver and scheduled nine treatment sessions. What exactly did this new regimen involve? Well, the physiotherapist, of course, a pair of gentle hands, a vibrator… and a big bill. The vibrator gets those little crystals shimmying and shaking, and the gentle hands execute the Epley maneuver (or the similar Semont maneuver, named for Dr. Alain Semont), which guides them back where they belong. After each session, I spent the next forty-eight hours in bed with my head at a forty-five-degree angle - leave out that part of the process, and the crystals swirl right back towards forbidden territory.

In addition to all of that, there were some circus exercises that made me feel completely ridiculous, plus the Brandt-Daroff home exercises, a habituation therapy that helped reduce the symptoms of vertigo and allowed me to function normally. It was a lot to deal with, but so be it: it really helped. When I asked my physiotherapist if I ought to buy my own vibrator, he grinned in amusement.

Relapse. But that wasn't the end of it. Because I continued to experience occasional episodes of dizziness, my physiotherapist recommended additional treatment. 'This is one for the textbooks,' he said. At my age, I really shouldn't be having these continued issues, and I had to do something about it. Some sufferers, he said, were helped by surgery - but he didn't know what sort of operation was involved or where to get it. So back to Google I went!

A little cyber detective work, and I dug up several articles about something called 'canal plugging,' a surgical procedure that blocks the most sensitive part of the inner ear, preventing the little crystals from drifting into the posterior canal. To me, this seemed to be a last resort - it's not used very often and involves a certain amount of risk, such as possible hearing loss.

Seek, and ye shall find. Further investigation led me back to AUREA, this time to Dr. Paul Van de Heyning, a colleague of Professor Wuyts and head of the ENT department at the University Hospital of Antwerp. Dr. Van de Heyning has spent years studying the pathology of balance, and he is the one who performs the surgery. He seemed to be the man I was looking for.

Another e-mail, again presenting my tale of woe. Might I be a candidate, I asked, for the canal-plugging procedure? I had other questions, too. According to my research, the operation was only performed after other treatment protocols had failed – on approximately 1% of patients diagnosed with BPPV. What were the criteria for being accepted into that elite circle? Was it true that the procedure is successful in 90% of cases, and that only three percent of those undergoing the surgery suffer permanent hearing damage or loss? Was it true – as some sources suggested – that the operation was no longer being performed, and, if so, why? In short, was posterior canal plugging a good bet for me, and, if so, was his team available to perform the surgery? I could have said all of that, I suppose, in a single four-letter word: 'HELP!'

In due course, Dr. Van de Heyning replied.

As it turned out, canal plugging was in fact only recommended in about two percent of cases. Before I could be approved for the procedure, all possible other explanations of my condition had to be one hundred percent excluded.

So I was yet again subjected to countless new medical exams. The doctor examined me, I redid the tests with the video goggles and endured the nausea-inducing caloric stimulation (with cold and then warm water sloshed into my ears). There was the swivel-chair test, the X-rays, an MRI. And finally the discussions of the procedure itself and the final green light, with surgery scheduled for July (another year has passed and we are speaking of 2008).

This top surgeon was prepared to solve my vestibular disorder for once and for all. How? Simple: by sticking an ordinary plug in my ear. I decided to hold off for a while. We were understaffed at work at the moment. I had already waited so long – what was the rush? Things would slow down around November. Let's do it then.

Fixed! It was a long and even a little scary countdown. As we neared liftoff, the surgery had to be rescheduled for a week *earlier* than planned. Just as well, since my situation had taken a turn for the worse. All of a sudden I found myself plagued by issues I had never before and had to deal with: knee trouble, mouse arm, a throbbing headache, a terrible sore throat, a night-time cough.

That last one turned out to be a serious problem. 'You're coughing? That's a shame: we will have to postpone the surgery.' Thus spoke the anesthesiologist, my last appointment before the big day. In a state of panic, I ran to the doctor and wailed, 'Now what?'

None of these last-minute ailments were imaginary. I really did have an inflamed knee, a heavy tingling in my wrist, swollen glands and a raw throat. With a spoonful of cough syrup, though, I figured I could handle the surgery. But: 'No medication before the operation!' the doctor ordered. 'Just relax and stay calm.' That was easier said than done, but starting the countdown all over again was unthinkable, so I forced myself to chill out.

As D-Day dawned, I was filled with doubts. I hadn't had a dizzy spell in weeks. Lying in the hospital in my surgical gown, I felt guilty for wasting the medical team's time. For a moment, I considered getting out of bed and going home - but I am glad I decided to stay put.

Since they were operating on my head, they gave me enough anesthetic to put me way under. I was unconscious for two days. I had not anticipated how much of a toll the surgery itself and then the recovery period would take. Probably just as well: if I'd known, I probably wouldn't have dared go through with it.

Is there a Dr. House in the house? After the surgery, I was so full of chemicals - antibiotics, cortisone, IV drips to prevent dizziness, pills to sooth my stomach, pain meds, a salve to prevent ear and IV-related infections - I was reduced to a pathetic little pile of Tania, sort of like Gregory House without the rudeness and sarcasm.

The poison, the IVs, the irritating pressure bandages wrapped around my head, the muffled roar in my ear… all that led to a feeling of claustrophobia, high blood pressure, heart palpitations, even hallucinations. My room was too small, the bed was driving me crazy, the TV volume was far too loud, the hospital smell, and some nurse shining a flashlight in my face every hour… ugh, it was awful!

Top Gun. But I was lucky to wind up in the care of a true professional. I don't think anyone else could have done as masterful a job as Dr. Van de Heyning. And the care and dedication of my dozen nurses was beyond reproach.

At last I was released from the hospital. Clutching a puke bag in my hands, I stared straight before me, afraid to tip my head up or down. I huffed and puffed, every step a challenge. But I got through it, and made it home without using the little paper bag.

There is nothing better than being home, staggering clumsily from chair to sofa! I looked like a corpse, but there was no pain. Aside from my appearance, the news was all good: according to the doctor, the operation was 'a technical success'. And what a relief: my auditory nerve came through undamaged. When a vibrating tuning fork was held next to my ear, I could hear it clearly!

Light at the end of the tunnel. The point of the operation was to release me from my dizzy prison, but relief was neither instant nor complete. For the first few days after I returned home, I reeled from room to room like a drunk in an amusement park - but apparently that's normal. The ear is full of blood and fluid, and my vestibular organ needed time to adapt to its new piercing. I went on popping pills and holding my head as straight as I could manage, hoping that, in time, my condition would stabilize. A little rest and rehabilitation and, sure enough, it was back to business as usual: back to work, back to taking care of my kids, back to life the way it's supposed to be lived.

So it only took fifteen years for this little guinea pig to get a proper diagnosis, and I did it all by myself! Well, with Google's help, of course. Thanks, Google, for guiding me toward a new and improved life!

**I am lying in a room,
surrounded by people in
green scrubs.**
***One watches me,
one jabs me with a needle,
one - the anesthesiologist -
holds a mask at the ready.
A whole team, all of them
working for me.
Just before the lights go out,
a computer screen blinks on.
I see my own head on the screen,
and then I vanish into
nothingness.***

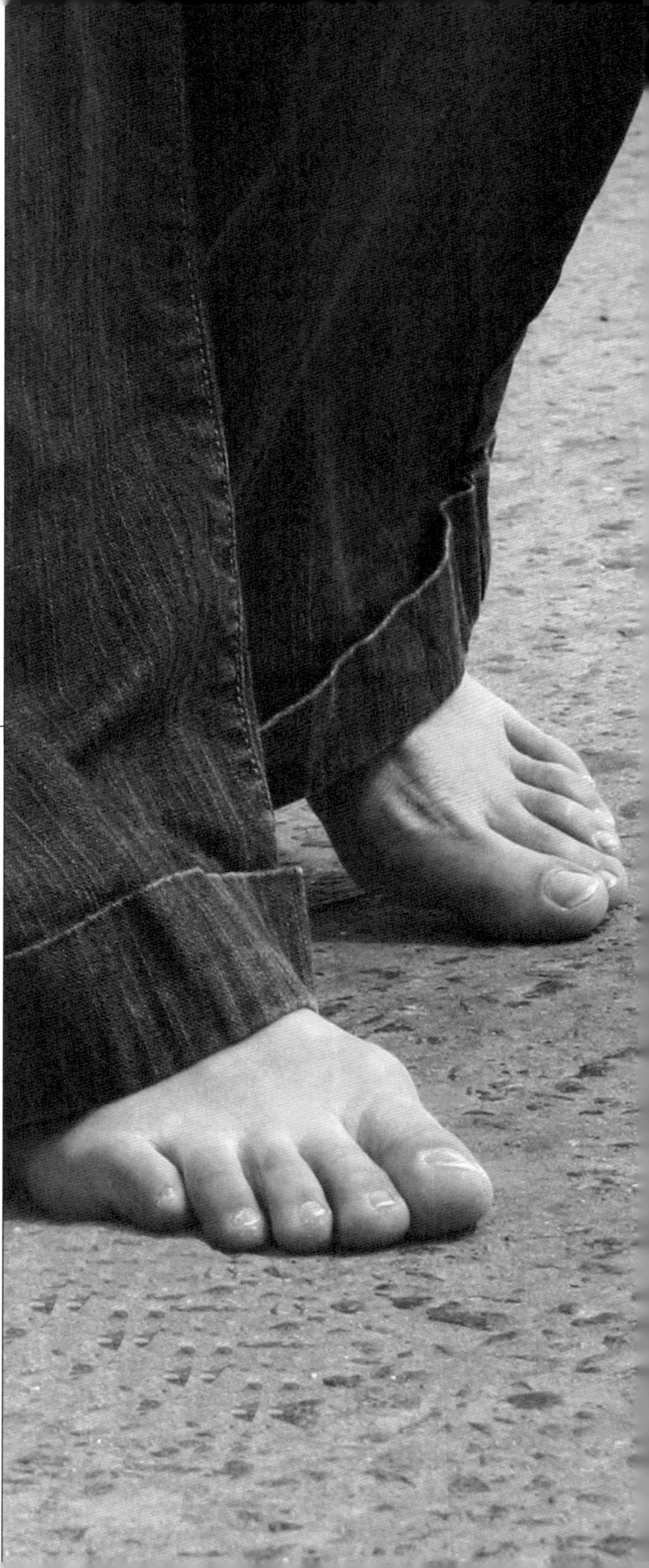

Chapter 2

Step by Step

As soon as I came out of the hospital, I felt a fierce desire to write about my experience. I sat at my desk, booted up my computer, and began a blog - a sort of postoperative diary. Because I was concerned that discussing my situation so openly might put my job at risk, I decided to blog under a pen name, and so 'Dizzy Me' was born.

Like a woman possessed, I launched into the story of my recovery as it progressed from day to day, interrupted by flashbacks that revealed what it had been like for me to live with - and, now, what it was like to live without - my compromised vestibular system.

Every day I hunted for relevant web links, hoping to set others like me on the road to relief. Writing about what I had been through, I found, helped me to process it and move past it. It wasn't until two years later that I had the idea of turning my story into a book.

What follows are my blog posts - my diary - complete with flashbacks. I am sure many readers will recognize their own stories in the pages of mine.

> November 5, 2008

The pajama game. Third day home. I am not allowed to wash my hair. My ear feels like there's a mile of cotton ball stuffed inside. That's just my imagination, I know. It's probably just the accumulated fluids. It's uncomfortable, but in a way handy: when Thomas' alarm goes off in the morning, I don't even notice!

I am still clomping around like a zombie, but I can manage. I am weaning myself from the pills. Don't like the way they make me feel. Thomas says I look haggard, ten years older. He is right: this is definitely not me at my best. But enough about that.

Later, I will try to take a shower. Maybe cleaning up will make me look a little younger. And then I will try to walk next door, see if the neighbor can take me to my check-up in Antwerp on Friday.

I struggle to my feet and get started. Okay, I admit it: I am enjoying the idea of being a blogger.

Stand on your own two feet. Have you ever really *looked* at your feet? Me neither, not until today. I know I take a size 7½ shoe – but I would have been better off with a pair of swim fins when I got into the shower. There is no way around this: if I am not super careful, I will fall right over. Good thing we have got an ultramodern bathroom that can handle an occasional collision. And now I am clean, the last remnants of my stay in the hospital washed down the drain.

The doctor warned me not to wash my hair, but I took his prohibition as a dare. And the Klorane dry shampoo just wasn't doing it for me any more. Speaking of which, I have to tell you what happened yesterday. I sprayed the Klorane – a white aerosol powder – all over my head, and then I saw myself in the mirror and called my long-suffering husband: 'Thomas! Come see what I am gonna look like in twenty-five years! What do you think?' He told me it wasn't all that bad, but he was being kind. Frankly, I looked ridiculous. Hmm, not a bad idea for Halloween!

Anyway, washing my hair was a challenge. Washcloth behind my ear to keep the skin dry, careful not to bump into the faucet and knock the water temperature up to scalding – and all the while trying to remember which direction was the ceiling and which the floor. My hair dryer roared loud as a helicopter, but that was due to the weird echoes inside my head. The whole process took a while, but I did it, and I am proud of the accomplishment, so proud I must have taken twenty-five pictures of myself. At this rate, who knows? Maybe tomorrow I will be ready to cook dinner for the family!

Nightmare on Elm Street. I walked a little today, even tried a few steps on high heels. In for a penny, in for a pound, right? I got out of my pj's and into a skirt and – my head held stiffly motionless – tottered next door to ask the neighbor for that ride to the hospital I mentioned. No luck: each of us has our own cross to bear, and as it happens she has a doctor's appointment on Friday. It's okay, though, I will figure it out. And I was glad to have a little human contact.

'Can I offer you something to drink?' she said. In my circle, that means a glass of wine or something stronger. But this time I had to decline. I am already wobbling around like a drunk, what do I need a drink for? We talked about my condition, and about several other people in the neighborhood who are also dealing with health issues. I need to pay a visit on my neighbor on the other side. She is very sick, not long for this world, and I know she can use a friendly visit. But not yet; I am still too weak.

My neighbor agrees with Thomas that I look awful. I can't seem to focus my eyes in one place; they wander lazily around the room. She decides to dub me the neighborhood scarecrow. That doesn't sound very nice, but, the way she says it, it's really sweet!

> November 6, 2008

On the straight and narrow. Day 4. I get up with the children and join them at the breakfast table. My voice sounds a little better, according to my mother, who checks in every day. I think she is right. My head is still swathed in bandages like a mummy. And I tip over at the slightest misstep. But if I hold myself to a straight course, all is well.

I carefully rinse off a few dishes and pick out clothes for the kids. This helps me feel at least a little useful. Thomas is good at most things, but hopeless at dressing the children. 'Let's hope you don't stay like *this*,' he told me yesterday. I hope so, too - and I am pretty sure I *won't*. The word of the day is patience. I don't really complain, but a hundred times a day I catch myself groaning, and if you add all these little mini-complaints together...

I bow my head to kiss the kids goodbye, and the motion brings me to my knees. I fight not to capsize and moan myself back to my feet. The children are gone. But here I sit.

The real world. Yes, here I sit. It's misty outside. And I can't leave. I am all alone. I can't handle the real world. Not yet. But I have got two weeks before I can expect to be back up to speed. It's funny how something like this changes the way people relate to you: the nicest reactions come from unexpected places, but some friends and colleagues simply drop off the face of the earth.

I shouldn't complain. I have seen it happen before, and it doesn't bother me any more. Everyone is leading busy lives of their own, and people are scared of illness. Now I have a new addiction: my blog. I can't get out and about the way I used to, not yet, so my virtual self assumes a new importance.

Greetings from Virtual Me. My blog has become my anchor. It's funny, looking at the world through the lens of my computer's screen. For the sake of honesty, I changed categories this morning: I am now listed under 'Health'. I didn't want to do that at first; my original tag was 'General'. But what does that even *mean*, 'General'?

This morning I checked out the listings of 'top blogs' – the Top 30 from yesterday, from this week, the Top 30 new blogs, the ones with the largest number of hits, the largest number of comments. All those statistics! It's almost frightening – some of my competitors rack up *millions* of visits. I think I am up to about one hundred and fifty or so, but that includes the eighty times I clicked on the page myself. You can even vote for your favourites, and it looks like I have actually gotten a vote: '100% good', the ballot reads. I haven't got the energy to tackle self-promotion. People who are interested in what I have to say will find me. 'If you build it, they will come.' And anyway, I am mostly doing this to help myself deal with the post-surgical trauma, right?

I'd like to thank my physiotherapist... Suddenly I feel like shouting '¡Olé!' I am walking on air, unstoppable. I have to call my physiotherapist right away. If he is busy with another patient at the moment, that's just too bad for her. Because I have urgent news I need to tell him – and I need to thank him, too.

These last months, I have been practicing the Epley and Semont maneuvers on my own. Driving fifteen miles to put myself in his hands had become too much of a strain. But he doesn't know what I have been up to. Maybe he thinks I am angry with him, when the truth is I owe everything to him. Okay, fine, that's perhaps a bit of an exaggeration.

Another therapist might have rubbed his hands in glee at my need for extra help, cackling 'Cha-ching!' every time I walked through the door. But he is the one who first recommended I look into the possibility of surgery. All those years, and I had never heard that from anyone else. I am so grateful for his advice. For now, I don't need him any more. Well, not at the moment. Maybe I will come back some day for help with my knee or my poor mouse arm...

I will e-mail him the link to this blog. I wonder if he remembers telling me, 'This is one for the textbooks'? Well, here we are! Anybody in the mood for melodrama can log on and enjoy the middle section of my page. Those wanting information only have to look off to the left or right. Not as easy as it sounds, by the way, if you're suffering from dizziness. Anyway, who knows, maybe next week I will try getting in touch with a publisher. I am serious: if I were a celebrity, I surely would have signed a book contract by now. Cha-ching!

Today I feel kissable. Starting right now, I am going to take a selfie every day, a visual record of my evolution. Today I feel attractive enough to kiss. Really! Although I will have to blur the image a bit: I don't like the way my eyes look.

I ought to clean up and get dressed. 'You'll feel better after a shower,' my mother used to say. That was good advice. I think I will take it.

Oxygen and the shivers. I am feeling stronger, strong enough to venture outside. The fall colors are gorgeous. I go out to the backyard to have a look at our bunny and bring my camera along. Maybe I will sit on the swing for a bit. No, I don't think I am ready for that. But I will liven up my blog with some pictures of myself. I am not sure Thomas will notice the difference just yet, but I believe my sex appeal has increased by at least five percent since my shower!

As I head back indoors, I see my nutty neighbor Marcel. He is descending slowly into dementia and stands there trembling. The last few weeks, he is almost always out in his yard. He shuffles around, fiddles with this and that - the other day he actually spat at me. Sometimes he calls the police and, when they come, he can't remember why he summoned them. I am the one who has to explain the situation to the officers.

The last time I saw him was right before my surgery. When I spot him today, I am startled, and my head jerks off to one side. Ouch. The motion almost knocks me off my feet. Careful, girl, you're still not ready for prime time.

Piano Girl. I am going crazy. Sitting here the whole day blogging is probably not the best idea I have ever had. Let me try the piano. The last time I practiced was three weeks ago. If I don't get my fingers on the keys, I will forget everything I have learned. I plan to resume my lessons sometime next week. I ought to be able to handle half an hour. If only I can get a taxi to pick me up. Eek, I hadn't thought about the transportation issue. Any volunteers?

So, the piano. Beethoven's *Für Elise* and a Bach prelude. The sound hurts my ears, echoes like I am in a huge cavern. And I have lost all sense of tone and rhythm. I can concentrate and play, that's no problem. But there's no pleasure in it. Even less, I am sure, for anyone unlucky enough to have to listen. I hope these aftereffects are only temporary.

A little while ago, I heard that someone else here in Belgium had the same surgery a week or two before me. I wonder how he is doing. Felicien, my dear father-in-law, can you check in on your friend Herman, the man you told me about, and let me know?

Tomorrow is my check-up, and I can ask if all this is normal. Hang in there, Piano Girl. Patients must have patience!

Deep-sea diving. Thomas comes home, looks me up and down and says, 'You've got this scary look on your face. Sort of, *Watch out, I am gonna get you!*' But I am right, he says, about my sex appeal. Maybe if I put a paper bag over my head? I know the scary look will eventually go away. It's not my biggest worry at the moment.

There is something else that's been bothering me, though, and now I realize what it is. It's not that I feel like I am in a cave, after all. It's as if I am under water. Everything sounds unnaturally loud, out of proportion, but at the same time muffled. That's it exactly. It's really annoying. I wish this deep-sea sensation would go away.

I get my father-in-law Felicien on the phone and ask him to call his friend, find out if he has had to deal with the same sensations – and, if so, how long they lasted… or is he still dealing with them. Felicien calls me back: 'He has had a relapse. He is in bed, feeling sick and throwing up.' This is not encouraging. But

Herman had his surgery in Louvain. And I am not sure if it was the identical operation or something different. One piece of good news: he did have that divers' experience, but it went away after a while. When he is feeling up to it, he is going to read my blog and get in touch. I wish him a speedy recovery.

Sleepless in Herne. Ugh. What time is it? Only 3:15? Thomas and I are both tossing and turning. I think he is even groanier than I am. I tell him that the sleep specialists recommend getting up after twenty minutes, doing something, then going back to bed when you are tired enough to close your eyes. 'I just went to the bathroom,' he mumbles. He must be exhausted!

I roll out of bed and check my e-mail, am delighted to find a message from the Avenue Louise in Brussels, which is where I work when I am able to work. But uh-oh, my blog has gotten another vote: 0 stars out of 5. Shit, is my writing really *that* bad? When you only have a couple of ratings, one bad one can ruin your average.

> November 7, 2008

The hour of truth. Three little mouths kiss me awake. 'Huh? What? Is it time for breakfast?' 'No, mum, we already ate!' I must have slept right through the clatter. So I have my own breakfast alone. I try to log in to update my blog, but I mistype my user name. I am really out of it this morning. Ditzy Me!

Today is my check-up. My sister-in-law Liesbet is driving me. I am due in at 11 AM. I suppose they will take the stitches out and test my hearing and balance. Actually, I am not really sure. It's a good thing they are following-up with me.

I am doing a little better. My voice is stronger, although it occasionally deserts me without warning. I can walk in a straight line more quickly, and with more confidence. But I still have to take it slow and easy when turning, and when looking up, down, or to either side. That's probably why I come across like some kind of alien life form. I still feel the pressure and that underwater sensation. I am eager to hear what they have to say about that. My head feels so heavy! Maybe I can order a new one?

Another five percent improved! 'You will feel better after a shower, Tania.' Thanks, Mom! I spruce myself up and get ready to go.

Rrrright as rrrrain 3 PM. Finally home from my check-up. A different doctor, this time. He's an R-roller: 'I am Doctorrrrr Zwarrrrt. Nice to meet you. Now, young lady, arrrre you rrrrready? Lie down and rrrrest yourrrrrself. That's rrrrright. You'rrrrrre doing verrrry nicely! All rrrrrright, upsy daisy! Feeling all comfy cozy now, arrrrrren't you?'

He is a typical good old Dutchman. But verrrry frrrrriendly. He launches into a series of questions about how I am feeling. I soon turn the tables on him and start firing my own questions in his dirrrrection.

I describe the deep-sea sensation I have been experiencing, the pressure, the buzzing in my ears, the fact that I am having trouble hearing, and ask him if all of that is normal. Do other patients report similar side effects? Will they eventually go away - and, if so, when? He excuses himself and leaves the office for a moment. When he comes back, he retakes control, and I do my best to cooperate.

'I have rrrresearched yourrrrr questions, and what you'rrrrrre rrrrreporrrrting is quite norrrrmal. You've got nothing to worrrrry about. Now, let's have a look-see.'

Um, it's the other ear, I tell him. 'Yes, of courrrrrrse, but firrrrst I need to examine yourrrrr good earrrrrrr, so I can comparrrrrre it with the one that underrrrrrwent the surrrrgerrrrry. Now, this instrrrrrrument is a bit too larrrrrrge. Let me find a smallerrrrrr one.'

And then he pokes arrrrround inside my 'abnormal' ear.

'This looks rrrrrather good. Of courrrrse, it's still inflamed, a lovely shade of rrrrred. But no sign of infection. Still earrrrrly days, though. Let's find some scissorrrrrs and get rrrrrid of some of these bandages.' *Snip snip snip!* 'That's betterrrrr. Verrrrrry nice, in fact! So, you head on out to the counterrrrr and make an appointment with the doctorrrrr who perrrforrrmed the surrrgerrry. Make it forrrr a week frrrom tomorrrrrrow. And be carrrrreful in the meantime, all rrrrright?'

If I win this lottery… I promise! I will treat myself to a ride in a hot-air balloon. I will go to every carnival I can find. First I will gobble down an order of fries, with a big apple beignet for dessert. My stomach full, I will ride the rides – they can bounce me up and down and spin me around as much as they want. I will brave a haunted house and bungee jump from a bridge and loop the loop in a stunt plane. From that day on, I won't just sit on the sidelines feeling sorry for myself!

No, Adele, I am not coming back. Not until a week from tomorrow, anyway! Thrilled to have my ear free of its prison of bandages, I went to get a coffee from the cafeteria. It's a nice little spot, and they even serve a tasty plate of spaghetti. I know, because that's what I ate the evening before my surgery.

I had dinner at 7 PM, but then I wasn't allowed to eat anything after that. I ate beforehand, though. First pancakes at the Wijnegem Shopping Center. I had never been there before, and I wanted to see the famous playground. An hour after that, a big order of spaghetti with lots of grated cheese. I was afraid I would be hungry, so I stuffed myself. That should keep me going for the next day and a half. That is how long I was going to have to fast – I wouldn't even be permitted a sip of water. The only 'nourishment' I was going to get was my Dr. House cocktail in a glucose IV.

So, a nice foamy cup of coffee, with a croissant and a cookie. My server wrote 'Come back soon' on the bill and signed her name. No, thanks, Adele, I will not be back.

Mirror, mirror, on the wall. Who's got the fairest ear of all? When we got back to Dimitri and Liesbet's house, I asked for a mirror and took a good long look. Not bad, really. Could be worse. Could definitely be worse…

Party time! Excellent! Oh, my dear Charlotte, I almost forgot! Tomorrow is your third birthday. I didn't bake a cake, I don't have any candles … and you are five hundred miles away. But every day is party time at Gramma and Grampa's house in France. What's on the menu, I wonder? Cake and waffles, buckets of fruit salad, a big bowl of ice cream? I know you are enjoying this time with your grandparents. And on Tuesday, Uncle Dimitri will bring you home. Happy birthday, Charlotte!

The secret of my success. I admit it: I am a little superstitious. My birth sign is Gemini, and we twins are known for being lucky. We can bump our heads ten times in a row, but our eternal optimism guides us onward. We stand up straight and keep on keeping on, heads held high.

Song of myself. Yes, I deserve a round of applause. It has been a week since my operation. I get out of bed feeling strong. I am spending a little less time on the internet. I have stopped taking all those pills. I am regaining my independence, even beginning to raise a bit of a racket. Tonight I did what my husband has been secretly rooting for: I cooked dinner! I feel steadier on my feet.

I am ready for the next part of my journey. Tomorrow I will be feeling fine and drinking wine! (Hey, that rhymes! Here's to good times!)

> November 8, 2008

Wait until I am myself again. I celebrated too soon. Yesterday, after I worked my way up to what I hoped was the top of the mountain, I suddenly found myself slipping back down from the peak. Pain and cramps. *Now what?* Ah, my antibiotics. They make me have to go to the loo all the time. Last night, I staggered out of bed and dragged myself to the bathroom at 4 AM.

'Good morning, Scary Face!' says Thomas. I tell him, 'You know what? Some idiot on Facebook says I am not a perfect lover.' He smiles. 'You are a perfect lover. It's just right now I am not making use of your services.'

Take *that*, Steven Haneca, whoever you are. I admit it: I am no sexy Bond babe. I don't have those Botoxed lips, and I will never have that 36-24-36 Barbie body. I haven't even shaved my legs this week. No, I am nobody's wet dream at the moment, not even my husband's. But when this girl gets herself back in shape, watch out!

The owner of my ear. For years, I was nothing but an ear. A body part with its own personal illness. 'Hello, Ear, come on in!' 'See you next time, Ear!' Electrodes attached to my head, bandages across one eye, headphones on and off, cycles of

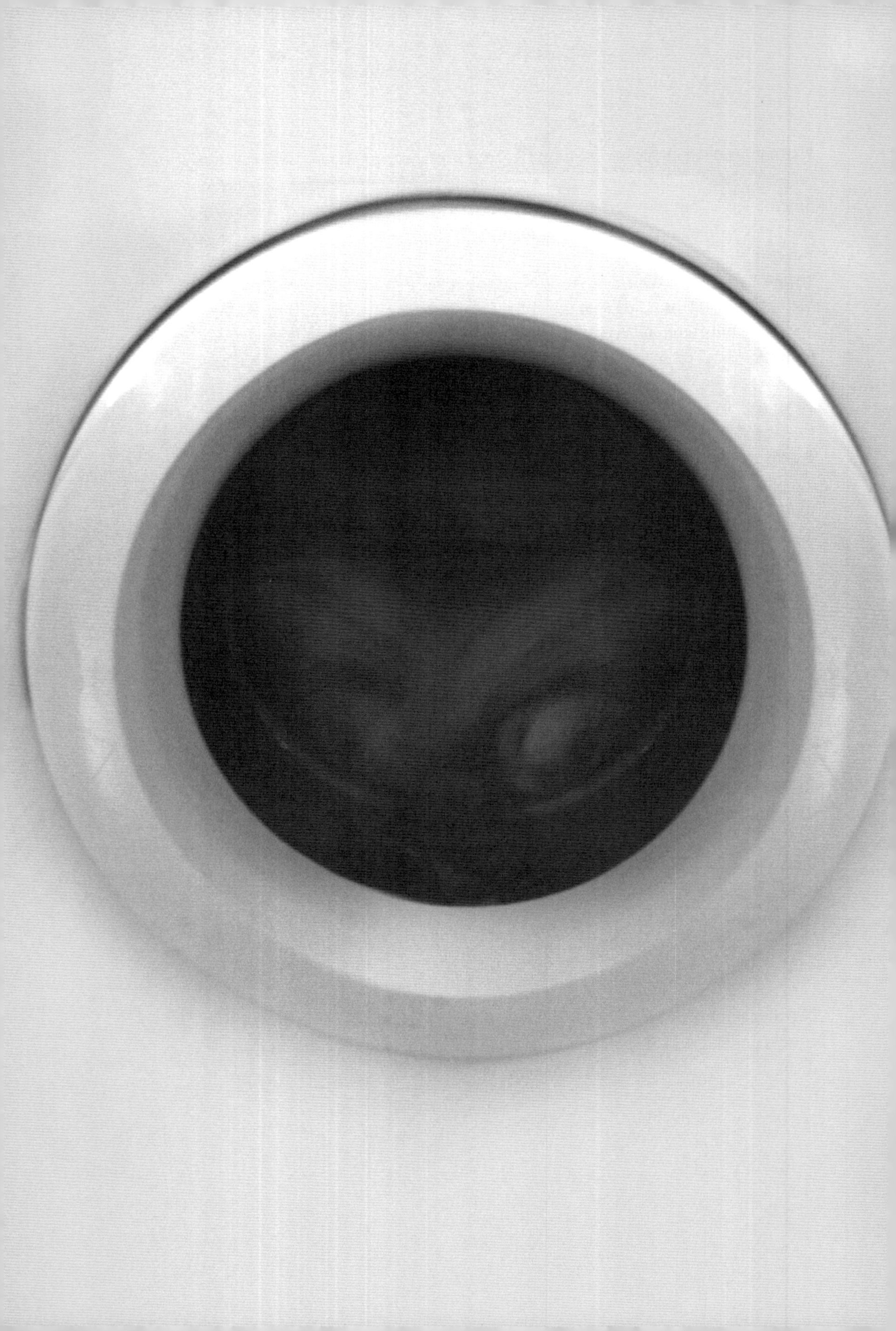

warm and cold water, a pail to puke in. That was all the doctors had to offer me… for years. Nothing but clinical tests and the unintelligible mutterings of the doctor *du jour*. Useless diagnoses, unnecessary pills.

But now I have taken charge of my own condition. From now on, I am not just an ear: I am a person *with* an ear, and I am much more than just a subject for medical investigation. 'Hello, Tania, come on in!' Still not a lot of frills, but at least a friendly look in their eyes, a measure of understanding, a willingness to listen and a few sentences of clear explanation. What a difference! Thanks, gyneacologist! Thanks, physiotherapist and Professor Wuyts and Dr. Van de Heyning! And thanks to the various office staff members, too.

Being sick is an inspiration. Hey. Dizzy Me here. A newbie amongst the blogging sickos. For the last week, I have kept pretty busy working on my online diary. At first, very carefully, I categorized it as 'General.' Then, a little grudgingly, I admitted the truth. And now here I am, already in the Top 10 under the rubric 'Health.' But blogging is dangerous, they tell me. Imagine this scenario: 'Hello, I have BPPV and I am looking for a job.' First thing a prospective employer does nowadays is look you up online. And Google sees all, knows all, tells all. One embarrassing Facebook photo, one ill-considered angry rant, and that's all she wrote.

But I am willing to take the risk. I have got nothing to hide. Honesty really is the best policy. That's why, early in my probationary period at my current job, I went to see my boss.

'I have got something to tell you,' I said, and I filled him in. 'I have got BPPV. I might have an attack tomorrow, and I might not.' His reaction wasn't all that bad. And then, in July, I told him I was scheduled for surgery. But I hadn't caused them any trouble for the year I had been with them. And the surgery wouldn't keep me out of the office for long. If the doctors and my own optimism were right, I would be back before they had time to miss me – and that would be the end of it.

I am feeling better, spending less time focused on myself. Since yesterday, I have begun paying more attention to the rest of the world. As long as things are going all right for you, you don't really understand what it means to be sick. But it's funny how quickly your perspective can change. Since I am thinking more now about other people still wrestling with my condition, I have begun adding relevant links to my blog. Being sick can be an inspiration!

> November 9, 2008

I write a book every night. I can already lie on it, my ear. Not that it's comfortable, yet, but I can do it. It feels like it's full of novocaine. You know the sensation from your sessions at the dentist: you can sort of feel it, but sort of not. I suppose it's not all that strange, really, but it feels strange. Anyway, that's how my ear *feels*. I wonder if Vincent Van Gogh felt like this, after… well, I don't really want to go there.

I can do it, but not for long. I toss and turn like a drunkard, but I can make it through the night. With every turn, though, I get these little shocks, just one or two seconds long. It's not that awful washing-machine effect that goes on and on without a break. I don't feel nauseous any more, don't have to throw up.

But I do get this peeeeeeping in my ear, all night long. When the house is quiet, I really notice it. I have been told that this is what a Ménière patient experiences. I will have to put up with it for a while, as long as the pressure is still there. But it'll go away, eventually. Won't it?

So I do it, lie in bed on my ear. Which means I lie there awake. Thinking, thinking, thinking. After years of keeping silent, now I need to let it all out. And it keeps on coming. It's not that I am making notes, but I just lie there thinking: *I have to write about this insight, I had better pass on that piece of information.* So I write it down, I pass it on… in silence, at night, in my bed. It's enough to drive you crazy. The parts of it I still remember, the following day, those parts wind up online. And for everything I forget, I am sure to come up with something else to replace it.

The stream of thoughts never dries up. I don't know where the ideas come from, but they keep right on coming. I have got a pad on the night table and from time to time I roll over and scrawl a few words - when it's something especially important. *I will have to tell them more details about the surgery. How they do it.* Things like that. Every night, I write a book.

No, I am not going to America. Canal plugging. It's been on my mind for months. Once I first heard about it, I couldn't stop thinking about it. Lots of research, a number of appointments. Would this procedure be my salvation?

I didn't have much to lose. The small chance of hearing loss was troubling. But I knew my kids would be better off with a mother who sometimes had to ask them to repeat themselves than with one who wound up shivering in pain and fear in the gutter.

The worst thing was everyone else's fear. My mother, for example: 'Oh, Tania, you're not serious about this, are you? Have you really given it enough thought? Maybe you're just overexhausted. I was talking with someone yesterday, and she's got the exact same symptoms, but she says it's just stress, and it'll go away on its own.' Yeah, sure, like that will happen. 'Don't you think you should go to America for treatment?'

Excuse me? After fourteen years, I finally get a sensible diagnosis, and now you expect me to go look for answers on the other side of the ocean? What am I supposed to do with my children, lock them in a closet while I am away? And what do you want me to say at work? 'Hey, I am taking off for a while. Going to see a doctor in America.'

No, thanks. My answers are right here in Antwerp. I have made up my mind. I am not going to America.

Oh, come on! First came the misunderstandings. Canal plugging - how does that work, exactly? The phone calls from my mother and brother were always the same: 'They're not going to cut into your brain, are they?' I can understand why everyone was worried. They were probably thinking the doctor would saw off the top of my skull and stir the contents of my head with a big slotted spoon.

'No, no,' I assured them. 'It's more of a back-door thing. They will just jack my little brain up and out of the way and do a little cutting and pasting - it won't take more than an hour or two - and then they will sew me back together. I might have a headache for a while afterwards, but that will pass. They are specialists, it will all be fine.'

In truth, I was a little scared myself. But I couldn't tell anyone that - they would have tied me down to keep me out of the hospital. So it's understandable that I kept my concerns bottled up. That didn't make the situation any easier to deal with, though.

Relief! Another doctor's appointment. When it ended, I left the building thinking, Canal plugging, hmm… And then suddenly my knees were knocking. I went back to the counter and said I had another question about the surgery. 'Take a seat, please, and I will get you back in with the doctor as soon as I can.' I sat, I waited, and eventually I was admitted to see a different doctor - or an assistant, I am not sure which. Whoever it was, he carefully explained the procedure to me yet again - with diagrams and everything - and calmed me down.

Apparently they really do use a back-door approach. Or at least a side-door approach. An incision behind the ear, and they go in that way. No jacking up of my brain? 'No, no, nothing like that. We will go in from the side.' All righty, then. And that three-percent chance of permanent hearing loss or damage? That's a chance I will have to take.

On my side, on my back, on my belly. Ten weeks on my left side. And at regular intervals I sat up at a forty-five-degree angle. During the bad times, I slept that way. If I tried to lie on my back or my right side, everything went topsy turvy, and I felt deathly ill.

So I slept on my left side. A night like that really takes its toll - and ten weeks of it is hell. But what other choice did I have? When the worst of it was over, it was still several weeks before I dared change position. Inch by inch, day by day. I was always frightened: scared to turn my head to the right, scared to glance up at the ceiling.

It's hard to believe, but sometimes I had to cup my head in both hands and force it to turn. Otherwise, I just couldn't do it. It's only now that I am telling anyone this. Only Thomas knew.

Because, you see, what if it all comes back? This is why it was so important I work with the physiotherapist. Habituation exercises. Basic Body Control for Dummies. Sometimes I can go ten weeks without a problem, but then there it is again. Every good night, I am full of wonder and happy as a child: 'Hey, I can turn my head!' Today, I can do it all: on my side, on my back, on my belly.

You will figure it out eventually. I have gotten smarter over the last year. I finally have some insight into the labyrinth, some understanding of when and why my attacks occur. Though vertigo most often strikes when you are lying down, I can be afflicted while sitting, standing - in any position at all, really. And now I know exactly what positions, what movements, will bring on an episode. I think I have even learned to recognize the warning signs. It's hard to describe, but it's as if there's a little propeller inside my head that begins to spin.

Even in 'normal' people, those little crystals shake loose every once in a while, then settle back into place. It's completely natural, as natural as the ongoing renewal of your cells. It's just that, in my case, they take a wrong turn on their road trip through my head. And that throws my entire vestibular system out of whack.

I was becoming more familiar with the map. Bend down to kiss my kids goodnight? Boom! Stand at the foot of the stairs and tip my head back to yell something up to Thomas? Boom! It was as if someone grabbed the back of my head and yanked me down into a huddled heap on the ground.

So I learned to compensate. Need to fetch that jar of peanut butter from the kitchen cabinet? Stare straight ahead, girl, and find it by touch. Time to pick out a T-shirt to wear? Remember: don't turn your head to the right. Just use your hands, and feel your way through the pile. Have to cross the street? Be extra careful when you look both ways.

The people who know me best can see it: my behavior has become a little strange, my eyes are open wider than they used to be. No, mom, I haven't been crying; this is just the way my eyes look, now.

For the last year before my surgery, I learned to outwit my system, which resulted in a lot less vomiting. But I was always aware of the possibility of an attack lurking there in the background. The worst of it was the constant need to treat my own body with suspicion.

Dizzy Me tricks. As I got cleverer, I began to develop a series of tricks that helped to keep me going. Time to get out of bed in the morning? That's a tough one. But if I take it very slowly, lying on my side with my good ear facing down, the risk is minimized. And so on.

If you have got vertigo yourself, you might like to give some of my discoveries a try, see if they work for you. To get up from your bed, for example, first roll cautiously onto your belly. Slowly bring your knees forward. Then very carefully rise up to a kneeling position. Sounds goofy, I know. But it works for me!

My physiotherapist also shared some tricks with me. We agreed that I tend to hold my neck tipped slightly to one side, which interferes with my blood flow. Even if this theory doesn't hold water, your posture is definitely relevant. When an attack strikes, you will automatically tighten your muscles in response, and that just makes things worse.

Here are some of the tricks I have learned:

- The Blood-Pressure Cuff Trick: I went out and bought one. Inflate it, not completely full, and lie down with your head resting on it. Tuck in your chin and curl your tongue up toward your palate. Then bob your head gently up and down against the cuff. This will improve the blood flow in your neck.

- The Towel Trick: I got this one from my physiotherapist, and it has really helped. You take a bath towel and roll it up from one end until you have a tight little cushion. Hold that behind your neck, your hands gripping it right below your ears. Then pull up and forward with both hands. Release, and pull with one hand, keeping your other hand still, first one side and then the other, so that your head shifts slightly to the left and right. This will stretch out your neck muscles.

- The Shower Trick: This one is simple. Stand under a hot shower and let the warm water work its magic on the back of your neck.

These three tricks really help to stimulate blood flow. They are a sort of first-aid kit for the neck, and certainly better than doing nothing pro-active and just lying helplessly in bed! In addition, I learned the Epley and Semont maneuvers, and I have gotten to be pretty skilled in their use.

Will the strategies which have worked for me be of any use to you? Please consult your doctor before you begin to experiment. Remember that you are *not* a doctor, and neither am I. You need to get a professional opinion before taking my advice!

A bump in the road. It happened this afternoon: I hit a bump in the road. Haven't seen a soul all week, haven't heard from anyone, my computer is acting up so I can't send or receive email or work on my blog. I missed my music lesson on Wednesday, and I can't face driving. My good mood is gone, and all I can do is crawl into bed. Half an hour goes by. Then I struggle to my feet. I want French fries. I want human company. Thomas takes me out for a snack. Not far, just five minutes from home. There is a whistling in my ears like the wind whipping around my head on a ski lift. But those fries taste great and, when I get home, the phone is ringing. A voice! Hi, Kristien!

When I paint my masterpiece. I am lying in a room, surrounded by people in green scrubs. One watches me, one jabs me with a needle, one – the anesthesiologist – holds a mask at the ready. A whole team, all of them working for me. It's all so professional. So precise. It's a little scary, the realization that this surgery is so uncommon. Just before the lights go out, a computer screen blinks on. I see my own head on the screen, and then I vanish into nothingness. With a clear view of my skull and his extensive training, the man who's working on my insides makes an easy job of it. And the outside? The doctor respects my appearance. He doesn't shave my head. And his stitching is perfect.

> November 10, 2008

Fire! Today I want to add tags to my blog. They will make it easier for lazy web surfers to find what they are looking for. And they will attract new readers. But the internet is not cooperative. *No signal*, I am told.

All right, then I will play my piano. I will try my prelude again. My teacher says it's supposed to sound like a rippling stream. Good luck with *that*, Tania, with one ear spelunking through a cave!

Rhythm, tone, and a feel for the keys. If I can't get those things back, I will grieve the loss. My playing is worthless, so I try again. The stream swirls. I pummel the white keys, firing cannonballs hither and yon.

A standing ovation for... My Happy Homemaker of a husband! He is just what the doctor ordered. He works all day, and then comes home to tackle his second job. He does the laundry. He irons. He cooks. He cleans. He gets the children dressed in the morning and puts them to bed at night. He drives them to school. He visits me every day in the hospital. He endures my low points, and ducks out to the neighborhood snackbar when I have the munchies. He lies awake at night when I flail around in bed. He somehow manages to keep on smiling.

Today, I will rinse. I drink a glass of wine. Then another. Maybe I will have just one more. 'The kids are a lot of work,' I say, 'but I am glad they are here.'

Arthur is a little teddy bear. Every day, he asks me how I am feeling. Am I still sick? When will I be better? Such a touching little boy, so incredibly sweet. He is four years old. Now Matthias: that child needs a good scolding. If he doesn't stop yelling, he is going to get sent to bed early. And then I will sit at my computer and tell the world all about him. He is eight. He doesn't understand what's going on. I think I have hurt his feelings. I probably should have been more patient. Charlotte comes home tomorrow. We will see how that goes.

The day drags on. Our internet still isn't working, and there hasn't been a single phone call. So I crawl beneath my blankets for a nap. I have got a music lesson on Wednesday. And a doctor's appointment a week from Monday. I don't want to leave the house for either reason, but I will have to set my hesitation aside. That doctor's appointment - I just don't know. I don't want to be a bother. But how am I supposed to get there? I am too proud to ask for help. I will have to take the train and then the bus.

'It's all so depressing,' says Thomas. I bite my tongue. I am always the one who is trying to help. If someone is feeling lonely, I invite them over. I visit the sick, day after day. And now it's my turn to need my friends and family. I check my hospitalization insurance. Maybe it will pay for a cab? Okay, enough self-pity. The phone rings - it's Katrin.

> November 11, 2008

Ground Control to Major Thomas? I wake up full of energy. That's another step forward. By 8 AM, I am showered and dressed and ready for whatever the day may bring. I break out the vacuum and push it straight ahead. I don't worry about the nooks and crannies, but the house still winds up looking much nicer.

Matthias and Arthur will be off playing at Aunt Josiane's this afternoon, and I am expecting company. Then our sweet Charlotte will be coming home from France. My natural good humor bubbles up to the surface… though my ear control and, as Thomas good-naturedly reminds me, my 'ground control' lag behind.

Body Worlds. We never go to the cemetery. It's just not our thing. Competing to see who can lay the prettiest flower arrangement on a grave? No, thanks, I pass. I show my respect to people while they are still alive. In my opinion, we only truly die when we have been forgotten. So I would rather swap happy stories about the dearly departed's lives than shed tears over their final resting places.

I was fascinated by the traveling Body Worlds exhibit, Gunther von Hagens' collection of plastinated human bodies. It's truly spectacular. Of course, I was mostly interested in the ears. They don't have a specimen with a canal plugging, though - at least not yet. They *would*, if I had anything to say about it. Maybe not *my* body - or not my whole body, anyway. Just my ear. I'd like to see my ear in Body Worlds.

The Row Models and the Mud Girl. A lot of traffic through the house this afternoon. Matthias and Arthur can't wait to be off for their play date. I warned Josiane she'd better put in ear plugs. Over lunch, I remind the boys, 'Be good! No shouting and running, no fighting, no teasing. Matthias, are you listening to me? I want you to be a good role model for your brother.' Arthur wants to know what a 'row model' is.

The boys leave, and Kristien and Johan arrive. I have got a cake in the kitchen, but first a little aperitif. My colleague Hilde is also supposed to stop over, but where is she? Half an hour later, the phone rings. Her car is stuck in the mud. Can someone come help her? 'I am not ready for that, yet, Hilde. But Johan and

Kristien will come. When you get here, I will have coffee and cake ready, and that will perk you up.'

Evening, and we are all together: Liesbet and Dimitri, Charlotte and her cousin Louise, Matthias and Arthur, Thomas and me. The perfect end to a lovely day. My nicely vacuumed living-room floor is littered with plastic tanks and a whole army of toy soldiers. I have to be careful where I step. The soldiers are shooting at each other, the air is filled with the roar of plastic airplanes. And of course one or another of the kids gets bumped or poked, and the sound of wailing briefly adds itself to the mix. The chaos actually does me a world of good. All these people in the house are helping me to heal.

And finally the children are in bed. Our family is complete again, and it's back to business as usual.

You complete me. It's a week, now, since I started my blog. This was new territory for me, and I had to take it one step at a time. It's been a lot of fun, and I have been able to get a lot of things off my chest. I set out hoping I might help a fellow sufferer or two, but I never dreamt I would reach so many people so quickly. The best part of the experience has been the comments. You readers bring my blog alive!

> November 12, 2008

Charlotte's birthday. An exciting morning at the breakfast table! On November 8, Charlotte's birthday, she was still in France with her grandparents, so we decided to celebrate it today, a few days late. We sing both the traditional 'Happy Birthday to You' and our own Flemish take on the song – 'Happy birthday to you, in the meadow there's a cow, and the cow says "I love you!" Happy birthday to you!' – at least a dozen times. Hip hip, hooray, and our little girl is delighted. Given my condition, I haven't been able to go out and get her a present. But she doesn't seem to mind: she has got a pile of cards, a pretty scarf, her family around her... and some birthday money to spend on whatever she likes. We will let her choose for herself. She is three, and that's old enough. There are balloons, and there is cake, and today is her chance to be the queen of the family. We even got a little crown for her. Everyone has the right to be silly sometimes - grownups, too!

The plug. My new right ear is now twelve days old. The scar remains sensitive, but otherwise all seems well. Still a little numb, like my lip after a trip to the dentist. A scuba diver under water, a spelunker deep in a cave, a skier riding the T-bar to the top of a mountain. I can feel my heartbeat inside my ear. That funny peeping sound is still there. Is there actual water inside? I gingerly poke around with a Q-tip. No, it comes out dry. But my, oh, my, does that feel strange!

Tania's ear is doing its best. It's searching for balance, but there is a little remnant of a spin. It's deaf, and yet it hears. The pressure remains. I have to be patient. Healing takes time. The plug will do its work.

Music to my ears. Wednesday is music-lesson day. Matthias is getting the whole nine yards: music theory, piano, violin. When I was a child, I took piano for a year or two, but then I gave it up. Three decades later, I regretted that decision and started in again at the ripe old age of... well, never mind that! Now that things are going so well, it's time I get back to it. And we are in luck: Thomas is home today. And I am in the mood, even though I am not very skilled as yet.

We agree to take it easy, this first time back in the musical saddle. We will do the piano and violin lessons but skip the music theory. Everyone comes along, and we bring a coloring book for Arthur. Papa takes Charlotte to the toy store to spend her birthday money, and the boys go in with me. Playing is odd, since I can't really hear myself. Duets with Matthias will have to wait. But all things considered, the lesson goes well. On the way home, my ears whistle a tune.

> November 13, 2008

Mind in a bubble. Here is how I lived for all those years. Husband, children, career, friends, hobbies, self-image and health - all apparently in perfect balance. No worries. That's the way society wanted me to be, and who was I to argue? I even went the extra mile. Because I was Superwoman, a whirlwind of talent and efficiency. I had energy to spare, running hither and yon, up and down, left and right, doing five different things at once and always hungry for more. Don't waste a minute! Charge straight ahead! Keep all those plates spinning!

I hid my handicap from the world, but I was a ticking time bomb - and eventually I simply couldn't go on. It was hard to admit that to myself, but there came a time when I had no choice. They did a scan of my head, stuck a scalpel in my ear, and *freeze*. Everything ground to a halt.

Right now, I am feeling down. I have got a blog, and that's about it. Well, okay, three darling children and a loving husband. The occasional e-mail, a phone call asking me how I am doing. A piano downstairs. And, really, how much more than that do I need? I have got a carefree little life. My needs are met. All I have to do is heal. I could get used to this!

I found another blog I like: *Mind in a Bubble*. It's really well done, and right up my alley. I will link to it.

Elmo's got the moves! Things are looking up. Except for my hearing. Well, and that whole keeping-my-head-in-balance thing. But I am fine if I stand up straight, and I can handle lying down. If I tip my head to the side, though, that still feels weird. So I walk with a metaphoric brick tied around my neck to hold my head in its proper place. It's a crazy image. But it helps. I wish I had more self-confidence.

We are out of peanut butter, and the store seems far away. The car is parked right out in front of the house, but I am not ready to drive. We have got three bicycles, so there are plenty of options. But I pick none of the below. I'd rather walk. But it's raining. The wind whistles in my ears. I will wait a little. Time for my Elmo dance. I turn on the radio. First my arms, then my legs, then at last my head. Let's go, girl, shake that money maker! Come on, everyone, dance with me! Tania's got the moves! Have *you* got the moves? Anytime, anywhere, on the floor, in a chair, Tania's got the moves!

Around the block. The sun is shining. I go for my very first walk. I am looking a lot better, so I figure why not take a stroll around the block? Or maybe I shouldn't. There's a dog roaming free in the street. I am not usually afraid of dogs, but this one makes me nervous. Her name is Tessa. Sounds sweet, but she has got some wolf in her, I think. No, better go the other way. My neighbor Herman's wife passed on, not too long ago. I should pay him a visit.

I am not exactly steady on my feet, but the fresh air does me good. The road slopes upward. It's muddy. I take a few pictures. My heart pulses in my throat. Made it! All I have to do now is climb the front steps. I ring the doorbell. Wouldn't you know it? Nobody home. So I head back down the hill. That's enough for today.

> November 14, 2008

You get no praise with one meatball. A bit of staggering and half deaf, but I still managed to get a lot done yesterday. Played the piano. Went for a walk. Wrote a little. Danced the Elmo dance. Taught my lovely friend Guy Minnebach, who's fifty years young and about two hundred pounds, to chat online. Got a couple of big hugs. And Hilde and Ronny, two of my colleagues at Manpower, came up with a solution to my HTML problem.

Still no peanut butter, though, and I am not yet ready to risk driving. Sorry, Arthur, but you will have to settle for a slice of cheese on your bread. Maybe I will be up for a drive by tomorrow. And there are things I am doing in the kitchen. Today, in fact, I am cooking! Spaghetti and meatballs. I even set the table myself. Unfortunately, the reaction wasn't what I had hoped for. 'I don't like it!' said Arthur. 'You're entitled to your opinion, young man. But you will have to eat it, anyway.' Matthias cleans his plate. Charlotte's with Arthur. At least two of us liked it.

Say what, now? Look what I just found, thanks to my buddy Google:

> Semicircular Canal Plug – Ewald introduced a surgical procedure in the late 1800s termed 'Canal Plugging' where the slender duct of a semicircular canal is occluded in an attempt to block sensitivity of the associated ampullary organ to angular motion stimuli (Ewald, 1892).
>
> It has since been shown, by direct afferent nerve

recordings and alterations of the vestibulo-ocular reflex (VOR), that plugging can be effective in attenuating the sensitivity of individual semicircular canals. It is also known that plugging, as opposed to labyrinthectomy, maintains spontaneous discharge of primary afferent inputs to the brainstem - a property that is believed to explain marked differences in vestibular symptoms following the two types of surgical procedures (Goldberg and Fernandez, 1975).

Since its reintroduction by Money and Scott (1962) Canal Plugging has been used for the treatment of vestibular disorders such as benign paroxysmal positional vertigo and to study the influence of individual canal and otolithic afferent inputs to the vestibular reflex systems.

Until recently it was presumed that Canal Plugging completely blocked the sensitivity of the occluded canals and that partial recovery of the VOR following surgery was the result of adaptation by the central nervous system to use inputs from the remaining functional end organs.

We now have overwhelming evidence that residual angular motion sensitivity by the semicircular canal persists even after complete surgical occlusion of the canal duct (Yakushin et al., 1998; Rabbitt et al., 1999; Lasker et al, 1999; Hess et al., 2000; Broussard et al., 1999). The magnitude of the plugged-canal response increases with increasing angular acceleration and, hence, is largest for rapid or high frequency head movements."

That comes from the University of Utah's Department of Bioengineering website (*bioen.utah.edu*).

The Ten Commandments for BPPV Patients. Use two pillows when you go to bed. Don't sleep on your bad side. Don't jump out of bed: get up slowly and then sit for a moment. Don't bend over to pick things up. Don't stretch your neck too far forward. Don't look up at the ceiling. Be careful at the dentist. The beauty parlor, too. No African dancing. And go to the physiotherapist even if you are not convinced it's a good idea.

Is that a Ginkgo biloba in your pocket, or are you glad to see me ?
The organic butcher called yesterday. He calls every Thursday: steaks or sausages, anyone? So I rattle off my list. And then he treats me to a joke. Yesterday, he had three of them for me.

When he thinks of it, he adds a few leaves to my order. Leaves from his tree, a *Ginkgo biloba*. Do you know what that is? I learned about it, once upon a time. In a former life, I was trained to be a herbalist.. It has been claimed that Ginkgo biloba stimulates the blood flow to the brain and improves the functioning of the nervous system. It's also used to treat memory loss and dementia, deafness, dizziness, headaches and even depression, cold feet and hands. According to those who believe in it, it's a magic bullet for many conditions. But it has also got its downside. Although the herbalist I learned from insists it helped restore his deaf children's hearing, many researchers say it's nothing more than a placebo.

One thing seems certain: a little bit of it will not hurt me. So leaf me up, Scotty: I will steep the butcher's leaves in a cup of tea and see what happens.

Victory is mine! That empty jar of peanut butter! Replacing it is my mission for today. And not just any peanut butter, but extra crunchy. The brand we buy makes a small charitable donation for every jar sold. So we don't buy it just because we like it. We buy it to guarantee poor children have the right to an education and to support organic farming. I can't think of a better reason to pick one brand over another.

It's quiet around the house today. Kind of boring. For the sake of those impoverished children and needy farmers, I will drag myself out the door.

It's only two miles to the store. Still, the idea of the journey is daunting. But I make it, I defeat my enemy: I pull out of the driveway, and off I go, destination the organic grocer. I look left and right when I need to, brave three intersections along the way, even manage to parallel park on the street. Yes, I feel like I am floating, but otherwise all goes just fine. I load up on peanut butter and ready-to-eat pancakes, and toss a couple of packages of modeling clay into my basket for the kids. They will have a fun weekend, for sure!

I am not ready to return home. It's too quiet there. You know what? I will buy a cake and pay someone a call. Why not? So I head over to my old college friend Ilse's mother's house, my second test drive of the day.

But she is not home. Now what am I supposed to do with this cake? But I am proud of myself, and I head back to Chez Dizzy feeling happy about my accomplishment. Arthur's peanut butter glitters on the cabinet shelf. I turn on the radio and make coffee. And the cake? I eat the whole thing, all by myself!

> November 15, 2008

Weekend at Dizzy's. I was surprised and pleased yesterday to stumble across the Dizzy Lounge, an English-language online support group for people with inner-ear and vestibular disorders. It's full of information, and there is also a forum and a chat room. You can find it at *http://cqcounter.com/site/thedizzylounge.com.html.*

And I want you to see this, too:

> The Vestibular Disorders Association (VEDA) is a non-Profit organization that serves people with vestibular disorders and the health Professionals who treat them. VEDA provides information, resources, support, and advocacy. VEDA strives to elevate public awareness about vestibular disorders in order to promote understanding, access to diagnosis and treatment, research, and help for those facing the challenges of living with a vestibular disorder.

They have got lots of information and a network of support groups, mostly in the United States and Canada, but also a couple of chapters in England. Here's what they have to say about canal plugging (or, as they call it, canal partitioning):

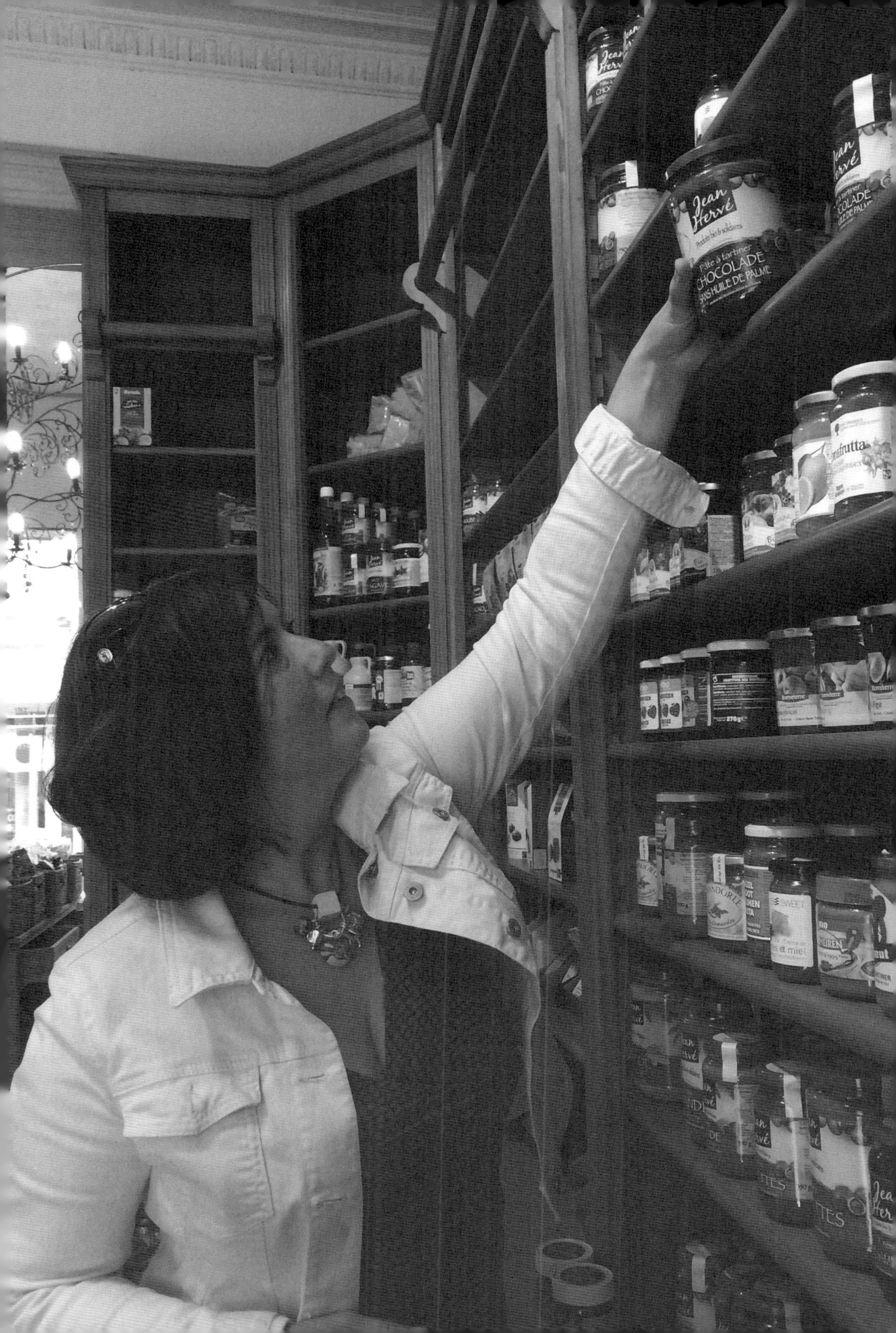
Jean Hervé
Produits bio & solidaires
Pâte à tartiner
CHOCOLADE
SANS HUILE DE PALME

```
The posterior semicircular canal is partitioned or plugged
with small bone chips and human fibrinogen glue to stop
the movement of endolymph and foreign particles within
the canal so that the canal no longer sends false signals
to the brain due to BPPV.
```

You can find them at *vestibular.org.*

Ping pong and the loss of balance during sex. I am feeling a little weak today, so I sit myself down with my laptop. I wonder how people from around the world - Belgium, The Netherlands, a Californian who has apparently lost her way in her exploration of the interwebs - how have they stumbled across my blog? I get some answers from *feedjit.com*, which gives me live insight into my traffic.

Some of the paths people have taken to find me are surprising. 'Kissing someone else.' 'Beethoven inspires *Für Elise* joke.' 'Ping pong illness.' 'Obama joke.' 'Eye reflexes in cats.' 'Recipe for spaghetti and meatballs.' 'Loss of balance during sex.' Crazy as it may seem, all these roads have led, not to Rome, but to Dizzy Me, though none of them really relates to the condition that afflicts me. Maybe I am steering some people wrong with my tags. I might be able to help them, anyway, with my clever Dizzy Me tricks, but the more I think about it the more I wonder. Ah, well. Even if I am not in a position to help you, I can still wish you better health and hope you will recover from whatever it is that ails you. That's what all of us hope, isn't it?

Echo and peep. At Thomas' suggestion, the kids have all gone outside to play. I am not having a very good day. That brick around my neck, the tumult my children carry with them wherever they go, the echoing and peeping. My stupid ear feels cemented shut. I am deaf, and yet not exactly. Sounds seem ten times louder than normal, and yet I can't understand them. It's driving me nuts, and I keep asking myself, *How much longer can this go on?* It's enough to make me bash my head against the wall.

They have gone for a walk in the woods, which gives me a chance to rest. It's almost 3 PM. My computer is threatening to go on the fritz again. Maybe I should get out of my pajamas and into a refreshing shower?

DizzyFIX: finally an answer for vertigo? Well, well, will wonders never cease? Today is a day of discovery, and I have got to share the latest news with you. It's called DizzyFIX, and it offers 'Dependable Relief From Dizziness' with 'No Medication, No Surgery - Real Results.' Vertigo sufferers have to buy it, says the man in the white lab coat. I want to see for myself, so I click on the promotional video… but my computer will not load it. I will watch it later. Meanwhile, you can check it out for yourself at *dizzyfix.com*.

> November 16, 2008

The whole ear and nothing but the ear. A rainy Sunday. Here in Belgium, we celebrate a holiday called Sinterklaas on the morning of December 6, but the good Saint Nicholas arrives - by steamboat! from Spain! - a few weeks early, and today is the day he got here. The kids are excited to know that their Sinterklaas presents are on their way… and I have a present for you that doesn't have to wait for December! There is a lot of solid information about balance, Ménière and BPPV on the University Hospital of Gent's website. It's very helpful material, with lots of diagrams to help the layman understand. One thing that bothers me is the suggestion that 'cutting the vestibular nerve' is mentioned as a possible remedy, though other authorities very strongly recommend against that procedure. Who should I believe? Still, I think the website is worth a look, and you can find it at *een-en-al-oor.be*.

[Translator's Note: This website, unlike the others Tania mentions, is in Dutch only, so probably not of much value to readers of this English edition of Dizzy Me. Literally, 'een en al oor' means 'one and all ear,' and figuratively it means 'to be all ears,' but Tania agrees with me that 'the whole ear and nothing but the ear' is a nicer way to title this section of her diary. FYI, leaving out the hyphens in the URL will take you to eenenaloor.be, a completely different website, which focuses on protecting your hearing while listening to live and recorded music.]

Bah, bah, black sheep! What if I was a timid little lamb? I would still be sitting right here, with my incorrect diagnoses, my stress and hormones, my scandalously lazy vestibular organ, my Ménière's disease or other related syndrome, my aberration or imagination. To get rid of me, the doctors would have handed me some medical mumbo jumbo and scribbled a prescription for whatever wonder drug happened to currently be in favour. 'Thanks for coming in, Ear. Take care, now, and we will see you next time!'

I am not obsessive about my condition, but this much I promise you: I am not going to settle for anything less than a cure. If I was a timid little lamb, I would still be sitting right here, dealing with my difficulty as best I could. But lucky for me I am the stubborn type, and I refuse to be pushed around.

What exactly am I trying to say? It's not fair that we patients have to struggle to get an accurate diagnosis. We need someone to guide us. If we can't find the right specialist, we are lost - and we may lose years to a compromised quality of life. If the wrong doctor sends us off in the wrong direction, there is no-one to set us straight. And those doctors who fail to come up with a good solution for us are reluctant to refer us to anyone else. Are they afraid to admit that they are clueless? Or is all that matters the opportunity to keep on billing us for repeated fruitless appointments?

That's why I am here with this blog. Am I feeling a little better today? Have I taken a step backwards? Whatever happens, I have a need to share it with my fellow sufferers. We Dizzy Deans and Donnas deserve better than we are getting.

Canal plugging explained. On the Ear Institute of Chicago's website, I found the following information:

> Posterior semicircular canal occlusion (also known as posterior canal plugging) blocks most of the posterior canal's function without affecting the function of other parts of the inner ear. Occluding the posterior semicircular canal prevents the trapped crystals from moving inside the canal. If the crystals cannot move, the symptom of vertigo is eliminated.
>
> Posterior semicircular canal occlusion is performed under general anesthesia. An incision is made immediately behind the ear. The incision follows the natural curve of the skin crease where the back of the outer ear meets the skin

of the skull. While working under a high-power surgical microscope, some of the mastoid bone behind the ear is removed (mastoidectomy). Removing some of the mastoid is done to expose the bone surrounding the posterior semicircular canal.

Once the bone of the posterior semicircular canal is identified, a small amount of bone in this area is carefully thinned to an eggshell-like thickness. At this time, a laser is used through the thinned bone to partially seal the posterior semicircular canal membrane, which lies deep to the bone. The laser, in effect, 'welds' the walls of the membrane together. (Use of the laser has shortened hospital stay and reduced the amount of disequilibrium after posterior semicircular canal occlusion compared to treatment without the laser. [Antonelli, 1996])

After the laser is used, the thinned bone is carefully removed to expose the inner membrane of the posterior semicircular canal. The canal is then tightly occluded with a plug made of bone chips and a naturally occurring gel-like material known as fibrin glue. The bone chips eventually cause bone to grow in a part of the lumen of the posterior semicircular canal, which results in permanent occlusion. After plug insertion, a piece of tissue (known as temporalis fascia, obtained from a muscle above the ear) is used to cover and further seal the opened area of the posterior semicircular canal. The skin incision is closed with sutures placed under the skin, which will eventually dissolve. A surgical dressing is kept in place for one to two days.

Hospital stay after posterior semicircular canal occlusion may vary from one to five days. The length of hospitalization depends on the severity of dizziness and unsteadiness that occurs after this procedure. A feeling

> of unsteadiness may last for several weeks after hospital discharge. Patients may also describe a brief sensation of motion when positive pressure is applied to the ear canal or the area behind the ear. This sensation may last for several weeks. Vestibular (balance) exercises (also known as Cawthorne exercises) are started as soon as possible after surgery. These exercises speed up the body's ability to compensate for a loss of balance function in one ear, which occurs after posterior semicircular canal occlusion. Results: Immediate and lasting relief of positional vertigo is very high, ranging from 93-100% for posterior semicircular canal occlusion (Anthony, 1993; Hawthorne, 1994; Parnes, 1996; Antonelli, 1996).

When I read this, I realize that I am completely normal, and it looks like my prognosis is good. You can find further information at *chicagoear.com*.

Patience. My father-in-law came to visit today. I made coffee and pancakes. I was glad to see him.

Tomorrow is a big day. I am due at the hospital at 10:20 AM for an extensive check-up. Liesbet will drive me. I have been hoping my ear would click open by then, that would be lovely. But unfortunately it's still all stuffed up. I will have to be patient for a while longer.

> November 17, 2008

Checked and double-checked. So, that's all done with! I showed up this morning at 10:20 and was done by 1:00 in the afternoon. The hospital was crowded. So many patients! They didn't call me in until an hour after my appointment time, but that's fine. I was given a thorough examination. My ear is healing nicely. The doctor told me that the stuffy sensation I am experiencing is normal. It will last for six to eight weeks, as will my compromised sense of balance.

They tested my hearing. It's not great, but we had not expected it to be. It should also improve over the coming weeks.

From this point on, I have got homework! Enough sitting around the house doing nothing. They gave me some exercises designed to retrain my vestibular organ. Half an hour a day, every day - and they want me to resume normal driving. I have another appointment in three weeks. By then, I should be a new woman!

Down in the hospital basement, I recorded a CD. Well, 'recorded'. They took beautiful pictures of my skull and brain, and burned them onto a disk for me to take home. I can open the images on my computer and admire my cute little vestibular organs. They look like two ballerinas doing pirouettes.

Out for the count. It's 8:30 PM, and our Tania is tucked up in bed. Pretty early for a grownup! I don't understand it: spent the whole day doing nothing, and still I am out for the count. Perhaps it was the ride in the car: it makes my ears whistle, and it's a rough gymnastic workout for my eyes. Or were all those tests simply too much for my system? I had to wear a pair of headphones, with a murmuring on one side and a peeping on the other, both sides running up and down through a range of pitches. At first they seemed to be moving along the side of my head and then behind me, until I couldn't even be certain whether I was hearing them at all. It's been two and a half weeks since my surgery, and I really don't know *what* to think.

So I sit up in bed, semi-conscious, messing around on Facebook. I will add a few thoughts to my blog, then switch off the lights. I underestimated what it would be like to recover from this operation. But give me three more weeks of rest, and I will be myself again. I call work to pass along the news, both good and bad. My co-workers are keeping things running smoothly in my absence. It's a good thing they like me!

> November 18, 2008

Working on my self-confidence. They handed me a three-page document yesterday: an exercise plan to bring self-confidence to my walk. To reduce the visual illusion that I am floating. To bring my gaze under control. To stimulate my sensory organs. That's what it says on the document. To minimize the risk of falling, I need to start out slowly. A wall behind me, so I can't tip over backward, in a narrow hallway so there is support to the left and right.

I think I will skip Page 1 for now. I admit it: when I look down at my toes, I wobble. But I don't have any trouble going up and down the stairs. It's just looking around me, moving my head up and down, tilting it to one side and looking behind me - those are the issues I need to deal with.

A little later, I will go out for a nice long walk. Over the years, I have come to enjoy the behaviors that delay a BPPV patient's recovery: idling in bed, sitting still, swallowing pills. The right program for anyone with BPPV, though, is to learn the habituation exercises and then practice them. Ménière medication? No, thanks. That just makes you sicker. It interferes with your recovery.

I found it hard to master the maneuvers. You are sick, you can't stand up straight, you are throwing up and feeling miserable. So how are you supposed to even get to the doctor, to the physiotherapist? This is why I finally came up with my 'self-service' plan. I wish the medical profession would understand the challenges we face and let physiotherapists make house calls. As it is, a patient in this sad condition first has to get into the car and go to the doctor, in order to get a referral to a physiotherapist. Then you have to get to the next address and sit in yet another waiting room, barf bag in hand. And, oh, those awful car rides! I felt like I was a danger to everyone else on the road.

Ear training. An update on my hearing. The ear is still stuffed. But it will open up eventually. I have already felt a couple of tentative clicks. I get about a nanosecond of relief, and then it's back to abnormal. But I am taking advantage of my existing reality. At least it leaves me with lots of free time! I can sit at the piano and noodle on the keys as long as I like. I hope the noodling stimulates my ear, even though I can't really hear the notes.

Piano time is a good test of my balance: my eyes move up and down between the keyboard and the sheet music, left and right along the ebonies and ivories. The exercises I was given at the hospital are similar, though they involve using the newspaper instead of the piano. But it's really the same thing, isn't it? Or perhaps

I am kidding myself, and what I am doing is of no value whatsoever. But at least I am practicing my scales!

My music teacher has given me a new piece to learn. I like the score. So at least there's something I can enjoy. My piano is my best friend, my comfort. I relish our time together. Our relationship is growing passionate.

An appointment with the Saint. A busy day today. Someone from the power company comes out to check our solar panels and certifies us as a 'green energy' household, good for twenty years. I have to remember to file the paperwork for our rebate at the town hall, but that can wait. Josiane stops by, ostensibly to talk about buying my Charlotte - her goddaughter - a Chérie Camille doll from Corolle, basically the equivalent of the American Girls dolls sold in the US. Josiane shows me a newspaper article about Chérie Camille, and she's decided that Charlotte simply has to have one. But the company is French, and the dolls are apparently impossible to find in Belgium. We poke around on the internet, make a couple of phone calls - and, bingo, we manage to locate one.

Josiane insists I join her for a little stroll. Two women in alphabet-soup recovery, her from CVA (a cerebrovascular incident, better known as a stroke) and me of course from BPPV. Each of us has been told to walk for half an hour a day. I am not sure shopping really counts, but that's what we decide to do. It's almost Sinterklaas, and there are presents to buy. We wade through miles of aisles at the toy store, and before we know it the afternoon is over. With all the things we pick out for Matthias, Arthur and Charlotte, I am going to need that energy rebate!

> November 19, 2008

Back to my future. Today I am writing about making history: I find myself feeling comparatively normal. Yes, that is history in the making. I don't know a soul who's had a successful recovery from my surgery. That makes me an interesting object for study, if I say so myself. I was still a little wobbly yesterday, but today I stand firmly on my feet. When I say 'normal,' by the way, I am not counting my hearing. That's going to take more time. But my courage is back: I can scurry around, on foot and in the car, running my everyday errands.

My everyday errands form a lengthy list, and today I checked off quite a few items. Maybe too many.

But I want to *count* again, to make myself useful, to re-engage with people and with my life. By the end of the day I am exhausted, but I am glad I got out of the house. Yesterday I gave Thomas the green light to go back to work in the mornings. I can handle the kids, I promised him. So this morning he hands me back my taxi-driver's cap and off he goes - and I am responsible for getting my effervescent trio to school. It's not far. I stick to the back roads and have no trouble. I have to concentrate, especially on keeping my gaze stable. Matthias isn't ready to trust me, yet, but I reassure him.

We get there, safe and sound. And now I am beat. Wednesday is normally my day off, but sometimes I wonder what 'off' really means. I volunteer at the elementary school in the morning, helping the children with their reading. Since my surgery, I have had to beg off, but today I am back.

Manhunt. I think I have found someone else who has suffered from my complaint and undergone the same operation. There are so many variations of dizziness, so many possible treatments. But, according to my sources, this man's case is quite similar to mine, although he is several decades older. I am very curious, intrigued. He had his surgery in Louvain and, from what I have heard, it didn't go as well as mine. He has since relapsed, though I don't know how seriously. It has to be pretty serious, since there is talk of a second procedure. I want to hear about it from *him*, not second-hand. Comparing our experiences should be interesting.

> November 20, 2008

Three weeks on. Tomorrow it will be three weeks since my canal plugging. My ear really seems to be adjusting to the plug. The only problem comes when I tilt my head to the side, and even that's not so bad. I took a brief drive to mail a letter and submit my energy-rebate form, and that was about all for today. In the car, I kept being startled by oncoming vehicles. Very strange.

I am going to give up on the 'homework' exercises. They're so boring! I have worked out my own training program, and that I will stick with. I spent some time playing the piano today. Now I need to change the bedsheets and maybe catch up a bit on my housekeeping. But the sun is shining, so I will definitely have to find time for a good long walk. I need that. I am coming down with a bad cold, though. Thanks, kids! My ear remains stuffed up.

Dear Diary. Here is what I did today: piano, cleaned the house a little, took a walk, saw some people. While walking, I ran into several of my neighbors. Herman made me a cup of coffee. I chatted with Bernard, and also with Johan, my neighbor Marcel's son. His mother is back in the hospital: cancer. Maybe I will go see her.

I cooked dinner this evening, but the kids didn't really like it. A brief visit from Inge, who used to share an office with me, and day was done. Oh, I made a yummy chocolate mousse, and *that* was a hit.

Who's that knocking at my blog? Who visited my blog today? Several people hoping to win lottery numbers or a good recipe for spaghetti and meatballs. Statcounter and Feedjit see all and tell all. Not who you are, exactly, but where you come from and what brought you to my URL, the search parameters that led you to me and the length of your visit. I can also see where you go when you leave me, which of my links you follow. The information encourages me. The fact that you are making use of the links I provide is a good sign.

Did you find something useful? If so, then I have done my job. Oh, by the way, I have discovered another website that gives handy tips for living with BPPV: *mtchuizen.com*. Lots of good information and illustrations, but it's all in Dutch.

> November 21, 2008

Blood, snot and tears? Well, no blood, really, but you could definitely rename us the Snotnose family. We have all got the same lousy cold, and it's a tossup which of us is suffering the most. Charlotte is certainly making the biggest fuss, but she is the youngest, so she has got an excuse. My throat is prickly. My ears are stuffed. At least Bartolomeo Eustachi's tube protects me from Charlotte's howling. With a lot of drama, I get the kids into the car so Thomas can drive them to school. In all the confusion, one of them forgets to bring a jacket, and Thomas has to turn around and come home to get it. Some calves have broken out of their corral, forcing him to take a detour. Lady Luck is certainly frowning down on him today. He is on his way to work, but running very late. I hope his co-workers will be patient.

Cuckoo for Koocook. Yesterday's experience in the kitchen was less than satisfying. Today, I am simply not in the mood. The kids settle for sandwiches, and I decide to try something special for my better half and myself. I consult *koocook.com*, a French-language recipe site, for inspiration. They ask me to identify three things I have got in the fridge: a zucchini, an eggplant, and some mushrooms, all of which really need to get eaten before they go bad. Sure enough, the website comes through, and I prepare a lovely Gratin Saveur du Sud:

> *Grease a baking dish with olive oil. Cut the vegetables into slices and layer them in the dish, seasoning each layer with salt, pepper and herbs. Top with mozzarella cheese and a can of tomato juice. Bake at 400° for about 40 minutes, then broil for an additional 10 minutes. Serve with bread.*

That sounds pretty good. I will try it!

Give us this day our daily walk. Josiane comes by to tempt me out of my cave with an offer of lunch. And who do you think our server turns out to be? My own uncle! I hadn't seen him in ages. No family squabble or anything like that. It's just that my extended family doesn't really go out of our way to stay in touch.

After we eat, Josiane and I pick up Charlotte's doll. Our daily walk, remember? Bend over, look up, glance to each side … second nature for most, still a challenge for me. But at least it doesn't make me sick. Every once in a while I put my foot down wrong, like a drunkard. We both find that funny, and I say, 'I hope I can do better than this when I am old, otherwise I will fall and break a hip!'

> November 22, 2008

A bitter pill. Pfizer has come up with a new stunt. They have placed a banner on the health blogs, with a flock of flying pills and this message: 'A thousand thanks. Without you, there would be no such thing as medicine!' On some blogs, that slogan will be a bitter pill to swallow. What if the reader is suffering from an incurable illness? Advertising can be a dangerous business.

One of my blogger colleagues, who identifies herself as 'livingwithlupus,' had this to say:

> How am I supposed to respond to this, Pfizer? Am I supposed to be happy? There is no medication specifically for lupus. It's an 'orphan' illness. We rely on medicines developed for other illnesses that coincidentally happen to help us with our symptoms. And why is that, would you say? Because you refuse to fund research into lupus. You could, but there simply aren't enough sufferers to make it worth your while. Of course, you could make a world of difference to us. We would be thrilled to say 'Ten billion thanks. Without you, we wouldn't have a cure!' Sorry, but I had to get that off my chest.

She has got a point, in my opinion. Sick people are consumers; the pharmaceutical industry is the last business that will ever go bust. As long as they invest in research into the 'big' diseases, the ones that will make their cash registers overflow with profits. For BPPV, of course, medication is pointless.
I agree one hundred percent with a very interesting article I found on *azlink.be*:

> There's little point in trying to treat BPPV with pharmaceuticals, since the condition has a purely mechanical cause: crystals drift to the wrong part of the vestibular organ, and must be returned to their proper position with specific spiral or swaying movement. When the proper maneuvers are practiced, the success rate is 80-100%.

As my neighbor Herman says, the doctors have become technical experts - lucky for me! - but when it comes to personal chemistry they have little to offer, and they don't seem to be getting much smarter.

Our Dutch neighbors. In The Netherlands, a dizzy patient can find help at the Apeldoorns Duizeligheidscentrum (the Vertigo Center in Apeldoorn). The ADC is a national resource for people complaining of dizziness. Various disciplines work together there. Such collaborative practice increases the chance of identifying the cause of the complaint - which in turn makes more effective treatment possible. In addition to the usual protocols, they have experience with more specialised therapies, such as the canalith-repositioning procedure for BBPV, gentamicin therapy for Ménière's disease, and vestibular rehabilitation for failures of the vestibular organ. The ADC conducts ongoing research into the vestibular system, and has recently been working with posturography, a new investigatory technique. Theirs is yet another Dutch-only website, but if you are interested in taking a look you will find it at *duizeligheidscentrum.nl.*

Write your own adventure. I found the following at *kennislink.nl*:

It's hard to describe how dizziness feels. One person may say he loses his balance, feels drunk. Another may call it a sense of lightheadedness and say she sees black spots before her eyes. Still others may experience whirling around in a circle - or seem to see the world spinning around them. These varied reports are due at least in part to the fact that dizziness can have various different causes, each accompanied by its own distinct set of symptoms.

An important part of the process of bringing your dizziness under control is the telling of your story. Often, your personal narrative can help your doctor to diagnose the cause of your condition - and suggest which tests are appropriate in your case. So it's a good idea to make notes about your experience before you go to see your doctor. That will simplify the search for an explanation.

When you write your story, consider the following questions:

- What does your dizziness feel like?
- Does it feel like your head or your entire body is spinning?

- Are your surroundings revolving around you?
- Do you have a tendency to fall, or do you feel as if you're falling?
- Are you lightheaded?
- Do you sway or wobble when standing or walking?
- What effect does the passage of time have on your symptoms?
- Did your condition appear suddenly or develop gradually?
- How long ago did you first experience the dizziness?
- Is the dizziness constant, or does it come and go?
- Are there circumstances the cause the symptoms to develop or get worse?
- Does the dizziness depend on how you move your head?
- Do the symptoms appear in bed, when you stand up, or while walking?
- Do you experience dizziness in crowded stores or at work?
- Are there other symptoms, such as problems with your ears?
- Have you experienced hearing loss on one or both sides?
- Do you have tinnitus?
- Is your ear sensitive or painful? Are you nauseous?
- Do you experience vomiting?
- Do you suffer from headaches?
- Do you feel like you're going to faint?
- Do you have heart palpitations or excessive sweating?
- Do you have trouble talking or swallowing?
- Do you see double or experience a reduction in your field of view?
- Do you feel claustrophobic or frightened?

Be aware that you may be asked these and other similar questions. It's a good idea to compile a personal 'dizziness handicap inventory.' You may also be asked about your medical history, and about what medications you are taking.

In other words, it's a good idea to be well-prepared for your initial consultation with an ENT specialist. By then, you will probably already have been examined by your regular doctor, who will have measured your heart rate and blood pressure, checked your ears, evaluated your eye movement, posture and balance, tested your reflexes and ordered blood work. If necessary, you may be subjected to specialized hearing and balance testing - and in some cases to a CT scan or MRI.

Step by step, the doctors will track down the cause of your dizziness. That's what happened in my case, too.

Crystals on parade: suspicious minds. *They are at it again*, I thought this morning. It's a feeling that often used to creep up on me, a day or two before an attack. I could feel them coming, thanks to a hard-to-describe sensation of there being something rotten in the state of Tania. It wasn't awful, but it left me with a certain uncertainty. And then the suspicions began to gnaw. In retrospect, I believe that those were the moments when the crystals lined up and began their parade through the labyrinth of my vestibular system.

And this morning, there it was again. Okay, I get it, it's the March of the Crystal Soldiers. I don't suppose I will ever be totally immune to that. But the parade route that led to the worst of my illness has been plugged. So from now on, I may feel the occasional bizarre sensation when they suit up and set off on their trek. But if all goes well, I will be spared the worst of the symptoms. I hope my theory is right, but my suspicious mind is churning.

Conny's Corner: an unusual case. I get to know Conny Kapitein today. She is a very special vertigonian. Compared to her, I had it easy. Reading her story makes me count my blessings. At first, her doctors thought she had BPPV, but it wasn't that simple in her case. After a series of misdiagnoses, the villain of her piece turned out to be chronic ear infections, which ultimately compromised her vestibular organ. I wish you could read her story yourself, but her website (*www.connyshoekje.nl*) and her 2003 book (*Van Horend tot Doof*) are only available in Dutch. I will tell you, though, that her case is unique, far from the norm when it comes to diagnosis and treatment. But Conny plows straight ahead, sharing her story online, presenting useful information and links to her readers. Her courage and strength are an inspiration.

Posturowhatnow? Posturography! It's a technique I had never heard of until I found the Apeldoorns Duizeligheidscentrum's website. How does it work?

> The conventional videonystagmography test (VNG) examines the vestibular organ and nerve. VNG, however, fails to take into account several additional factors critical to maintaining balance, such as the visual contribution made by the eyes and the proprioceptive information provided by the mechanoreceptors in the feet. The posturograph measures postural and balance disruptions, using a

footplate containing pressure sensors, and checks the patient's ability to maintain balance under an assortment of conditions.

The posturograph records failures and compensations of all components of the vestibular system (vestibular organ, eyes, mechanoreceptors in the feet).

In addition, posturography can help with balance training, vestibular rehabilitation, and the consequences of the results achieved via such therapeutic measures. In the future, we believe that Computerized Dynamic Posturography (CDP) will play an important role in the treatment of balance disorders resulting from neurological disorders, and in the prevention of falling.

And there is another test that can be used in cases where it's suspected that there is a problem with blood flow to the vestibular organ: vascular ultrasound.

The carotid arteries and several other arteries in the same region can be visualized with the help of Duplex, a combination of echography and Doppler. The artery's vascular wall is checked for irregularities, and it is also possible to check the speed and direction of the blood flow.

Mirroring. Thomas gives me a present today, a mirror I can use to check the scar behind my ear. All this time, I haven't been able to see it, and I have been pestering him: 'Look at my ear! Does it look okay?' One little mirror, and he is released from my whining. But the gift was sweet of him, I think. He tells me that my standing horror face is gone, though I still have that piercing gaze. We agree that I am about 80% of the way back to the old Tania.

> November 23, 2008

A day of rest. No big plans for the blog today. It's Sunday, and I am enjoying a day off. Croissants with lots of coffee, some caterwauling on the violin and a little tickling of the ivories… and in response to a general request from the more sensitive amongst us, I have removed that awful searchlight illustration from my home page. Apparently it was a problem, especially to Ménière's sufferers.

> November 24, 2008

Calling all triggers! I used to have a lot of triggers for a severe attack: rolling over in bed, lying down, standing up quickly, turning my head to the right, looking up at the ceiling, sweeping spider webs from the overhead light fixtures, vacuuming the corners of the room, bending down to load the washing machine, tilting my head while selecting clothes from my closet, washing my hair in the shower… and there were others, too. Basically, the problem was moving my head from its straight and narrow path. It generally happened when I was simply living my life, busy, not paying attention - and, boom, suddenly it was Dizzy Time.

The day before yesterday, I felt that horrible premonition of coming disaster when I woke up. Today, though, two days later, it's gone. All I feel is that slight spinny sensation that is still with me, three and a half weeks after my surgery. It doesn't really bother me. I have actually gotten used to it - that and my cardboard ear and partial deafness. Thanks to the stuffiness in my ear, I often misunderstand things people say to me, especially when my kids address me from across the room. It's kind of amusing, sometimes, but I hope it passes.

Now that I am leading a more balanced life, I am beginning to test myself. Last night, I tipped back my head and looked up at the ceiling for quite a while, just to prove that I *could*. Today I am pulling every trigger in my book. I clear away a spider web in the bathroom and scrub the tile floor on hands and knees. This is the first time I have dared to tackle that job. Now I am taking a break, sitting at the computer and listening to Paolo Conte. In a while, I will get back to it.

The silver envelope. Tonight we empty out the mailbox. Haven't done that in a while, and it is practically invisible under a thick layer of snow. Inside, the mail is soaking wet. One of the envelopes, a silver one, is addressed to me. Thomas finds it intriguing, so I open it first. A card from my colleagues at work! Get well soon and come back happy.

Well, of course I will! Give me two more weeks, and I will be good as new. I will just grin and bear it for a while longer, and then heigh-ho, heigh-ho, it's back to work I will go! My goal is to be in the office on December 11 – all recovered and standing firmly on my own two feet.

The Brainport balance device. I just got a call from my colleague Linda. She knows someone else who suffers from a balance disorder, and she has apparently been wearing a tongue stimulator that seems to help. I have never heard of this! I look it up and discover an entirely new category of dizziness: people with a neurinoma or schwannoma, which is a tumor on the peripheral nerve sheath.

The tumor itself is benign, but it can make you quite sick and *can* become life threatening. A Dutch-language website and associated forum – *brughoektumor.nl* – introduces me to the Brainport balance device. Here is what a contributor to the forum has to say:

> It's used by people with balance problems, but at the same time we work on improving both our posture and our gait. Most of our patients have chronic balance problems and have gotten all the rehabilitative benefit they are going to get from physiotherapy and medication. The Brainport offers them a faster and more effective solution. Reported benefits include: improved balance when standing and walking, lasting effects with regular use of the apparatus, improved quality of life, it can be used at home without assistance, easy to transport, absolutely no negative side-effects.

And how does the device work?

> The apparatus informs the patient of the position of the

> head by electrotactile stimulation of the tongue. This information allows the patient to maintain perfect balance during therapy. The primary advantage is the retention effect: continued usage of the device results in continued benefit. In addition to improved balance and gait, most users report significant improvement in their involuntary eye movements, improved sleep, and a reduction in dizziness and headache. Each patient's case is different, but most users report significant improvement within five days.

No idea if this will help *all* dizzy patients. But the device is manufactured and sold by an American company - Wicab, Inc. - and their UK website presents considerable evidence that the device has worked for many sufferers, including those with Ménière's disease. There is lots of information available online in English; for example, you can read an article aimed at laypeople at *science.howstuffworks.com/brainport2.htm* and judge for yourself.

Have mercy! I am hearing regular clicks in my ear this morning. A good sign, I hope. Maybe my auditory canal is getting ready to open. That would be so welcome! Patience, Tania - you will get there!

Meanwhile, I have made some changes to my blog's color scheme. Some readers have told me that three columns of text is too 'heavy' for them, making it hard to read and causing eyestrain. I can't change the number of columns, but white text against a colored background is distracting, so I have flipped the colors. Maybe the green background I was using isn't the dizzy-friendliest color, so I have gotten rid of it. And I have also dumped the animated illustrations and JPEGs.

Chatting with a chum. I have already mentioned my father-in-law's friend Herman, a fellow sufferer who has gone through the same surgery as I had. Finally someone with whom I share a common history! We agreed to talk on the phone, so I could get his story straight from the horse's mouth, and today was the day.

Perhaps it's premature to call him a fellow sufferer, since it turns out he probably *doesn't* have BPPV and did not in fact undergo canal plugging. But it was still an interesting conversation. His attacks last for hours and are accompanied by severe vomiting. We are in agreement that, unless you are very careful, such an affliction can take control of your life. You don't know when it will strike, and you have to fight to avoid a state of constant suspicion. He is still waiting for a proper diagnosis. Meanwhile, he got a gentamicin injection in Louvain – in, if I understood him correctly, his ear. Gentamicin is an antibiotic, injected via a very long needle; gentamicin therapy is mainly used in Ménière patients. It puts your afflicted vestibular organ out of commission and therefore usually takes away your dizziness. After six weeks, though, he relapsed. Sad.

I have found contradictory opinions about this therapy: one source says it's ototoxic and will eventually damage your hearing, while another recommends it. I wonder what exactly the pros and cons of the treatment are. I wish him luck and a speedy and accurate diagnosis.

> November 26, 2008

The death of me. Time flies: I have been home from the hospital for four weeks. And now it's time for an unavoidable chore: I am sitting in the waiting room at my health-insurance company, where I need to apply for a subsidy, given the amount of time I am spending away from work. For a while, now, the very thought of this has made me shudder. I am not worried about paying my medical bills. It's the feeling of shame and uselessness that bugs me. At least that's how I feel at the moment. Well, it's only for another two weeks – after that, I will be right back in the rat race.

My wait turns out to be fruitless: I am required to present a note from my family doctor, verifying the length of time I will be unable to work, and of course I had no idea this would be needed. What a nitwit! And I will lose 10% of my subsidy for every day the form is late. 'You'd better hurry on over to your doctor's office and then get it in the mail,' they tell me, 'or else come back and deliver it in person.' I call the doctor, arrange an immediate appointment, and zip off to collect the paperwork.

My new doctor wants to hear all about this rare operation I have had. It could be useful to other patients, so I give her the complete story. She agrees with me: it's practically impossible for a doctor to have contacts with every possible type of specialist, so it's often better for the patient to do her own research, as I have done. Back home, I practically keel over when I realize I have forgotten one page of what I need. So I have to go back. Bureaucracy, you will be the death of me yet!

Useful, usefuller, usefullest. To compensate for the uselessness of my existence, I volunteer again this morning at the elementary school. For half an hour, I give each of four children a turn to read aloud. My job is to encourage them to enjoy reading, and to evaluate their ability.

One of the mothers tells me that her daughter finds this the most pleasant activity of the school week. That's enough right there to keep me coming back: the appreciation, the happy expressions on the children's faces, the progress I see them make.

It's Open House at the music school today, and I almost forget about it. But I go, and listen to the toots, whistles, plunks and booms of the recorder, the triangle, and the other instruments.

For just a moment, my ear opens op. The clicks are coming more frequently now, more and more of them every day. That keeps me going, today - but I wind up with a throbbing headache.

Don't just say 'dizzy.' Please! There are quite a few different types of dizziness, although the symptoms at first glance are somewhat similar: BPPV, Ménière's disease, inflammation of the vestibular nerve (vestibular neuritis), a viral or bacterial infection of the inner ear (cochlear labyrinthitis), a leakage of fluid into the middle ear (perilymphatic fistula), a neurovascular conflict, a tumor on the hearing and balance nerve (such as acoustic neuroma)... the list goes on. So dizziness doesn't necessarily mean that there is something wrong with your vestibular organ; the problem may be cardiovascular, neurological, metabolic, even psychological. There are plenty of possibilities. (And remember, not all dizziness is vertigo!)

> November 27, 2008

How does a caterpillar walk? Let's see who has visited my blog today. Feedjit shows me the search terms that have brought people to me. Most of them were looking - more or less - for what I have to offer, but once in a while Google delivers someone who was really looking for something else. This morning, one visitor typed 'How do caterpillars walk?' and wound up at the Dizzy Me blog! Well, this particular caterpillar's taking her time emerging from her cocoon - but once she is out, she will be the prettiest butterfly you have ever seen!

Four weeks post-surgery, the sensations I am experiencing have gotten a lot less sensational. I can even stay firmly on my feet after two generous glasses of wine! I still feel a little funny when I am lathering shampoo into my hair in the shower, but I prop one elbow against the tile wall and feel confident I can keep myself right side up.

Little tricks. I imagine I will continue to rely on them for some time to come. Once you have learned to expect your body to behave a particular way under particular circumstances, you don't *unlearn* those lessons easily. But the pressure in my head is ebbing, day by day. I can feel my scar pucker, but that's really nothing to complain about. The clicks in my ear are signs of progress. At this point, it's just a question of time: my next exam will be on December 3.

Thomas took my picture first thing this morning. I wasn't fully awake, but the 'horror face' is gone. My cheeks have filled out a bit: I have put on some weight.

Apropos of nothing, my piano teacher is a slave driver. He piles on too much work!

A happy ending for Wim. Wim is a Ménière's patient, and he posts to the Ménière's forum. A while ago, he had some very good news:

> After 16 gentamicin injections and a hopeless existence, I finally found the courage to let them cut my vestibular nerve. The first months after the procedure were difficult, but recently things have been going incredibly well. I feel able to engage in my life again. I am back

> behind the wheel of my car, I am out in the world and enjoying myself. Next week, I am going to spend five days hiking the Rheinsteig Trail, fifteen miles a day beside the Rhine River. I have my life back. I want everyone who has got Ménière's to know about this. If you would like to be done with it, once and for all, this is your chance. It took me years to get up the courage. I was more afraid of the surgery than of the affliction. But now, after a forteen-year hiatus, I was finally able to do the thirty-five-mile seven-village Oud-Vossemeer volksmarch again. Who could manage that wearing prism spectacles, sticking to a potassium-rich diet, or taking betahistine dihydrochloride? It's simply wonderful! I wish I had had the courage much sooner.

That was what he posted last summer. I was surprised, because I too was sceptical about the wisdom of cutting the vestibular nerve. So, how is he doing now, half a year later?

> I had my surgery a year ago, and I continue to be extremely happy with the results. My life has changed as dramatically as it changed when the attacks began, though now in a positive direction. I am back to work full-time, and I recently traveled to Israel. It was a tiring vacation, but I did it and I truly never thought I would be able to handle such an experience. If only I had had the operation sooner all those wasted years I can never get back. But be aware: it's not a walk in the park. The first months of my recovery weren't easy. It took time to get me back on my feet, but it was time well-spent.

> November 28, 2008

Back off, blogaloo. Today I begin backing away from my blog. I am not shutting it down. But I am going to start posting less often. I can't keep up the pace indefinitely. At this point, I think of myself as almost completely healed, and I have said much of what I have wanted to say. It's time for me to stop focusing so much of my energy on what used to be wrong with me. Plus I want to give myself the chance to really enjoy the next couple of weeks before I go back to work at last. But don't worry: the moment my ear pops open, I will be sure to let you know!

So it's your turn now, fellow sufferers, to share your own experiences. If you've got news to report, or links to add, go right ahead! Meanwhile, I am going to make the house all cozy for the weekend. I am going to get a Christmas tree for the living room and crawl up into the attic to fetch the lights and ornaments. Maybe tomorrow, when it's all set up, I will stop by and post a picture…

> December 1, 2008

The Tania goes zoom-zoom. A new month, wow! I'd just as soon forget November, the sooner the better. Surgery and sick leave have left a bad taste in my mouth. So let the hectic times roll, I am ready for them: back to work, the busy holidays, lots of family visits and meals to cook, presents to wrap and unwrap and all that jazz!

What's that? You're wondering if I feel inspired? You mean right now? Well, I am sorry, but the zooming in my ear doesn't do my creativity any good. *Zoom zoom zoom… zoom zoom zoom…* the blood rushes through my head. *Zoom zoom zoom…* that's the only thing I can think of to write. Jeez, does this happen to you sometimes, too?

The ear mechanics. You really ought to get a sense of how many of you there are. Under your various online aliases, you key in the same search terms and wind up here. Greetings, Gent! Lovely to see you, Louvain! 'Morning, Mechelen! And *kaif halak*, Cairo! I hope your dizziness doesn't ruin your holiday season.

So, tell me, has Google helped you deal with your vertiginous darkness? Just as you have been following my adventures, I am interested in following yours. This isn't an ivory-tower medical site – it's just real people sharing their real stories.

And that can be fascinating, don't you agree? It's almost funny, this ongoing search for a little understandable information and empathy.

It's snowing today, and the sky is depressing. Why in the world would anyone venture outside? I can't think of anything I feel like doing. So I will sit here and go on a scavenger hunt, scavenging for information. Hmm, here is an article on an American website, the National Institute of Deafness and Other Communication Disorders' *nidcd.nih.gov*: 'Innovative Surgery on the Ear Bone Relieves Rare Form of Severe Dizziness and Hearing Loss.' It's about a unusual disorder, superior canal dehiscence syndrome, in which a thinning of the canal bone at the top of the inner ear's three semicircular canals causes deterioration of hearing and balance.

The strange thing about the condition is that patients report that their dizziness is a reaction to the sound of their own voice echoing inside their head. The canal can also react to pressure changes caused by such physical activity as coughing or sneezing. Researchers aren't completely sure of the cause, but they believe it may have to do with improper development of the canal bone, or it may be brought on by head trauma or barotrauma (changes in air pressure between the inside and the outside of the body). Abnormal eye movements are also noted in these patients, a reaction to auditory stimuli or pressure changes. Really odd, but very clearly explained in the article.

And guess what the NIDCD recommends?

> The symptoms that accompany superior canal dehiscence, a rare hearing and balance disorder, can be treated successfully by a single operation that plugs up a thinning layer of bone in the inner ear.

Their surgery is a little different from ours, but the similarities are remarkable!

All presents and accounted for! Tomorrow is my checkup. Well, doctor? Is my balance pretty much back to normal? That woozy sensation, is that on its way out, or will I have to carry it around for the rest of my life? And what is going on with my ear? The zooming and clicking, are those signs it's getting better? Is it preparing to open up? Not that I am complaining, you understand! These are all minor inconveniences. I would just like to know. Arthur is quite worried about me. Every day, he asks if I am better yet. He says, 'I think you are, mommy, and I think Santa Claus is nice, 'cause he brings lots of presents!'

> December 3, 2008

The Good News Show. Welcome to today's episode of *The Good News Show*. I am your host, Happy Me!

I may have to change the name of my blog. Or, no, better not: if I do, my fellow sufferers won't be able to find me.

But here is what I came online to say today: I have been to the doctor. There was a mob of people in the waiting room, and a long wait to get in. That comes with the territory, though, when you want to see the right specialist.

But the news is that the wait - for me, at least - turned out to be worthwhile. I chatted with a woman whose condition was as bad as mine was before my surgery. She had also been recommended to look into canal plugging. By the way, I asked the doctor how many of these operations they perform in a year - and the answer was two. 'It's a very delicate procedure,' she explained. It works, though, and I am better! The results of my hearing test were solidly positive: three weeks ago, my right ear was a mess, but today my score was significantly improved. Dr. Van de Heyning was very pleased!

And my balance? Well, at times I still feel a little strange, and when I drop into my chair I am clumsy as an elephant. But that, too, will improve over time. My body has got a built-in computer with its own memory, and that memory remembers how proper balance feels. Now that I have been plugged, my internal memory has to reprogram itself for this new reality. And that takes time. We'll have to see if my system is sufficiently dynamic to make the adaptation.

> December 4, 2008

All right, Mr. DeMille, I am ready for my close-up. As of today, I am actively preparing for my comeback, because I return to work a week from Thursday. Thanks to the cold, wet weather, I am staying indoors now that I am home from the doctor. I check a blog I have been following, take a few selfies. The difference between four weeks ago and now is remarkable. Then, I really was a horror, but today I am satisfied with the way I look. The alien appearance and piercing stare are happily gone. I am still working on my behaviors, which are not yet hundred percent back to normal.

In the waiting room, I could pick them out, the BPPV'ers. It's strange to recognize the condition in someone else. You are confronted with your own case. *Do I act like that, too? I don't want to!* 'Typical,' my doctor told me. 'Those odd mannerisms, and the longing to recapture the ability to move normally.'

So, what exactly do we do? If we want or need to look off to one side, we don't turn our heads. Instead, we swivel our torsos, keeping our heads perfectly aligned. Our necks seem frozen in position. Our eye motions are bizarre - very wooden and suspicious. We *look* stiff, but we don't *feel* that way. And half the time simply shifting position in our chair is an invitation to an attack.

'Have you been doing your exercises?' the doctor asks. 'Um, I read the instructions, but, I will be honest, they seem ridiculous. Does playing the piano count?' The doctor understands. And agrees that my way should be fine.

I was awake at 5:15 this morning. Arthur was coughing so severely he threw up on his pillow. I had to give him a bath - and when I dropped back into my bed, Matthias, disgusted by the smell, crawled in with me, clutching his stuffed animals. I rolled over to hug him, and I could feel the fear stirring between my ears.

Fine, I know what I have to do. When I go back to work, I want to be an ordinary employee, not some 'special case.' I have to get beyond all the odd reactions and behaviors. To get myself in the proper spirit, I start by vacuuming the house, then give myself a vigorous shampooing. I put on some New Wave music and practice moving my head to the beat. The downside is that I spot a spider web on the ceiling. Yuck!

For a change of pace, I play two pieces on the piano. My Russian music teacher is really pushing me! According to him, I play too quickly. I hadn't read a note of music in thirty years, and now I am attacking the keyboard with two hands at top speed. The results aren't exactly pleasing to the ear – especially since I have been practicing with compromised hearing. But he is pitiless and gives me four pieces to work on at home: two by Bach, and two Russian folksongs.

The rest of the day has me doing a lot of bending and stretching. There are five people living in our house, and that means six or seven loads of laundry to be done. Plus a mountain of ironing, because I don't want to *look* at an ironing board over the Sinterklaas weekend. Oh, and then there are the beds to make…

And the beat goes on. While I work, I play records I haven't listened to in years. Boney M's 'By the Rivers of Babylon' and 'Ma Baker' cheer me up. *Freeze! I am Ma Baker, put your hands in the air, gimme all your money.* Music to iron by. My third load of laundry is percussion in the background. I have brought the clothes rack in from the garage; it's too cold out there. Outside, the birds haven't yet noticed the goodies I have left for them. *Here is a special bulletin: Ta 'Bader is the FBI's most wanted woman. Her photo is hanging on every post office wall .*

Yes, Tania's back! Although there is more of me than there used to be: according to the bathroom scale, I have put on almost nine pounds. I was going to make cauliflower with béchamel sauce for dinner tonight, but I am not in the mood. Tomorrow I am going to visit my mother-in-law. She has been in the hospital for half a year with MS, which can also cause dizziness. What should I bring her?

Drunk as a skunk? Ever heard of CVD? Central Vestibular Disorders are disruptions of the vestibular system that result from physical injury. CVD patients often seem to be drunk, even if they haven't consumed any alcohol whatsoever. Their disorders often involve hearing loss, and their speaking volume is often compromised. Causes of CVD may include vascular deviations of the brain stem, acoustic neuroses and tumors on the brain stem and/or the cerebellum, multiple sclerosis, and various forms of migraine. Charming, right? Those interested in learning more can find lots of information online, for example at the American Speech-Language-Hearing Association's website (*asha.org/aud/articles/CentralVestib/*).

> December 5, 2008

What a difference a month makes. I am suddenly reminded of my Dr. House period: groggy from the surgery, puffed up from the cortisone, piercing horror gaze, dizzy dizzy dizzy. But now, four weeks later, I am an entirely different Tania, almost ready to return to work.

> December 8, 2008

BPPV ≠ Ménière's. A visitor to my blog has asked me if my canal-plugging operation is also an option for Ménière's patients. Be careful! Although our complaints are similar in many ways, there is a difference between BPPV and Ménière's disease. Dizziness in BPPV patients, remember, occurs when the crystals in the utriculus - a small part of the vestibular system - drift out of their proper position. This problem can in many cases be treated by simply training the patient to perform certain precise maneuvers - most commonly either the Semont or the Epley maneuvers - which send the crystals back to where they belong. Vestibular habituation therapy - the Brandt-Daroff exercises - are also often recommended. Only in cases where these non-invasive treatments are ineffective, or when the patient relapses regularly, might canal plugging be advisable.

Ménière's patients resemble BPPV patients at first sight, but the mechanism is actually entirely different. It's generally agreed that, in Ménière's patients, an excess of fluid in the inner ear creates pressure that may in turn cause a tear in the canal wall. This leads to an acute attack of vertigo that closely resembles a BPPV attack. When the tear in the canal wall heals, the pressure can again begin to build. The exact cause of the increased pressure is unknown, but ultimately fluid is accumulating when it should be draining. Other symptoms that differentiate Ménière's from BPPV include hissing in the ear and hearing loss, which are at first temporary and observed only during an attack but may later become permanent.

Because these two conditions are different, different treatments are indicated. Medication that would be ineffective if administered to a BPPV patient may help a Ménière's patient. Gentamicin injections or the cutting of the vestibular nerve may also be indicated in Ménière's cases (*see* **A happy ending for Wim, November 27**).

A bit more explanation about my surgery. On the one hand, canal plugging is a delicate operation, since the surgeon has to go in through the skull, which encapsulates the vestibular organ - and the organ itself is quite small. On the other hand, the success rate for the procedure is very high: it proves effective in some ninety-five percent of cases, and partial or complete hearing loss on the side of the surgery is reported in only one to three percent of cases, when the auditory nerve is damaged or becomes infected.

Still, the procedure isn't performed very often, since many BPPV patients suffer an attack no more than once a year and most patients receive sufficient relief from the Semont and/or Epley maneuvers and the habituation exercises. Given these realities, canal plugging is rarely indicated. In the University Hospital of Antwerp, for example, an average of only two patients a year undergo the canal-plugging surgery.

It's almost six weeks since I took my turn on the operating table, and I haven't had an attack in all that time. I experienced some partial hearing loss at first, but that has almost completely gone now. I still feel a little strange from time to time, but that's because my vestibular organ is still being 'reprogrammed' to compensate for the plug. My ability to function is completely normal.

My cautiousness is another matter: that attitude is hotwired into a long-time BPPV patient. It will take months before my self-confidence is fully restored. But that's an issue that really only affects me when I am lying down; it has no consequences in my daily life. Like my self-confidence, this too will improve with time and training.

Given my years of experience, this is the key piece of advice I have to offer: the most important thing a Dizzy You can do is seek out a conclusive diagnosis of your condition. Your best chance of getting one is to go to a state-of-the-art medical facility that specializes in treating balance disorders. Hospitals that don't have the proper diagnostic equipment often wind up misdiagnosing vestibular problems, which of course then leads to unhelpful treatment. Read everything you can find about the various possible explanations of your symptoms, and make sure that what you're experiencing matches what your doctor tells you is wrong with you. This is what helped me to realize that I had BPPV and not Ménière's.

Are you less than convinced that an accurate diagnosis has been made? Are you concerned that your symptoms *don't* match the condition you have been told afflicts you? Then it's probably a good idea to get a second opinion, since it seems that many doctors are under- or even misinformed about the workings of the vestibular system.

Once you are sure you have been properly diagnosed, it's time to shift your focus to the array of treatment options available to people with your complaint and weigh the pros and cons of each. There is a lot of helpful information out there, but you should avoid the trap of automatically believing everything you find on the internet. Blogs like mine and patient forums can be supportive, reassuring you that you are not the only person on the planet who is suffering. But for accurate *information*, you need to consult actual medical sources. Even there, though, you are likely to find conflicting 'facts' and opinions. Keeping that in mind, the better informed you are when you see your doctor, the more likely you will be to ask the right questions and understand the answers. Don't take my word for that. You will see for yourself: the communication process works better when the patient is well informed. They say that knowledge is power, and some doctors have a tendency to be abrupt and even unhelpful with patients who come across as unknowledgeable.

> December 9, 2008

All quiet on the blogging front. Another two days at home, then back to work. I really needed these six weeks away. I realize that I underestimated the challenges of recovering from my surgery. I thought: *Snip snip, a week to heal, and I will be right as rain!* The doctor must have gotten a chuckle out of my naiveté. 'At least three weeks,' he told me - and I think he was underestimating on purpose to convince me to agree to the operation. I should have known better, but that's all water under the bridge now. Back to work on Thursday, and I am ready.

Normally, I am a good-natured whirlwind of activity. I have had enough of this lazing around the house. I have reached all of my limits: my 'sickness' limit, my 'being alone' limit, my 'laziness' limit, my 'feeling like a prisoner' limit.

When you drop out of your usual world for a while, it's like you have been sucked into a completely other universe. What's a person supposed to *do* at home for six weeks, when all her friends have jobs? Blogging has helped me make it through. It's a shame that people like me have to get sick in order to take a break from the rat race. All things considered, has my experience been good for me? I think so. I have learned to appreciate what I have in life. To tell the difference between what's fake and what's real. To recognize what matters, what really counts, what's important - and what's too trivial to worry about.

Take, for example, the ability simply to walk a straight line, to function normally, to do whatever I feel like doing as a healthy member of a healthy family. Now *that's* what I call true wealth!

But the last of the limits I mentioned a moment ago proved almost too much for me. Especially these final days. I don't really have anything left to say. And neither, apparently, does anyone else. It has been remarkably quiet here in the blogosphere. Each in our own way, we have been mourning the loss of our two little stars, the youngest amongst us. So unfair. Impossible to understand. Seppe and Lotte, barely eight years old and four, have lost their battle with cancer. I have been wearing a black ribbon in their memory. How much sadness can a human being withstand?

> December 11, 2008

And now... heeeeeere's Tania! Thomas teases me today. 'Look out, world! Make way for Tania!' It's scandalous, the way he laughs at me.

I am out the door a little after 7. 'Do you have to leave this early every day from now on?' says our eldest. An hour and forty-five minutes in the car, and I arrive. Happy to be healthy again.

It's a normal workday for me. Except for the hearty welcome back, of course - complete with coffee, cake, a little gift from my colleagues… and an overflowing in-box. At 6 PM, I quit out of Photoshop. So much close concentration in one day has left me exhausted. I get in the car for the drive home. And guess what happens on the way? Flat tire!

> December 12, 2008

Dizzy Me's a Busy Bee! Now that I am back at work, I have lots to do. Your messages have been streaming into my mailbox, asking me if I recognize your symptoms, assuring me I am not alone. One correspondent quotes me describing my *own* symptoms and adds, 'I have got all the same complaints!' And then there is the very sad story of one reader who has been so shattered by dizziness that he has had to learn from one day to the next how to live without balance or hearing. That shouldn't happen to anyone.

But what really encourages me is the realization that keeping this blog up and running is doing some good in the world. Even if it only helps a few people, that's still *something*, right? So to anyone who's been sitting in front of the computer screen impatiently awaiting a response from me, please remember that I am now one of the healthy people and off at work during the day. In the evenings, though, I promise to make time for you. And that's a promise I am confident I can keep. Deal?

> December 14, 2008

Look, Ma, no hands! Have I got something to tell you! We live in a part of Flanders called the Pajottenland, and it's a pretty hilly area. This afternoon, Thomas and I put the kids on their bikes and aimed them uphill towards a neighborhood playground. We hurried along on foot behind them, helping them steer, giving them little pushes as needed… and calling out 'Car!' warnings at least a hundred times. When we finally reached the top, we all played together in the playground. Since the last time I was there, new trees have been planted.

It's mid-December, so the branches are mostly bare, but it should be lovely in the spring.

Well, I simply couldn't resist: I climbed onto the swing and pushed off, and I swooped back and forth, up and down, faster and faster, higher and higher. It was terrifying, but I did it!

Then, after that, the seesaw. With eight-year-old Matthias on one end, poor little Charlotte, who is three, wasn't getting much of a ride, so I clambered up and balanced myself in the middle and, by shifting my weight from one foot to the other, I helped the kids bounce up and down until we all were laughing like loons. I teetered one way and tottered the other - but I didn't topple!

I rode the swings and the seesaw, I had fun, and I feel *fine*!

> December 18, 2008

Oops, I blogged it again! My computer has given up the ghost. They are trying to revive it, at least long enough to save the thousands of photos I have taken of my kids over the last year. Every December, I make a photo album for each of them for Christmas, a pictorial journey back across the previous twelve months. This year, it will be a stretch to have the albums ready in time. I may have to give them as New Year's presents, instead.

I bought a new computer, of course, but I haven't been able to get it onto the internet until today. And it's inappropriate for me to work on my blog or respond to personal e-mail from the office.

This evening, I finally managed to connect to wifi, so I am taking advantage of the opportunity to report that my fellow blogger Flupque is doing better again and to pay a sad cyber visit to Seppe and Lotte.

I have been doing fine. My balance seems completely restored, enormously improved over a week ago. For those who like statistics, I estimate that I am about ninety-seven percent of the way back to normal. And I can put some of that remaining two to three percent down to my lingering uncertainty. But that is hardly even worth mentioning. In a way, it just makes me a teensy bit special.

> December 20, 2008

Tania's Believe It or Not. Yesterday was Friday, and my boss treated the office to pizza. Ten different people approached me with the exact same questions: 'So, how have you been? Weren't you out sick for a while?' And ten times I gave the exact same answers.

And now I get a week's vacation! Decadent, no? But the week ahead won't be exactly relaxing. Now that all the misery is behind me, I have got a lot of catching up to do, and every day is pretty solidly booked. Last night, there was a concert at our local church, and afterwards I stood around chatting with friends and neighbors - 'Can I see your scar?' - and drinking champagne, then cola, then coffee, then hot chocolate. This morning, I had a bit of a hangover, but I still went out shopping for last-minute gifts. And this evening our IT guy comes over, and I pour us each a glass to toast his successful surgery on our old computer! Still to come: the Samson and Gert Christmas show, the Antwerp Zoo, two holiday dinners, a lecture about bisons, and a visit to Plopsaland. [For the American and British readers, Plopsaland is an amusement park on the Belgian coast, about two hours west of where we live. And *Samson en Gert* is a popular Flemish children's TV program, featuring Gert Verhulst and his talking sheepdog puppet Samson.]

My mother calls and asks my better half how I am doing. 'Fine,' he tells her, 'if I can believe her blog.' Later, when he reports on their conversation, he laughs and adds, 'It's simple, all I have to do is check your blog, and I know what has been rattling around in your head.' I roll my eyes - I can roll my eyes! - and say, 'Hello, Thomas? I sit right next to you at the dinner table? We sleep in the same bed? You could just *ask* me, you know!' I guess it's a good thing I *have* this blog. Without it, my own husband apparently wouldn't know how I am…

> December 29, 2008

My ticking time bomb. For almost two months, now, Dizzy Me isn't Dizzy Me any more – step by step, I have been returning to the original Tania. It's high time I stop boring you with my daily comings and goings and with stories about my children. My last few posts have been fun to write, but they haven't really done what I originally created this blog to do. For fifteen years, I was a ticking time bomb that could go off at any moment. Now it's time to let it all out, after years of keeping it to myself. And if my doing so can help my fellow sufferers, too – well, that's a nice little bonus, isn't it?

> December 31, 2008

Thinking allowed. As 2008 draws to a close, I want to muse about the year that's ending. My thoughts are jumbled, and they tumble over each other so chaotically that even I have trouble following them. My dizziness is gone. Exiled from the kingdom of my head, defeated on the battlefield of my consciousness. Beheaded, in a manner of speaking. But the windmills of my mind continue to turn, like a circle in a spiral, like a wheel within a wheel. It's impossible to forget all that I have endured. I am not sure I would want to forget it, even if I could. It's all a part of who I *am*.

It's funny, I lived with vertigo all those years as if I was married to it. It was a mean partner, though. Deceitful. Not to be trusted. Crept up on me and attacked when I wasn't expecting it. It was stronger than I was. It had me in its power. I always had to cave in to its demands. That bastard! He came between me and everyone and everything I cared about. But he never made me give up. I kept the worst of my misery to myself. Only a handful of people knew about him – he was nobody else's business. As best I could, I pretended to be normal. I kept moving forward. All those lonely, frightening drives in the dark, my head spinning like a drunkard's, fifteen miles each way to my physical therapist. Hoping for relief from my umpteenth attack. Frozen with fear, my hands gripping the wheel. Praying the drive home would be easier. Then, when I *got* home, announcing that I wouldn't be joining the family for dinner, crawling into bed and under the blankets, sick to my stomach, unable even to *smell* whatever was cooking. Ugh. When I think back on the chances I took…

That was not a good marriage, and it lasted long enough. But you don't forget overnight a partner who has been at your side for fifteen years. Not a day goes by without my remembering him. Whenever I roll over in bed, or reach something down from a high shelf, or move in a way that used to be forbidden, memories of him course through me.

For years, I slept on my good side – I only had one good side, and it kept me turned away from my actual husband in bed. Now I have got all my sides back. I can turn, roll, sit up, lie down, sleep on my back or my belly, sleep *flat* instead of at a forty-five-degree angle. It's wonderful to have all these options! And last night, when I was lying on what used to be my bad side, spooned up against Thomas' warmth, my arms wrapped tightly around him, I made a resolution for 2009: from now on, what used to be my 'good' side is now officially banished!

> January 2, 2009

DizzyLAB. I found this online at the University Museum of Utrecht's YouthLab:

> Have you ever felt dizzy? Does the feeling come while you are spinning around and around, or not until after you have come to a stop? See for yourself with this simple experiment, and try to figure out an explanation by comparing yourself to a glass of water.
>
> Experiment 1
>
> What do you need?
>
> - A swivel chair
> - Someone to observe
>
> What do you do?

• Sit down on the chair. If you don't have a swivel chair at home, you can simply whirl around and around while standing. Either way, be sure to have someone else there to help you if necessary. If you spin too quickly, you might fall down!

• Spin around, and pay attention to whether or not you feel dizzy.

• Come to an abrupt stop. How do you feel now?

Why does dizziness happen? You have a 'balance' organ in your head, and it's full of liquid. Compare yourself to a glass of water: the glass is your balance organ, and the water is the liquid it contains.

Experiment 2

What do you need?

- A swivel chair
- A plastic cup
- Water
- Some scraps of paper

What do you do?

• Fill the plastic cup about halfway with water and drop in a few scraps of paper.

• Set the cup on the chair and spin the chair. Pay attention to how the scraps of paper move in the water.

• Bring the spinning chair to a sudden stop. The cup will also stop spinning, but what happens to the water and the paper scraps?

Now can you explain why you only feel dizzy after you have stopped spinning?

> January 6, 2009

That obscure object of study. Tomorrow I am scheduled for yet another visit to the hospital. They are going to check my vestibular organ. Is it working properly? How is my hearing? And so on. Wait for my turn, examination, wait some more, next test, wait again for the results… and then another wait to make my next appointment. The day will be over before I know it. That's how things work at the university hospital. And given the rarity of the operation I underwent, they had be crazy not to carefully monitor my progress. They only get two opportunities a year to do this procedure, so of course they want to learn as much as they can from each patient. In fact, I have become a pretty fascinating object for study, and it's all in the name of progress, right?

> January 7, 2009

Did I really win the lottery? Doctor's appointment this morning. I get there half an hour early, so I have time for a cup of coffee. And who do I bump into? The same two cool women I talked with last time. Like me, Marie-Thérèse has spent the last fifteen years wrestling with dizziness. Her friend has been at her side through thick and thin and serves as her chauffeur. We have a very nice chat about our balance issues and the surgery - it's possible she may wind up having the same operation. Everyone's situation is different, though, and first she needs to be thoroughly examined, to see if she is an appropriate candidate.

We enjoy our conversation so much that I lose track of time, and the doctor has to pull me away from them. Her examination confirms what I have hardly dared to imagine: I am cured! I acknowledge that I sometimes get the feeling I am on the verge of an attack… but the good news is that the attack never comes.

I wonder out loud if this is a sign of craziness, but she assures me it's perfectly normal. It takes time for the vestibular system to heal, especially after one of its canals has been blocked off. And according to her, it's *impossible* for me to experience any further attacks. In about four months, she says, she will give me a balance test to see how my vestibular organ reacts to stimulation under these new circumstances. Can it be true? Have I really won the lottery? These woods from which I am emerging have been scary, dark and deep – and I have promises to keep, and miles to go before I sleep.

A little nervously, I tell the doctor about my blog. I know I am *not* a doctor myself, but it's so difficult for patients to find good information. Why shouldn't I continue helping them? The doctor agrees it's a shame that even ENTs don't have enough access to knowledge. There needs to be a symposium, she says, and she is planning to organise one in the near future.

My exam takes about half an hour – record time! – and the doctor suggests a link I should add to my blog. It's one I have already got, though, and it's in English: *dizziness-and-balance.com*.

Did you know that Cathy Epley – Dr. John Epley's daughter – is manufacturing a chair designed by her father to help diagnose and treat BPPV? It's called the Omniax System, and unfortunately it's far too expensive for any but the wealthiest patients. But you can read about it at *vesticon.com/epley-omniax-system*. Maybe the time is right to start a charitable organization – like we have for cancer and other better known illnesses – whose goal is to make this amazing technology more available to people who could benefit from it. Can I get a volunteer?

> January 12, 2009

Tell 'em Dizzy Me sent you. I am back! Well, it's not that I have actually been *away*. I have just been busy with work, the holidays, my kids. So it's been several days since my last post. I still can hardly believe it: I am cured. Really *cured*!

I have been hearing rumors that things are changing in the medical community. Canal plugging seems to be becoming trendy. Tell 'em Dizzy Me sent you!

> January 24, 2009

Getting better all the time. It was a gift from two very wise friends: Louise L. Hay's *You Can Heal Your Life*, 274 pages of wisdom that comforted me during the lonely six weeks I spent at home after my surgery. For a while, now, I have been trying to think of the best thing I could do with that book, but I haven't been able to pin it down.

Life isn't something that 'happens' to you. Our thoughts and beliefs about ourselves and our lives are often the basis for our emotional and physical problems. When we learn to love ourselves more, we automatically become more successful. Every thought we think creates our future. We are one hundred percent responsible for our own experience. That is a brief summary of Louise Hay's philosophy.

I flipped through the book several times, and I paid some attention to identifying which bad thoughts were my pitfalls. But then I put it back on the shelf: I don't like being confronted with myself. So, no, I haven't read it all the way through. But I appreciate the gift, and I *have* gotten value out of it.

The fact is, here is what I have experienced: You are healthy, you work, you live. Everything is going just fine. You get together with friends. If someone is feeling down, you offer a shoulder to cry on. You have got a circle of people you know you can count on. And then the bottom falls out of your life. And things go from bad to worse, and then from worse to worst. A few good souls help you keep it together. But you're deeply disillusioned by too many of the people you were one hundred percent positive you could rely on.

Anyway. That book. In which of these affirmations, it asks, do you recognize yourself? 'Everyone is always helpful.' 'They are all against me.' And now I feel guilty. I start thinking: *It's my own fault*. I am the one with the negative attitude. And I am ashamed of the resentment I carry around within me because of those

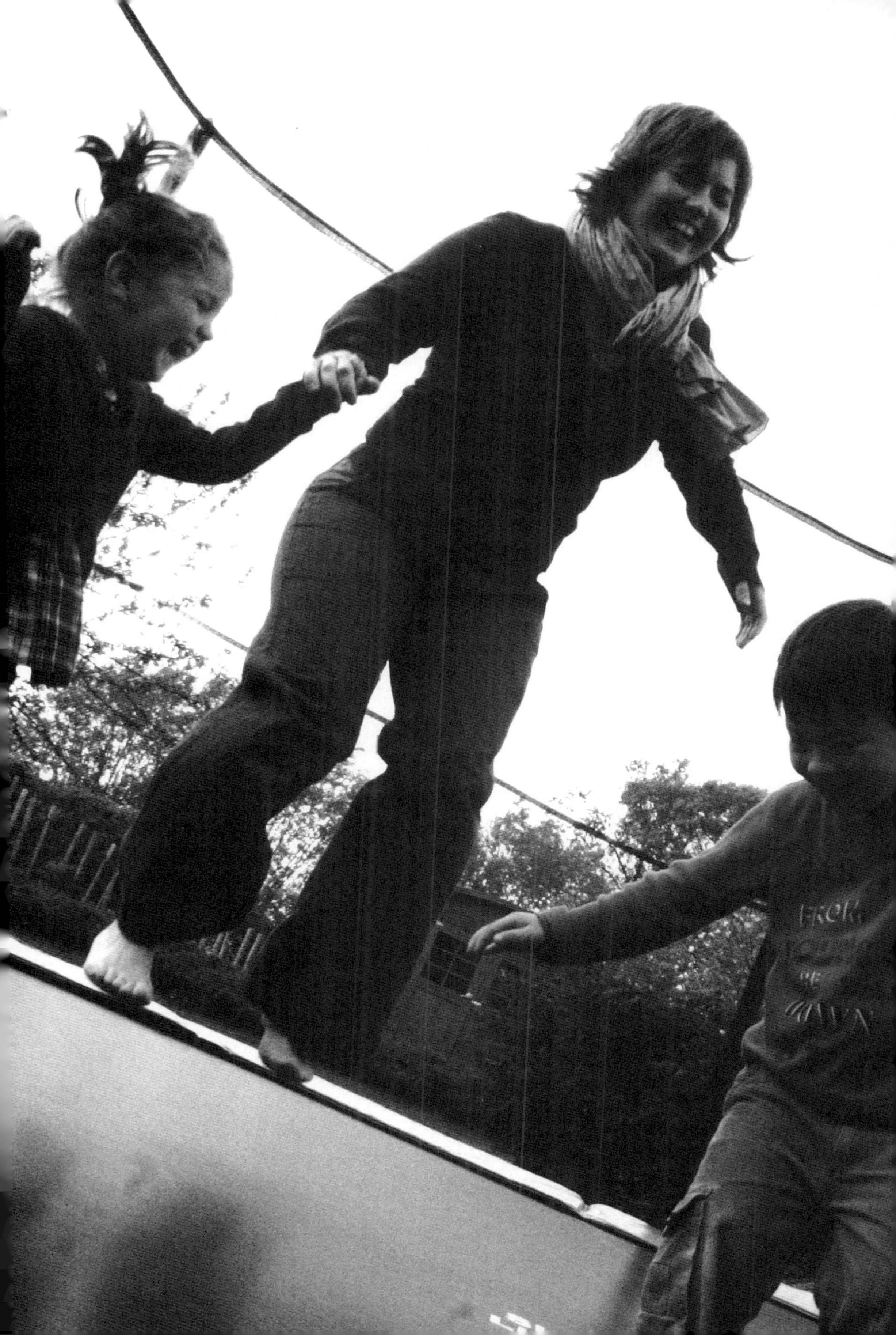

lonely weeks at home. I was always there for *them*, wasn't I? And this one time I really needed them to be there for me, even if it was just a phone call. 'Hey, we haven't forgotten you. How are you doing?' Sure, there were people who *did* call, but I was home for six weeks, and there was absolute radio silence from people I would have expected to hear from, people I thought were my friends.

According to the book, life is very simple: what goes around comes around. The book says I have to forgive, think positively, and most of all avoid the paranoid suspicion that no one likes me. The more happily you can live your life, apparently, the more you can count on success. So why do I walk around with a sour expression on my face? In fact, I have seen many older couples who clearly enjoy each other's company all the time, not just when they are engaged in some 'fun' activity.

But despite the book and the fact that I am healed, disillusionment gnaws at me. I have trouble with the idea of 'friends.' Well, I suppose there is room for me to work on myself. I will try to remember to think positively, to believe that people are inherently good. I will tell myself 'you are great!' and 'people *like* you!' Nothing to it. My so-called friends were just *busy* while I was sick, that's all...

For Yoghurt.

> Amsterdam – It was a passerby who called the police just past 11 PM on September 13, not one of the squatters' stronghold Vrankrijk's bartenders or managers. An unconscious man lay on the sidewalk in front of the Baroque-style building in the Spuistraat. He was bleeding from both ears, and there were wounds on his face; a trail of blood led from the Vrankrijk's bar to the body. The victim, who was apparently beaten with a blunt instrument, was a thirty-four-year-old man known only as 'Yoghurt' in the capital city's squatter community. The doctors who treated him stated that, given the severity of his injuries, he was lucky to be alive. In addition to the facial lacerations, the base of his skull was fractured.

> When he was released from the hospital, his face was partially paralyzed, his hearing was damaged, and he had partial amnesia. One of the victim's friends witnessed the attack and told police that three men in the bar beat Yoghurt 'with an iron object.'

That story was published in *Het Parool*, one of Amsterdam's leading daily newspapers. Mayor Job Cohen announced that Vrankrijk's operating license would be suspended. But Yoghurt will never walk again. He will never heal. He will receive reconstructive surgery to help his hearing, but for the rest of his life he will suffer attacks of dizziness.

> February 2, 2009

Anything you can do, I can do... half as well? Hans Beck, the inventor of Playmobil, is dead. In Europe, every house with kids in it is a house with Playmobil in it: those little 3' figures with moveable arms and legs and - what I find the most exciting - each topped by a head that can turn through almost 180°!

I built my own fantasy world around Herr Beck's creations. They were my knights and my rescuers, my sturdy policemen and dapper firemen. They were Farmer John and my neighborhood vet, my pirate, my playmate, my trapeze artist. I pulled their little plastic hats from their heads and peered into their skulls, switched hats back and forth between doctor, lawyer, Indian chief. Even today, we still buy new sets for the kids - and I still play with them myself.

More than 2.8 billion of the little figures have been manufactured, and we have got a nice collection of them in our living room. Although there have been more than 4500 different types of figure made since their debut in 1974, the basic idea has remained constant: little hard-plastic dolls without knees or elbows - but with heads that can turn almost a full half circle! Imagine: 2.8 billion little dolls, every one of them with a spinnable head. Compare all that with one little Dizzy Me, whose head can't even make a *quarter* circle without catastrophe. That's just not *fair*. So I went searching for a decent doctor, and look at me now: I am as flexible as a Playmobil figure!

> February 4, 2009

Healthy, but oh so tired. I am exhausted! It has been three months since my surgery. No more attacks. I can sleep normally, work normally, live normally. But I am so tired! And I can't use my dizziness as an excuse any more. No, now it's the microorganisms. Viruses, flu, stomach bugs, runny nose, sore throat… they come at me from all directions. Friends, family, colleagues… everyone is sick, and, oh, how their misery loves company! I have been trying to resist for weeks now. I ought to keep my distance. But I can't always avoid them – and the result is that I crash into bed at night and wake up *just* capable of making it through another day. And rinse and repeat.

By three in the afternoon, there it is again: headache, right at the edge of a fever, pressure behind my eyes. It makes me cranky, and I start to complain about too much time behind the piano and the consequences to my right wrist. I take a paracetamol, and it gets me through the rest of the day. At five o'clock on Friday, I finish the workweek's last creative-marketing effort, wish everyone a half-hearted happy weekend, and get in my car. With three kids at home, all needing my attention, the drive home feels like a journey from the frying pan to the fire.

Thomas is out tonight, so I am a single parent for the evening. I pick my three little angels up from their after-school program. All week long, they have been agitating for a trip to the snack bar. Even when I am feeling at my best, that's still an episode of *Survivor.*

By the time we get home, we have already weathered three or four crises: the squabble over who gets the front seat, the hissy fit because a book bag that's supposed to be on the *back* seat has been moved to the trunk, the whining because 'he got out on *my* side of the car,' the fury when 'she cut in front of me!' And that's just from the day care to the snack bar – a distance of less than a quarter of a mile.

In we go, and now they are hitting each other with their jackets as they wait impatiently for their cones of French fries, spinning around on their squealing metal stools, dropping their plastic forks, moaning that their fries are too hot, spilling their apple juice, pelting each other with wadded-up paper napkins… and then of course there is Arthur's endless burping. And of course Charlotte has to go to the bathroom the second *my* fries are ready, and she is mad at me for making her take off her skirt, and outraged when I flush the toilet instead of letting her do it.

Fortunately, the woman behind the counter gives each of them a lollipop before we leave, and at home everyone behaves while I read them Disney's *Lambert the Sheepish Lion*. It's a peaceful ending to a long day - but, oh, am I tired!

> February 11, 2009

Seven times yes, four times no. My surgery was at the end of October. Three and a half months later, yes, my balance seems fully restored. No, I haven't had any more attacks. No, no more staggering around as if I am drunk. Yes, I occasionally feel the slightest bit strange, but that's hardly worth mentioning.

So, yes, my vestibular organ is functioning normally, even though that one canal has been plugged. Yes, I can sleep on either side, on my back and on my stomach. Yes, I can probably even dance, although I haven't tried that yet. No, my ear doesn't hurt, and my hearing is perfect again… although, yes, if I rub my ear, it still feels like cardboard. And yes, I haven't been able to shake it yet: I lie on my back in bed, I look to the right, and there it is, the awful sense that 'here it comes again.' But does it come? No!

> February 20, 2009

Once I had a secret love. I hadn't played for thirty years, but six months ago I resumed taking lessons. I still make mistakes. There is lots of hesitation. But I am on the right track. I don't always read the notes correctly. I am too slow, so it takes a lot of effort. 'Feeling! Play from your gut!' orders my teacher. I will get there, eventually. No matter how many times I have to back up and start over.

I had promised myself that I would return to the piano some day. My ear surgery, the temporary deafness, those things motivated me to stop waiting for 'some day' and gave me the perseverance I needed. And now I am making progress. So far, I play only for myself. But soon I will be ready to make my secret love public.

> February 21, 2009

Three-point snot. Yesterday, 10:15 PM. She shoots - she misses. Bad aim. I was lying down, nothing really wrong, an innocent abed. I pulled my covers up a little higher. The expression on Thomas' face spoke volumes. He picked up my misguided missile. Amused, teasing... and also a little annoyed. He is wearing the sort of long-suffering smile that tells me he is feeling - I know, shame on me! - a little henpecked.

During the day, I am something of a perfectionist. That's the way I was raised. Everything in its proper place. Keep a step ahead of the dust. Meals on the table at set times, the ironing done on laundry day, and so on. That's Daytime Tania. Evening Tania likes to shoot baskets with her snotty tissues.

I can usually sink a three-pointer from across the room, but sometimes I toss an air ball. Oops! Even more fun is shooting rolled-up pairs of socks at the open washing machine - though it's probably not a good idea to actually *wash* them rolled into balls. But best thing is trying to rebound a wadded pair of underpants off my husband's head. I am just playing, Thomas! And then I drop back onto the bed and snuggle into my covers, as if I haven't done anything wrong. Who, me?

Now that I think about it, though, and begin to analyze my actions... well, okay, this is probably not the nicest thing to do. But what of it? That playful spirit is, after all, the real me. Nothing's better than to cut loose with a casual 'Fuck you!' against the trials and tribulations of an overloaded day. Or, what with work, the kids, my household chores and health problems, against the trials and tribulations of an overloaded *year*. Add all those overloaded years together, they make quite a pile. The occasional swearword is a ritual I use to help keep my head above water.

And today I am tired tired tired and, truth be told, sick sick sick. I have run out of pills, and they weren't helping, anyway. It feels like somebody is pounding on my head with a mallet. My nose is full of snot. My eyes are beady. My throat is raw.

My glands are swollen. And on Monday I have to go back to work, whether I feel up to it or not. Because everyone else in my department has the week off, so I don't have much of a choice – *someone* needs to be there.

I suppose my immune system is still feeling the aftereffects of the surgery. But what about all those antibiotics I had to take?

Anybody in the market for a house full of germs? I will be happy to make you a special price.

> February 24, 2009

To market, to market. How can one nose have so much gunk in it? But I am alone in the marketing department this week, and I have got a ton of ideas to work on. No time to whine. The work is going well, and I am happy with the results. And a bonus is that there hasn't been any traffic on the roads. On the way in, I have time to stop off and pick up some goodies, and then I can work without the usual interpersonal distractions, head home early and relax. For a change, I am working every day. No piano time tomorrow – the only thing on my calendar is marketing.

> March 3, 2009

I contain multitudes. At 8:48 AM, I crawl with the best intentions back into bed and bury myself beneath my blankets. I lie there, tossing and turning, the thousand chattering voices in my head demanding my attention. They are impossible to ignore: 'I'd better add that to my to-do list' and 'I absolutely *have* to give so-and-so a call' and 'How could I have made such a foolish mistake?'
I beg the voices to talk about something more pleasant. I argue with them, plead for them to permit me some balance between my work life and home life. For a moment, they seem willing to co-operate and begin to fade.

But their army is too strong, and my defenses have been weakened for weeks.

And the work-life voices are joined by the housewife voices – I have so many silly little obligations, so many chores I have fallen behind on, and the voices nag at me without pause: 'You need to find out what to do about that infestation of caterpillars in the garden, Tania' and 'There are crumbs all over the kitchen floor' and 'When are you going to get around to vacuuming under the stairs?' Not to mention the kids' clothing that – after buying the wrong sizes and going back to the store to exchange them for what turned out to be *other* wrong sizes and going *back* to the store to finally find the *right* sizes – still needs to be laundered and folded and put away in their closets. And the piles of adorable photos I want to frame as gifts for the grandparents. I am *so* overdue for an IKEA run!

Appointments and other obligations. You know the drill. And there are bills to be paid, can't forget about those! I still haven't paid off the hospital, four months after my surgery. Do they think I am made out of money? I wish I was! Not to mention all the health stuff I had to buy. Will it ever end? Apparently not: I am overdue for a mammogram, and what about Arthur's spots? The poor child swears they don't bother him – but I know they're itchy, and I feel guilty I haven't gotten him to the dermatologist. And of course I have another balance test coming up. But I just don't feel like making the appointment. It can wait. But when was I supposed to take the kids to get their hair cut? I know I have it written down somewhere. I'd better find that note – otherwise, I will look like a terrible mother.

And I have to feed the rabbits, and the mailman is due any minute. Jesus, how will *that* look, if she rings the bell and I open the door in my pajamas, my hair a disaster area? And why is this stupid *cold* not better yet? My own sniffling keeps me awake. My nerves are shot. It's sadomasochism, that's what it is. And finally I fade away into dreamland…

The piano store is calling my name. I am not going to fritter away this rare sunny day in my pjs, am I? Although the predicted sunshine hasn't broken through the clouds just yet. And my current piano beckons me. I had better do something about that. So up I get! I noodle around on the keys, which is quite enjoyable. And now it's time to do some writing, to get rid of some of the weight I have been carrying around. Otherwise, those voices will *never* leave me alone. My online to-do list is a useful tool. It helps me keep all the plates spinning.

Oh, lovely: an e-mail from my former colleague Inge, asking me to help her transplant a chestnut tree on Sunday and take a walk in the woods and go out for pancakes. 'Yes,' I reply, 'that sounds like fun.' And then I write again: 'Did you mean just me, or the whole family?' I am tired and sick, and I have got that mountain of ironing to climb. But Inge's always good to be around.

Take a deep breath. You know what? I think I will do a mental body scan, then get into the shower. And after that, we'll see. Do you have mornings like this, too, or am I just crazy?

> March 4, 2009

Marching forth. Am I feeling better? No. Is my voice back? No. Has my snotty nose dried up? No. Have I had a good day? Yes! There are two straight crayoned lines on the floor: one almost five feet long, the other close to six feet. And then two decorative curves to the right. The table has been moved from its place. The cabinet, too. Took all my strength to do it. I was on my knees, measuring and drawing, figuring out where to put the new piano I have got my eye on. Crayon on the floor. The kids aren't allowed to do that, but I am! I can see it already. Which way should I position it?

Called my piano teacher for professional advice, emptied out my piggy bank, pestered the biggy bank with questions about savings plans, arranged for the neighbor to come over and give me *his* opinion. Sigh. I have gone and admired the new piano three times over the last two days. Our plans are marching forward swiftly. Even Thomas is on board. So what now? I am going to leave the crayoned floor plan where it is. To be continued…

> March 12, 2009

Fast forward. It's Tuesday. Traffic, work, traffic, cook, eat. Make plans for tomorrow's activities. I pay some bills – the correct amount this time, to make up for the mistake I made last time. After reading the kids a bedtime story, I am at my computer until 11, preparing some files for my brother. It takes too long to upload them, though, and I finally quit out of the program and save them to my thumb drive. That means more time behind the wheel and an extra stop tomorrow morning, but family is family!

Wednesday

02u58 AM A nightmare wakes Arthur: ants are eating Papa, and they are nibbling at Arthur, too! He crawls into bed with us.

04u00 AM Thomas has to get up - he is working the early shift today, and by 4:30 he is gone.

06u00 AM My turn to rise and shine, so I can be ready for my own day before the Three Musketeers roll out of bed.

08u00 AM Relief is in sight! Or maybe not: the cleaning lady's not here. What next?

08u15 AM I dash out of the house, forgetting my purse, sheet music and violin. But I can't be late to school. It's against the law to make a phone call while driving, but I do it anyway. The PWA's changed the time of my appointment without telling me: they are coming at 12:30. I call Thomas - against the law, but... Can he take care of paying the hairdresser, since I left my purse at home?

08u30 AM Perfect: I drop the two youngest kids at their nursery school right on time.

08u45 AM Perfect timing for #3, too. Today is my day to volunteer in the classroom.

09u30 AM I hand my evaluation sheets over to the teacher and bolt for my car, off to the hairdresser. Make a call from the car - against the… well, you know - call the PWA to say I am running late, can we push our appointment back a half an hour? They agree.

09u45 AM Perfect timing: I am at the hairdresser's. I am not sure about the coloring, since I have to be back on the road at 11 to collect two little heads that also need trimming. I ask my stylist if she can hurry things along. The hairdryer performs a miracle. At 11 on the dot, I am back outside. So far, so good!

11u20 AM At the main entrance. I can see their shaggy little heads, but I have to wait. First the whole school lines up, then the kids taking the bus are first out the door. I stand there patiently, watching the second hand on the clock.

11u50 AM Back at the hairdresser, my two towheads in tow. They behave beautifully.

12u00 PM Papa arrives with Head #3 and money.

12u15 PM The first two heads are ready. Papa leaves and takes them with him. I remember I need to go home to pick up my music and violin.

12u35 PM Head #3 is ready – and hungry. We race the fifteen miles home. 'Mama, you're a road hog,' he announces. He is right, it's awful. I will do better tomorrow, but today we are in a hurry.

13u00 PM Perfect timing: the cleaning lady is at the door. She doesn't have a key, and I am ahead of Papa. He had to stop at the grocery store for bread.

13u15 PM The table is set. I get a bit of ironing done and squeegee a dirty window. Everything else will have to wait: there's always next week. I grab a quick bite, and at 1:25 I clatter downstairs to get my music, the violin, a backpack and a pair of shoes.

13u30 PM We head off for music school – about twenty miles away.

14u00 PM Half an hour of piano and half an hour of violin. Everything else is cancelled – the teacher has exams.

15u00 PM Music lessons are over. Now quickly to my brother's – and I have managed to remember the thumb drive! A brief visit, and hurry back home.

16u00 PM Home again, home again, jiggedy jig! The cleaning lady is waiting for the cup of coffee I promised her. Papa reads the kids a story and falls asleep. I make coffee. The neighbor rings our doorbell. We all have coffee and then set off for the piano store: two cars, four children.

16u55 PM Made it – five minutes before closing time. They let us in. And forty minutes later, everything is arranged. I don't have time to process our decision, but I am thrilled – we have got something to toast tonight!

18u00 PM Does the neighbor want to stay for dinner? And his daughter and grandson, too? Yes, sure, and we pop a cork for the celebration. To music, and to our new piano! It's a pleasant evening. The kids are all wound up. Luckily, our guests are very polite: about 9:00, we're in the doorway, waving goodbye. And then? The usual: pajamas, children in bed, a little straightening up, and collapse.

Today

06u00 AM Back to reality. Get up, traffic, log on to computer, pour coffee, answer emails, meeting, files, meeting, another meeting, another half-hour working on the files. I have got two vacation days left over from last year that I have to use before the end of March or I will lose them. When? When? When will there be a slow week, so I can afford to be out of the office for two days? Well, I shouldn't complain: I have got it pretty good here.

17u50 AM The harried creature drops into her car and heads for home. Shit, it's Thursday, so Thomas is working late! At the last minute, I realize that I am supposed to pick up the kids. I will have to drive fast to get to them… and then drive-through fast food to feed them. Ah, well, they will be happy about that. I would really like to have a day to myself when the new piano is delivered. A day's relief from the rat race. Just one! But I still have to set up my next balance test and a mammogram. I suppose that can wait until the end of April.

If I were to go back and reread all this, I would probably find myself disgusting. So I think I will skip it. What good will it do me to reproach myself? Even after these last six weeks, I still haven't learned my lesson.

> March 16, 2009

The eensy-weensy spiders. They were high up on the ceiling beams. Deep in the slits in the wood. But turning my head in all necessary directions was no problem. One more to-do-list item checked off. Next? The vacuum cleaner roars, and I don't get dizzy. Four and a half months without a single rotten dizzy spell!

> March 19, 2009

Second life. Another half hour and the new piano will be here! I took two vacation days for this, because I want to be able to enjoy it. Well, enjoy? So far, today has been devoted to hours of anticipation, of pacing back and forth, of biting my nails. But the sun is still up, and the delivery guys just called to tell me they are only half an hour away. My second life is about to begin. I will spread my wings and caw a raucous 'Fuck you!' to the global financial crisis. One lesson I have learned: you only live once. And I want to feel every second in the tips of my fingers.

> March 21, 2009

Tonight's concerto: 'Third Time's the Charm.' Four hours with my kids, and Murphy's Law strikes again.

First movement: No money. Thanks to a bank error in connection with the new piano, my credit cards have been blocked.

Second movement: Charlotte suddenly comes down with a fever and I have to rush her to the doctor. Their bill comes to thirty-four euros, and all I have in my wallet is thirty. Fortunately, it's just the flu and nothing more serious. Relieved, we all troop back home.

Third movement: We aren't in the house for five minutes when there is a knock at the window. 'Matthias fell off the swing!' In the distance, I can hear his plaintive solo: 'I am dying! I am going blind!' What child in his right mind reads a book on the swing?! *My* child, naturally. So off he falls, and the swing swings back and hits him in the eye. I call the doctor and asked if we can come back, explain I don't have cash or a working credit card. 'No problem.' Back we go, and the doctor does what she can. The concerto comes to an end, and the gang returns home yet again.

So now there are three pianos in our street, and our neighbor drops by to test ours out and play a few pieces. With the kids in mind, he has even worked up a couple of Disney classics. We drink a toast to the new member of the household, and I whip up some dinner. It's a romantic evening, even with my three ruffians tearing around the place. And, oh, does the new piano sound lovely!

> March 26, 2009

Mother, may I? (Or *must* I?). I am permitted to stay home from work today. That is to say: I *have* to. Charlotte's flu has returned. And Arthur has got some sort of stomach bug. So we go to the doctor. Not bad. On the way, Arthur spots a blue road sign indicating that both bicycles and pedestrians are permitted on this particular stretch and educates me on his five-year-old's version of the rules of the road: 'You are allowed to bike along here, but you have to hold your mama's hand to cross the street.' To be honest, his lecture helps to calm me down.

> March 31, 2009

Bravo, Dizzy Me. They got me, too. Two days of fever, but I was determined not to let it slow me down. I finally had to admit defeat, though, and on the second day I came home from work early. I don't mean to toot my own horn, but I am proud that I finished up an important assignment before I staggered out of the office. Bravo, Dizzy Me!

On the way home, I must have pressed the gas pedal a little harder for every degree my temperature rose above normal. So the flu bug has *really* got me, and now I have a speeding ticket to pay. I should have just followed doctor's orders and stayed in bed this morning. Bravo, Dizzy Me.

> April 3, 2009

Six of one, half a bottle of another. I must have swallowed twenty aspirins, but my temperature just will not come down. So my nasty little mycoplasmas and I are under house arrest. I never knew a human being could get this sick.
I don't think I felt this rotten even after my surgery. It's truly debilitating. Five days of non-stop fever and counting. I have been gobbling pills like candy, double the recommended dosage. The effect thus far? Nothing.

But I drag myself groaning from the sofa and use this opportunity to add some actual *information* to my blog. Lately, I have been babbling about trivia, and I haven't had much of real importance to say.

'You don't think you returned to work too soon?' my doctor asks. 'It takes a good long time to recover from surgery. You jumped back into your normal life too early, trying to be the perfect mother, wife and employee, and you haven't given yourself the chance to fully recover. So look what happened! This time, you'd better take my advice.'

Okay, I grudgingly agree. But no antibiotics. That's where I draw the line. I will get better naturally – well, okay, except for the aspirin. I will take echinacea and iron pills, but no antibiotics. You think I want the nausea and vomiting they can cause? Well, think again.

She accedes to my demand. As long as the fever is gone by the end of the weekend. So, fingers crossed. My blood work says that, all things considered, I am in very good shape. Blood sugar, thyroid, liver, kidneys: all perfect. Cholesterol: I am a textbook case, despite the occasional fried-chicken dinner and my daily melt-in-your-mouth bouchée à la Reine

I hate being inside on such a pleasant day, but I need rebuild my resistance. So I lie here suffering, taking my temperature, knocking back the aspirins, feeling sorry for myself – though I haven't forgotten my fellow blogger Flupque: I have got two candles lit for you, my friend!

My mom, who lives five hundred miles away, calls. She grumbles about my speeding ticket. But that's the *least* of my worries, and I really don't want to talk about it. She tells me to make myself some soup. As if I could eat. She tells me I can send the kids earlier than usual for their Easter visit, and they can stay for longer than usual. All three of them? Not a great idea. Before she hangs up, she reminds me to eat something.

I think I have lost a good six, six-and-a-half pounds, and it is weight I am certainly better off without. I just hope Thomas doesn't come down with this awful flu. 'I don't think I will,' he says. 'I don't have *time* to get sick. I have so much to do.' Oh, really, husband? And you think I *have* got time for this nonsense?

> April 5, 2009

Have no cell wall, will travel. They are no fun at all, my mycoplasmas. Six days of uninterrupted fever. And I am dizzy - although this time it has nothing at all to do with drifting crystals, just my very low blood pressure. I wasn't sure I would be able to make it through the weekend without a trip to the urgent care, but I managed. And now my temperature has come back down to normal. I am exhausted, my body feels made of lead, I have coughed myself hoarse. But I have a week off work to recover, and I think I am going to need it.

This afternoon, I am due for some R&R. Hubby Dearest is at work, and I am on my own. With a shawl around my shoulders, I sit out in the sun with a view of the kids' sandbox. By tomorrow morning, all systems should be go.

Mycoplasma. Those pesky little bacteria have apparently been tested for possible use as a biological weapon: in wartime, according to the theory, they would rob the enemy of his will to live and render him harmless. I can well imagine! And it's better not to speak of the long-term consequences. They are a little like a sunnyside-up egg: they have no cell wall and just sit there and tremble. Once they get inside you, though, they can do a lot of damage.

I think I will pour myself a glass of wine this evening. I am not taking antibiotics, so go ahead, Tania, knock yourself out!

> April 7, 2009

Fine, thanks, and you? I got an unexpected call from my old physical therapist today. He treated me when I was pregnant with Charlotte, still dizzy and at the end of my rope. How have I been doing lately? Fine, thanks. Great, in fact. Haven't felt dizzy in five months. On May 20, I am going to be tested in the balance chair.

What I completely forget to tell him is that I actually feel awful at the moment, still sick as a dog. But not dizzy! Just *sick*, wasted from the endless hacking. I try another brand of cough syrup, but nothing seems to soothe my aching throat.

If this keeps up, I will cough myself inside out. I try my hand at the piano, but halfway through the piece a big hack attack forces me to give up.

He is one of those super bikers, rides events like Bike-Aid to raise money for cancer research. Like Lance Armstrong, he has been there himself. But you would never know it to look at him - he is in incredible shape, and soon he will be doing a ride from Chernobyl to Brussels, a distance of over twelve hundred miles.

> April 8, 2009

Enemy Mine. Okay, the other side wins this one. I was hoping that the mycoplasmazoids would fold their tents and silently steal away by now, but I guess they are having too good a time inside me to leave. My ribcage has been refurbished into a twelve-story hotel for the occupying forces, and the mycoplasma pneumonia will not give me a moment's peace. They seem to be heading down to the basement, and I am not at all happy about that. As of today, I will start taking the damn antibiotics after all, and I have got two extra weeks of sick leave and an assignment to undergo altitude training at my parents' house in France. I hope it's healthier there than it is in this crazy country.

> April 10, 2009

What a difference a day makes. I would rather not know what exactly that medication is doing to my insides. One thing is for sure, though: it's helping me. In between coughing jags, I am actually getting a little rest, though the attacks themselves are still coming from way down deep. I have stopped feeling like smashing my head against the wall. And I am beginning to rediscover the joys of sunlight and fresh air. Of playing the piano. Of being alive. Of planning for the future. For the time being, however, I continue to take things slowly. First, I need to get better. Completely better. The information flyer that came with the pills mentions a possible psychological side effect: euphoria. Could that be it?

Next week, I am going to a sort of 'air cure' sanitarium with my parents. They have selected one of the better places, a B&B in Vergisson, in southern Burgundy in France, surrounded by vineyards and with a view of the Mont Blanc. The sunshine will load me up with vitamins, and hopefully I will come home a new woman.

> April 16, 2009

Elle dit beaucoup de bêtises. A five hundred-mile drive to better health. French air, French sun, French breezes, French clouds. Not to mention the French bread and French fashions. A week in wine's amusement park, and my cough is much better, thanks! Although, as my grandmother would have said, '*La lutte contre le champignon microscopique… ça dure et ça reste dure, mais la pharmacienne m'a bien aidé.*' The fight against those microscopic mushrooms is an expensive battle, but the drugstore can help you to win it.

Meanwhile, here is what Dizzy Me has to say: '*Je suis toujours fatiguée, mais pour le reste je tire mon plan. Salut et à bientôt!*' I am still exhausted, but everything is going according to plan. So cheers, and I will see you soon!

Of course we will be bringing some good French wine home with us…

> April 20, 2009

Snap, crackle, pop! Another five hundred miles in the car, and we are home sweet home. Suitcases unpacked and one of them repacked, because tomorrow our baby Charlotte is off again for two weeks with Grandma and Grandpa in their camper. Good for her, since, as soon as you come back to Belgium from the south - even though the sun is shining and the garden is lovelier than ever - your bones begin to crackle and ache. Mine do, anyway. It's almost funny, how your body reacts to the change in the air. The last lingering effect of the mycoplasma, I suppose. But I have still got a week to work through all that, and hopefully the sun will continue to play along. It's wonderfully quiet here, now that the kids are back in school. I am still crackling, but I will adjust.

> April 21, 2009

Flashback. Poor lamb! My colleague Linda was supposed to return to work yesterday after a long illness, but a serious kidney crisis has cropped up. Certainly not the nicest weather for an overnight in a stuffy hospital. So I figure, if she can't go out and enjoy the sun, I'd better deliver the sun to her: I bring her a gaily colored beach chair, a pile of graphic novels, and a pot of bright-yellow flowers. And now her room looks a lot more cheerful.

I feel for you, girlfriend! Visiting you gives me a flashback to my own time in the hospital. I have to keep it short, though: Linda is running a fever, so I can't stay long. After I leave, I roam around Halle – where once upon a time I used to live – for a while, and encounter memories on every street corner. And who do I bump into? My kindergarten teacher from thirty-three years ago! What a welcome coincidence! I recognize her right off, and she knows me, too. Miss Looza, I used to call her. I can't remember why. Because I was a five-year-old child, perhaps, and that was as close as I could come to 'Rosa', which was her real name?

> May 10, 2009

Daredevilly Me. It's Mother's Day, my day in the limelight. We have a tearful morning, though: Matthias can't find the present he made me. We search everywhere: his book bag, the garage, the car… that child is so absent-minded! Whatever it is, he apparently left it at school. So he weeps, and I sniffle along with him.

Charlotte's and Arthur's problems are of two entirely different types. They are always competing, and today is no different. Arthur has written me a Mother's Day poem, and he spits it out without a stumble. Bravo! Charlotte's not a poet, so she cuts to the chase and gives me a very pretty watering can for my garden. I sit there patiently until she finally stops insisting, 'It's mine! It's mine!' And this year I hit the jackpot: an electric toaster! 'Finally,' says Matthias, 'now we can have toast without setting the whole house on fire!'

At last comes the ultimate gift: I get to play the piano for an audience of seventy people. Today at last I can repay them for all the time they have devoted to me, this past year. I am nervous, I will not deny it: my fingers tremble, my head, my toes. But I play. I play *well.* And I survive! When I finish, there is rousing applause, and I get lots of compliments. So I guess the truth is you *can* teach an old dog new tricks. What was I so worried about? Matthias serves as my personal photographer. He practically lies on his stomach to get some of the shots he takes.

And that's not all! After my recital, we are off to the carnival! I skip the bumper cars, though. That's a risk I am not going to take until - soon, I hope! - my doctor gives me the green light.

> May 18, 2009

Bah, humbug. It's almost over. On Wednesday, I will flash back seven months to the days when I suffered sudden attacks of dizziness and nausea, to the feeling of the ground falling away beneath my feet, to uncertainty and countless medical tests, so many of them I felt like I was choking on them. This will be the last time, I hope. The nauseating caloric tests - the ones with cold and warm water - the classic balance test with the video spectacles, the moving balls and the swivel chair. And then the conversation with the doctor, which, to be fair, isn't as awful as all the rest of it. All this to establish, once and for all, that I am cured. And to help advance the medical profession's understanding of my condition, of course, since the profession has, after all, been helpful to *me*. But still, I am just not in the mood. Yuck.

No mercy. Morning, and I am on my way to the University Hospital of Antwerp. Here is what I have to look forward to: a mammogram, my hopefully final balance test, a hearing test, and one last debriefing with the doctor. A half day of scurrying from pillar to post. When I get there, I am in for a scolding - I am running half an hour late, I have forgotten my prescription, I didn't bring the results of my last mammogram, I think I would have forgotten my head if it wasn't screwed on. But that lies an hour in the future. Right now, I am doing fine.

So, on my way to the University Hospital. The speed limit is 50 miles an hour, and there are speed cameras at regular intervals. I am doing 53, 54, 55, 52… concentrate, Me, and keep it at 50! I am in the left lane, passing all the brave souls who are afraid to go faster than 45. It's a pleasant ride, not so much traffic, the radio on.

I am listening to a talk show, a discussion of solar panels and the VREG, which is the Flemish government's regulatory agency for electricity and natural gas. And then I notice the annoying tailgater who is apparently got it in for my rear bumper. I can see his face in the rear-view mirror: he is a scowling creep, somewhere in his late twenties. Riffraff, I decide. He looks angry, begins swaying back and forth across the lane dividers. He is trying to pass me on the right, and he shakes a fist every time he has to brake for the slowpokes in that lane. I don't have to be able to read lips to guess what he is muttering.

My heart shifts into a higher gear, but I maintain my cool. *You don't bother me*, I tell him inside my head. *But if that's how you are going to behave, there is no way I let you pass me*. I really hate his sort of arrogance. He snarls and curses and shakes his fist, changes lanes, speeds up, brakes. Just as he is about to do something really dangerous, we come to a red light. This is the moment of truth. A little communication via my mirror can't hurt. Not what you are thinking, though: instead of giving him the finger, I lift my hand and show him all five of them. *Fifty miles an hour*, I am warning him. And then I turn away and ignore him. But the young gentleman apparently misunderstands. The light turns green, and we resume driving. I keep to the speed limit and stay in the left lane. He tries again to pass on the right, but he fails to reckon with my girl power. I speed up and slow down in rhythm with the speed cameras, and time it out so that, just as he is about to pass me, we come up on one and he has got to hit the brakes. I can see him growing more and more angry, and I begin to worry about the next stoplight. And then a loud crash releases me from what could be about to turn ugly.

The idiot has rear-ended someone else. Pity for the someone else, but I am happy to be rid of him. I yell out a joyous 'Yes!' and turn up my radio and hit the gas. And I suddenly decide that it's time to ask my doctor if it's okay for me to ride the bumper cars with my kids.

Yes! Yes! Yes! I am cured! The canal plugging has had no negative impact on my balance, and it's freed me from my attacks. My hearing is perfect. And, yes, I am cleared to ride the bumper cars! From what the doctor tells me, it looks like canal-plugging surgery is slowly but surely becoming more common.

In the corridor, I run into Professor Wuyts. I thank him for the gift he has given me after fifteen years of suffering. He shows me a glass jar containing a tiny object: an adorable little vestibular organ. It's so small! That makes the precision required for the operation even more impressive. I have said it before: these doctors really are professionals.

> June 23, 2009

Back in the saddle again. It's been a while. I haven't been feeling well lately, and I have just been too tired to blog. I am still not at my best, but there is news today - so here I am!

A plug for canal plugging. Today was Marie-Thérèse's surgery. At least, if all went according to plan. She was pretty nervous about it - as was I about mine. We talked twice on the phone, shared our stories. I hope she will recover quickly, and that the operation will work as well for her as it did for me. Then there will be two of us properly plugged.

> June 25, 2009

She can hear clearly now, the pain is gone. Marie-Thérèse calls me today! She's out of the hospital and home, and everything's going great. Her hearing is fine. She feels good. I am so happy for her. And she is enthusiastic about the future. This should encourage those who have been sceptical about the surgical solution and could perhaps themselves benefit from canal plugging.

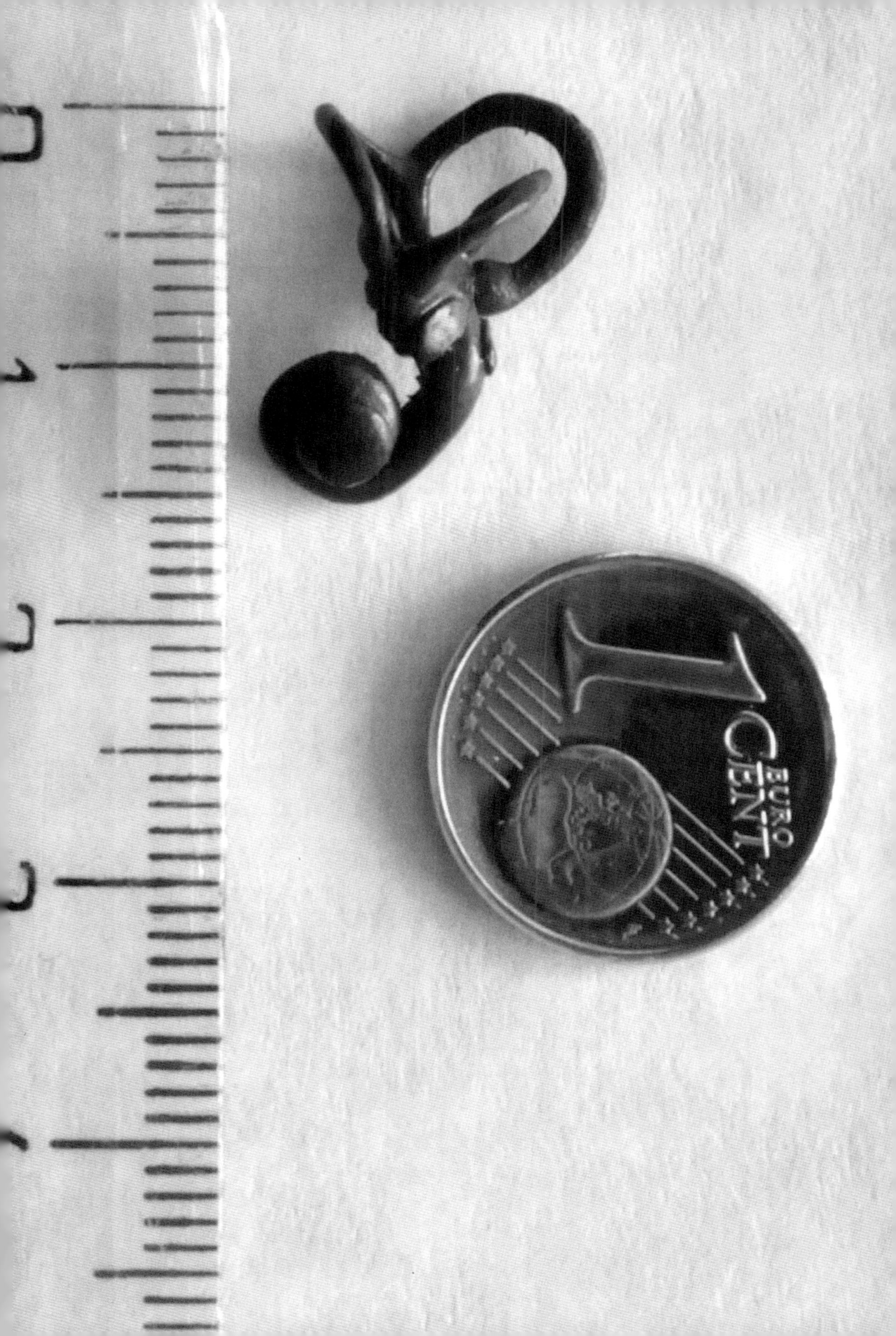
1 EURO CENT

>June 30, 2009

We don't need your stinkin' mycoplasma! It began around April 1, but it was no April Fool's Day joke. My mycoplasma bacteria have been bothering me for the last three months. I have no resistance. Antibiotics were my only recourse, so I took them. But they didn't help much at the time, and, three months later, I am still not operating at one hundred percent. I can't get a good night's sleep, and every muscle in my body aches. Wrist pain, nerve pain, bellyache, radiating back pain, runny red eyes. Not one of my molecules is behaving the way it's supposed to behave.

Living like this, the other people in the house have come to see me as a hypersensitive whiner. I am nagged by guilty thoughts: *What if they think I am a hypochondriac? Maybe I am just imagining things.* But my swollen lymph glands convince me there's an actual physical problem, so it's back to the doctor I trudge.

And, sure enough, it turns out that all of my big and little complaints stem from a single cause. After three months, those blubbery mycoplasmaniacs are still active and acute. That means another three weeks of antibiotics. I can hardly wait. Can't they just prescribe me sun, vacation, peace? Give me a year without anything going wrong, and I will be thrilled. But this? Another three weeks without a glass of wine? This is *such* bad timing: my vacation is just beginning!

> July 1, 2009

Super Stadsbader. In the doctor's office. My prescription is ready. We sit side by side, our noses practically touching the computer screen. Together, we are studying the results of my blood test. One number shows up highlighted in red. That's not a danger sign, just a way to draw our attention to a value outside the normal range. In this case, it's my hematocrit level - which reads far beyond those of mortal men… my secret superpower. Does this make me faster than a speeding bullet, more powerful than a locomotive, able to leap tall buildings in a single bound? No, none of that. But an elevated hematocrit is actually beneficial to people participating in endurance sports, and I decide I might as well do something worthwhile with this surprising finding.

> July 7, 2009

Ask Tania. I have been getting more phone calls than usual. Fellow sufferers about to go under the knife, or those who have already had the surgery. It's kind of nice, chatting with people who have had or are about to have an experience similar to mine. Today it's Marie-Thérèse, who was operated on two weeks ago, on the line. Her doctors are so uncommunicative, she says. She gets more information from *me* than from them. Is it normal that she hears a peeping in her ear, that she feels an attack coming on but it never arrives? Yes, indeed, I assure her, I felt the same way. Like I was underwater, wearing scuba gear. So don't worry about it - another couple of weeks, and all that will be history. Look at me!

> July 12, 2009

I want to ride my bicycle. Since yesterday, I have taken up a new sport. It may turn out to be just a passing fancy - we will see. But the fact that my hematocrit level is high has given me the motivation - well, that and the fifteen pounds I have put on since my surgery. Or perhaps it's got something to do with my giving up African dance? Now that I am no longer shaking my moneymaker, my moneymaker seems to be growing...

So I dig my exercycle out of storage and set it up on the patio, and I have been pedaling for the last half hour. The view is lovely! Thomas is shocked at the sight of me in workout clothes and suggests I might want to put on another layer. But I just continue pedaling. For this first session, my goal is seven miles at an average speed of fifteen miles per hour. My heart is racing: 180 bpm, which for my age is about as fast as I want it to get. According to the screen, I have burned 250 calories. I am dripping with sweat, since I am completely out of condition.

Bicycle races are coming your way, so forget all your duties - oh, yeah! Fat-bottomed girls, they'll be riding today, so look out for those beauties - oh, yeah!

> July 20, 2009

Ladies, would you care to join me? *This is working*, I think. Nine days, and my passing fancy has not yet passed. Actually, I am really getting into it. I get on my bike once or twice a day, preferably at the crack of dawn. At 6 AM I head out to the patio, take a deep breath of the morning air, and do thirty to fifty minutes of hard labour. Another deep breath, and into a cold shower. Afterwards, I feel wonderfully tingly. Why didn't I know about this long ago?

Today I do six and a half miles in the saddle, then six and a half miles on foot - walking shoeless by the water. The sight of the sea cheers me. I am turning into a fresh-air fiend. And when I see all the various shapes and sizes strolling by - big, small, slender, thin as a rail, the occasional 36-24-36'er, the stout, the XXL'ers, the ginormous - I realize my goal is a sound body to house my sound mind. All other positive consequences will follow naturally, I hope. In any case, by the end of Day 9 one thing has become very noticeable: my track shoes, which used to pinch my toes, are now a much better fit. So, ladies, would you care to join me?

> August 3, 2009

Chamois. A week's vacation in Vergisson. We teach Arthur to pedal a bike. Ride on donkeys. Climb rocks. Hoist a glass or two. Do a lot of hiking.

Back home, I break out my chamois and get to work polishing my exercycle, the windows, the inside walls of the closets. Tomorrow I go back to work. But first I will get up at six and hit the bike. For tonight, though, I am done. After four months, my mycoplasmatrons are finally beginning to give up the ghost. By September, according to the doctor, they should be gone.

> August 5, 2009

Rebranding. It's time to face the inevitable: the rebranding of my blog. I will soon hit ten months of dizzy-free living, and for months now I have been avoiding the issue. Many of my readers are getting tired of me chattering on about playing the piano, riding my bike, dealing with my kids - and airing my frank opinions. I am not really writing a health blog any more. I am going to have to switch to some other category.

One thing I don't have to worry about: Feedjit's tracking data make it crystal clear that people who are looking for information about vertigo continue to find their way to me. As long as I don't start calling myself Happy Me, they will stick with me. A full ninety percent of my readers are fellow sufferers - there are quite a few of us out there! Although I am going to have to make some changes, I will not abandon my friends.

If you were to go strictly by the number of comments posted, you would think I was talking mostly to myself. But nothing could be further from the truth. Other blogs get dozens of responses to every post, but - except for Flupque - mine come in almost exclusively via e-mail. Maybe that's because the subject matter is so sensitive? Anyway, my readers for the most part prefer to remain anonymous.

So, what category should I select? I could go with 'lifestyle,' but that label doesn't exist. Maybe 'daily life,' but that doesn't sound as hip. It's like picking a brand of bottled water to serve to company: should I select something simple, like Dasani, or something chic like Perrier? It's all a question of positioning. Where do I want to fit in? Where do I *belong*?

The die is cast. I am giving up my #6 ranking in the Top 10 health blogs and taking on last place in the 'daily life' category. So it goes. But who knows? Maybe I will change my mind yet again...

> August 6, 2009

Sometimes, sometimes I wonder. Sometimes I wonder if this biking thing is really worth the effort. It's been a month, now, and I have produced no noticeable results. Six AM. I pretend that I am having fun. The morning mist. The fresh breezes. The outdoorsy smells. It's *good* for me! Don't give up. But it's hard. Especially when my better half drops into bed at night, reaches for the alarm clock and - with a perfectly serious expression on his face - looks at me sideways and says, 'What time should I set it for, sweetie? Sex o'clock?'

> August 17, 2009

Apple jelly on wheels. It was July 11 when I decided to do something with my elevated hematocrit level. Until now, that has meant exercycling on the patio. But I have taken a next step: since Saturday, I have been venturing out onto the open road. Crazy, but it seems so *easy*. Going full out by myself, cruising around the neighborhood with the family, taking an evening ride with Matthias to see a good friend's organic garden, beehives and aquaria. Early mornings, I am still unfortunately stuck with the stationary bike. Thanks to the rush-hour traffic heading for Brussels, I don't really have any other choice.

It takes sixteen minutes before my legs start to burn. A month ago, I was exhausted after five. Given all the apple jelly I make, I need the extra exercise. Apply jelly turns out to be pretty dangerous stuff.

This morning I bring a jar to the office to share with my colleagues. Some fresh basil, too. It's got nothing to do with marketing, I know. But picture this: apple jelly, strawberry syrup and basil liqueur mixed together, spread on a piece of toast and topped with basil leaves. It's an experiment, and everyone agrees it's a success. After an hour, our tummies are rumbling for more. The aroma of it seduces a visitor to the office, who asks if he can try it. So of course we all have to join him.

> August 26, 2009

Fallin'-flyin'. This morning. Time to exercise. I bike between meadows and farmland. Cows, horses, donkeys, greenery. The smell of fertilizer and a tractor's exhaust but, all things considered, beautiful beautiful beautiful!

And then? Big white cloud at one o'clock! Fire? A pesticide drop? I take precautionary measures and pinch my nostrils shut. As I approach a curve in the road, the cloud grows enormously. Shocked, I jerk on my brakes. And every last ounce of me goes flying over the handlebars. One elbow and one palm make initial contact with the ground. I lie there, woozy, and the farmer goes right on spraying. I come back to my senses. Did I really take a fall because of a pressure washer? Five minutes later, I am still lying there. I must look a sight. I get up and right my bike, and the front wheel is now wobbly. The spraying stops. The farmer looks up. From his expression, I suspect he may be playing with only about 47 or 48 cards in his deck.

'You scared me,' I reproach him, 'but it wasn't really your fault.' Yet I am thinking, You stupid *f- armer*.

'You could hurt yourself like that,' he mumbles.

'I *did* hurt myself,' I say, and the tone of my voice is intended to encourage him to help me. But he doesn't take the hint. I wipe away a tear and climb back in the saddle again. And he switches his machine back on. How stupid can one human being *be*?

> August 28, 2009

Peeling potatoes in my panties. *How to Mess Up a Vacation in One Easy Lesson*, by Tania Stadsbader. And trust me on this: I am an expert. All the free time in the world, and what do I do with it? I change my mind a hundred times. I can't stand it, this eternal internal conflict between the voices in my head. Are all those voices really *mine*?

Here is an example: The other morning, I gave all my empty jars away, and by the afternoon I decided I wanted to make jelly. Except now I didn't have any jars, and I wasted two half days searching for the exact kind I had just given away, a search which kept me from doing other more important things. Sometimes I really annoy myself.

My heart says *Play the piano, Tania, go over your notes, break your biking record.* But my brain says *Clean the kitchen, do the laundry, iron the kids' clothing*. Because school starts in again next week, and everything has to be ready.

I slip into a pair of pants, realize they are too long for me and kick them off. I really don't know how to hem them, but I find a needle and thread and sigh.

Should I parade into the kitchen first and peel potatoes in my panties? Company is coming later in the day, and I have to go to Open House at the kids' school and stop at the drugstore. And I really need to pick up some paint chips - I have been thinking about a new color for the walls - but there simply isn't enough time.

Got to find that recipe! I want to make something special for our company, but I can't remember the details. I can see it all unfold: they arrive, the barbecue is not fired up yet, the dishes are piled in the sink. Oh, right: the neighbor brought over some tomatoes, and I have to return his bowl. So I had better tackle the dishes. But, no, first I need to hem those pants, otherwise I can't leave the house. I feel suspended in air… and I had better not forget to hit up the butcher.

As if all that's not enough, at 4 PM I have an appointment to see a podiatrist for the first time in my life - and I absolutely *can't* blow that off. Meanwhile, an e-mail dings for my attention, and I ought to answer it before anything else. But what about those pants? It's noon already, and I have gotten *anything* done. Sewing really isn't my thing…

> August 28, 2009

Oh, no: a toe show! Lieve, my podiatrist, can read toes. She took a class in it. Tonight, Thomas, I am going to put on a toe show, because mine turn out to be gorgeous! And you know what she says? The fourth toe on my right foot - the one just in from my 'pinkie' toe - is a whopper. It's even longer than my middle toe. That means that I am powerful, I know what I want, I am a woman with a plan. And I know how to explain things. That is what my relationship toe says about me.

The middle toe is a big one, too, which indicates that I am very sensitive. And the rest of them are nothing to sneeze at - definitely not ugly, like Thomas tells me.

Lieve says they are fine. 'Can you sleep,' she wants to know, 'with all those plans rattling around in your head?' Absolutely, I tell her. As soon as the light goes out, I am gone.

> September 2, 2009

Free fallin'. As of today, I can be clumsy and fall off my bike as many times as I want. I bought a helmet with lots of air holes and a two-year crash guarantee! Now I can relax.

> September 7, 2009

Boogie-woogie bugle girl. Another phone conversation with Marie-Thérèse. She had her surgery at the end of June. 'Everything is going great,' she says. 'Such a shame I had to wait fifteen years for this. What a waste of time.' Things are fine with me, too, I tell her. I also lost fifteen years of my life to dizziness. Those years are gone, though, and we can't get them back. At least we have our futures to look forward to.

Yesterday we could barely see straight. Today, I am doing Zumba and biking, and Marie-Thérèse is dancing the boogie-woogie! Amazing, isn't it? And people say there is nothing to be done about vertigo. It took us years to grope our way to a solution on our own.

> October 13, 2009

Hold your breath, make a wish, count to eighteen. We are almost there. Hard to believe, but I had my surgery on October 31, 2008 - almost exactly a year ago. I remember swearing, 'No, Adèle, I won't be back.' And now, just eighteen more days to count down, and I have won the lottery! Adèle, you can serve that cup of coffee to someone else. Because I have got my balance back. I can ride my bike and, if there isn't any traffic, still make it to Zumba. I can check the ceiling for spiders, vacuum all the way into the corners of the room, jump out of bed without a care.

I am willing to admit that I still worry just a smidge, but only first thing in the morning, my head still resting on my pillow. Turning to the right, I remain careful. But nothing bad ever happens. After all those years of trouble, it's hard to break myself of my habitual cautiousness.

Once again I think about writing a book. One day I really feel like doing it, the next day I wonder, *Why bother? Who would be interested?* In a way, I am searching for a more metaphoric type of balance. What am I going to do with my life? What course will my future take? But whether she has got a tailwind pushing her forward or a headwind holding her back, Tania will *never* give up.

> October 23, 2009

A plug of her own. The flu has invaded our house. Wednesday it hit Charlotte. Thursday Matthias. And today is my turn. It batters me, gnaws at me, makes it hard to find my way. And yet the day also brings a piece of wonderful news: there are now - to the best of my knowledge - *three* women in Flanders who have undergone the canal-plugging surgery. First me, then Marie-Thérèse, and a fortnight ago it was Ingrid's turn. The recovery period is challenging for her, but that is perfectly normal. Two weeks is still early days, and every day checked off the calendar is a significant step forward. I hope it will not be long before Patient #4 gets a plug of her own.

> October 25, 2009

Black beauty. I have been playing the piano for a year. In an indirect way, I owe that to my dizziness. Still, each time I see my new piano I am overwhelmed by the beauty of the instrument, its construction, the simplicity of its keyboard, the sound of every note. I have to remind myself to go on breathing.

Sometimes I actually pet it. To me, it's a piece of heaven, a drug. On the other hand, it can be hellish trying to teach notes, tempos and rhythm to five-year-old Arthur, to instill in him patience, to dry his tears and convince him to take the next step forward. And then there is the fury of his nine-year-old brother Matthias when the right notes refuse to come out of his fingers. Not to mention my own frustration when it takes me a hundred tries before I can finally get through a piece without a mistake.

But it's all worth it. Even after a thirty-year 'break', it's not too late. Week after week I remind myself: *Keep going, Tania. And don't forget to breathe!*

What lies beneath. As I count down the days – three to go! – to the first anniversary of my canal plugging and a long-anticipated celebration of my release from dizziness, a flood of e-mails flows into my in-box.

My blog still doesn't get many online reactions, and I haven't had much in the way of news to report for months, but I feel like I need to carry on. Because if you should do a search tomorrow on 'BPPV', 'vertigo', 'dizzy', 'Epley', 'balance disorder', 'crystals in the ear', or pretty much anything along those lines and find yourself linked through to my blog… well, almost 50,000 others will have landed there before you.

Most of them are searching for answers they haven't been able to get from their doctors. And most of their e-mails urge me not to retire the Dizzy Me blog. It apparently provides support to people who haven't yet been given a conclusive diagnosis, gives them information they would be hard-pressed to find elsewhere. Yes, it's information collected by a layman – but at least I am a layman with years of experience. I select my links carefully, avoid quackery and – I hope! – never steer anyone down the wrong path.

What I find so fascinating in these emails are the similarities between the writers' stories. Their journeys precisely mirror my own, down to the smallest details: the attacks, that awful 'it's about to happen' feeling (often followed by it *not* happening), the desperate uncertainty, the crazy behaviors that go along with the condition. Today, it's a blessing to be able to reach a jar of peanut butter down from the shelf like a normal person. And then there are the reports of disbelief and misunderstanding, even once the surgical procedure has been scheduled.

Oh, sure, I have got plenty of so-called 'friends' who tell me I am making a lot of fuss about nothing. Most of them, you see, only ever encountered me when I was between attacks. If you haven't been through it yourself, it's impossible to understand this invisible ailment and the impact it can have on your life.

Today I received an email from Viv that, a year ago, I could just as well have written myself. (You'll find Viv's story at the back of this book, in the appendix titled 'The Patients Speak'.)

> October 30, 2009

Spooning. 'Spooning' has its own interest page on Facebook. I am guessing that most of the people who have liked it are ordinary folks who simply happen to enjoy sleeping spooned up against their partners. After all, spooning makes both the spooner and the spoonee feel warm, happy and safe. Or maybe, for some, it's a way to avoid a spouse's morning breath, or to stop him from snoring? There are plenty of reasons to do it, I suppose. But I hope you will agree with me that, whatever your reason, spooning is *pleasant*.

For me, though, there is more to it than simple enjoyment. For years and years, I *could not* spoon with my husband, because that would have forced me to sleep on my bad side, and my dizziness would not permit that to happen.

Well, tonight, to celebrate tomorrow's anniversary, I am going to spoon with Thomas. And he had better not *dare* to deny me!

> November 22, 2009

Announcing *Dizzy Me: The Book.* After a year and 50,000 hits, after all my doubts and a lack of the appropriate tools… my new computer has arrived. Long live InDesign! Now nothing can stop me. I have shifted into overdrive and started work on my book. I have been sitting here writing and tinkering with layout half the night. And I am almost halfway done!

I have got 240 pages written, about my illness and my cure and my blog. My own story. My post-operative diary. My physical and emotional recovery. I put it all in there. In a way, I have made sense of my fifteen-year struggle. Meanwhile, several of my fellow sufferers have also had successful surgeries – after, like me, years of mistaken diagnoses. This book will be my 'and she lived happily every after'!

> December 11, 2009

The Rocky Horror Phobia Show. I used to be fearless. Children climb the tallest trees, ride the most dizzying carnival rides, jump around on the roof, ski straight down mountains – who needs to slalom? – and that's the way I grew up. It's easy to explain: young brains are remarkably flexible. They learn quickly… and forget with equal ease.

But adult brains? Frightening memories come back to haunt us. And when those fears are unreasonable, they can morph into phobias, which can require extensive intensive therapy. The problem is that a scary thought which suddenly pops up from your past can terrify you all over again. These memories can be erased with the proper therapeutic treatment, but that can take months or even years. If only it could be done in a day or two. I would sign up for that *Eternal Sunshine* treatment, if it were available.

Which brings me to my 'here it comes again' phobia. My own personal Pavlovian conditioning. I am cured of my dizziness, I know that, but the feeling creeps over me from time to time, even all these months after my last attack. I don't like admitting that, but I have to, if I am going to be honest. After years of Dizzy Me-ness, I can't just shake the feeling off when it comes. Instead, my neck quite naturally tenses. And a tense neck can cause – you guessed it! – dizziness. Or maybe first I had a totally innocent stiffness in my neck – after all, that happens – and it's the stiffness that subconsciously suggests an attack is about to hit me. Either way, this is still a bit of an issue, and I am not happy about it, not one bit!

I hate the feeling, the memory of dizzy spells past, the sensation that cautions me all hell's about to break loose. I have to regroup, remind myself that the nightmare is truly over. *Really*, I tell myself, over and over again, seriously. *That stiff neck is just playing a trick on you.*

By writing this book, I am reopening old wounds. And that's not a good thing to do. But it's a thing I *have* to do. It's my therapy. I have to figure out how to deal with my phobia.

New research suggests that it may be possible to erase fears much more quickly in the future. That youthful carefree attitude would be handy for adults dealing with PTSD or phobias. I heard it on the radio. It would involve surgically removing the perineuronal net, a special layer of the brain that surrounds the memory center. The experiment has already been done successfully on lab rats. I would volunteer to be a human subject, if they would take me. Then I could lose that terrible feeling forever.

> December 26, 2009

A promise is a promise. About a year ago, I made a promise. With that promise in mind, we got in the car this morning, and I rolled down my window and shouted, 'Bellewaerde Park, here I come!'

So. I ate the greasy French fries. The waffle, too. Even had several bites of cotton candy and a few cups of hot chocolate. More importantly, it's been years since I had the guts to ride anything more challenging than the kiddie cars. But today I let myself be scared in the Christmas Madhouse. I took wing in the Flying Carrousel. I looped the loop in the Crazy Coach - on a full stomach, no less! - and braved the Ferris wheel and spun around on the Snow Express and was shot into space on El Volador. I staggered around on ice skates.

Okay, I just missed a ride on the Boomerang, because I hesitated a moment too long at the entrance and the roller coaster rolled without me. But Thomas and the kids gave that one a miss, too.

I really *did* that amusement park, to the delight of my children. Matthias could not understand how I could be laughing when his heart was practically pounding out of his chest. But my vestibular organ knew exactly how to react to everything I put it through! It may be hard to believe that a dizzy patient could handle what I handled today, but the tests confirm it in black and white. From now on, there is no room for doubt: I am one hundred percent cured.

Oh, let me tell you about Marie-Thérèse, the second Belgian recipient of canal-plugging surgery. She called me on Christmas Eve, and she can hardly believe it: her life has completely changed. She is out dancing every weekend. She is busier than ever. She is happy.

But enough of this serious talk. You want *proof*, am I right? So let me give you a look at my first tentative steps in this amazing amusement park we call life!

Come on, turn the page and read on!

> 2015

Seven years later. *That is the way my online diary ended, a little more than a year after I had my surgery. That was the moment I finally dared to believe that I was truly cured, the moment I turned my efforts from blog to book. I put on my big-girl shoes, found a publisher, got some learned medical people from Belgium and The Netherlands to put their heads together, and encouraged a number of my fellow sufferers to share their own experiences.*

Dizzy Me was published in 2010 and quickly sold out. We expected to appeal to a small niche audience, but the need for such a book was apparently greater than we had anticipated. In 2014, six years after my operation and four years after my book's first edition, I remained completely free of attacks, and Floris and I agreed that it was time for an update. So we released Dizzy Me II *and even* Dizzy Me III *in 2015.*

And now we are putting together an English-language edition, with a translation sponsored by a successful crowd-funding campaign. This one is not just another update, we think, but an upgrade, featuring the newest medical and scientific insights into the causes and treatments of vestibular disorders and a number of brand-new personal stories from patients.

We hope you will enjoy this Happy Me edition of our book!

—Tania

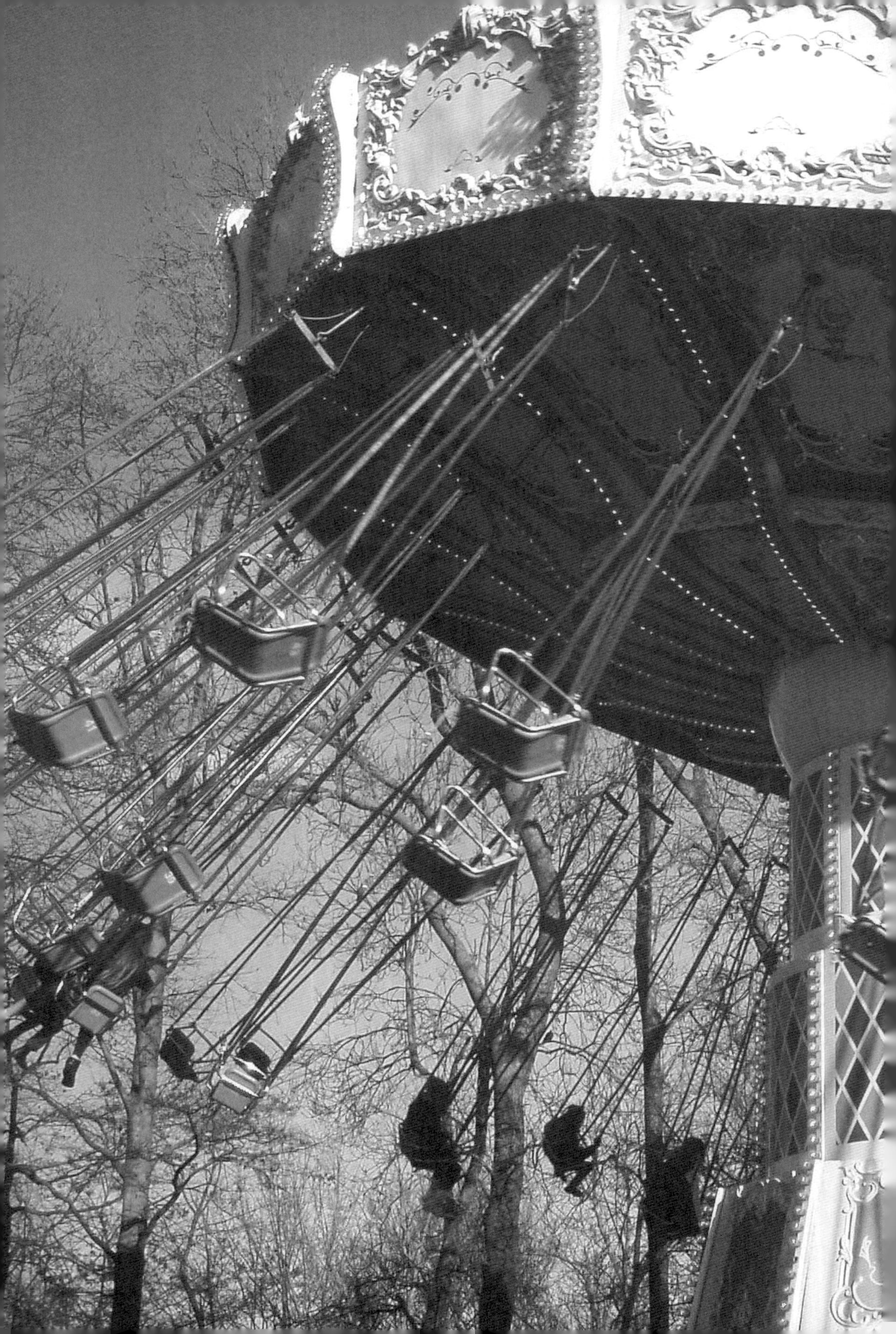

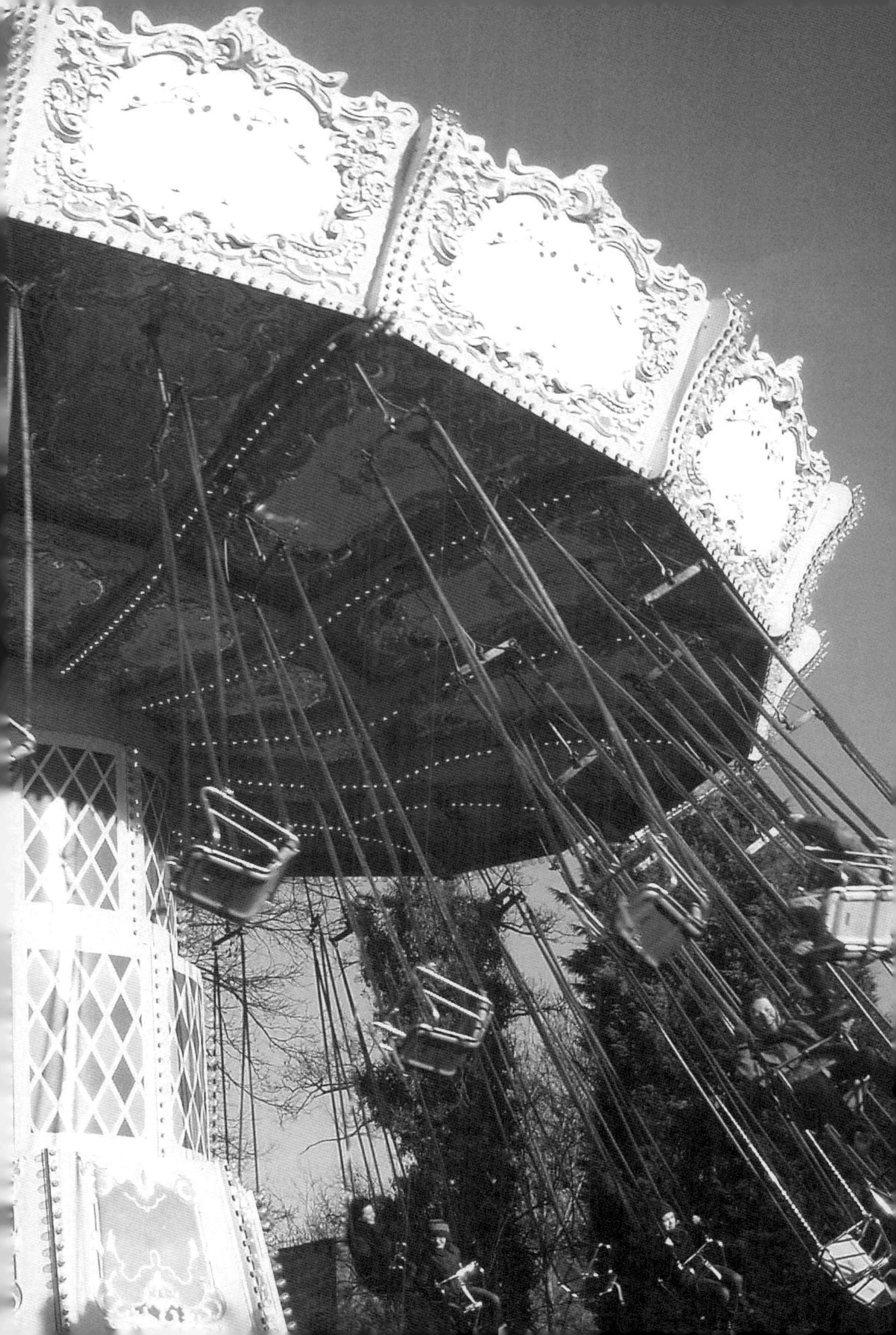

For a moment, he doesn't know what he sees.
Dizzy Me no longer exists. Today Floris meets a storm named Tania.
I sit next to him, the man who helped to cure me and who has become my co-author. After all this time, we sit together again, discussing strategy for the new edition of our book.
There is an amused expression on his face, and he jokes - half seriously - that I have become a bit of a MILF .
Yes, Floris, you are right, and I have worked damn hard to get here!

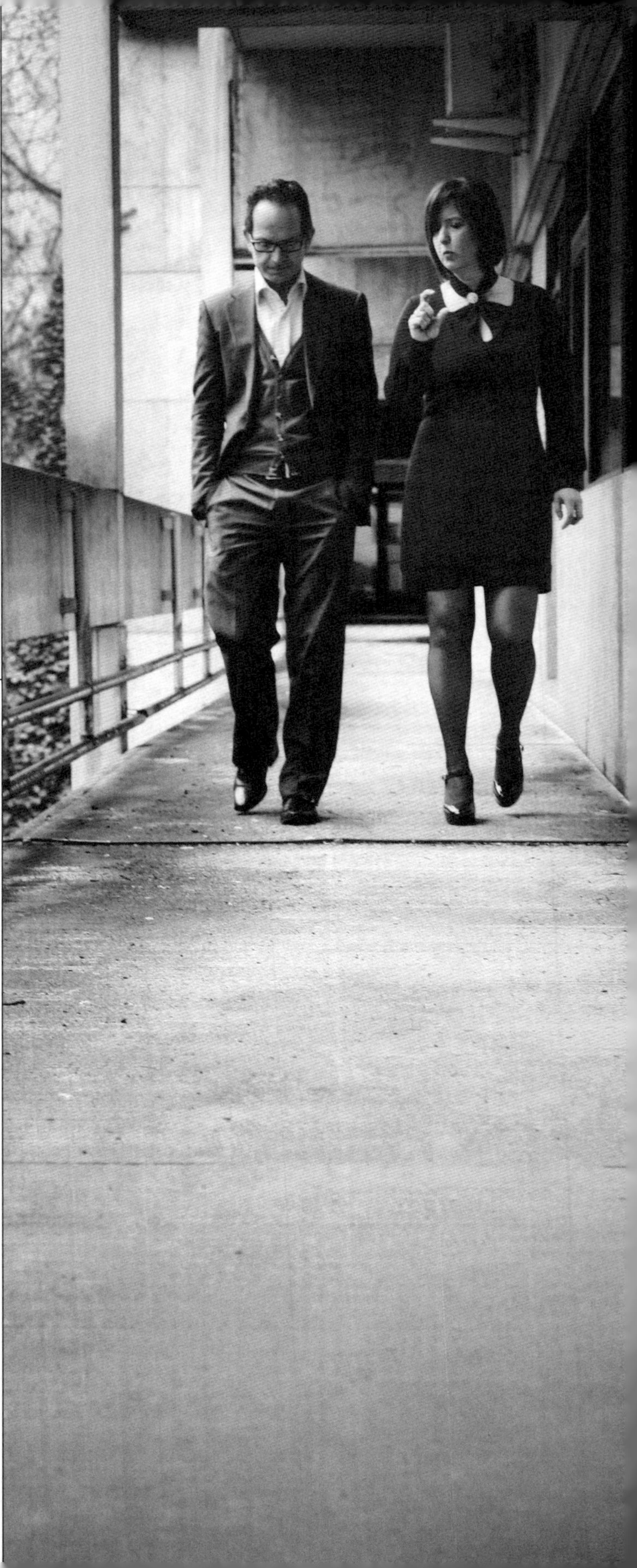

Chapter 3

Dizzy Who?

First I fell into a bottomless pit. Then I pulled myself back to the surface. It was a question of ctrl-alt-delete, and, after a lot of effort, I am back on my feet again. This brief follow-up to my online diary will tell you what I have done with my life since its final entry. I will share about my relationship with my doctor, about the silly everyday details of my life, and about the woman I have become.

Five years younger. It is August 14, 2013. My tablemate and I order drinks at an outdoor café at the Vrije Universiteit Brussel, which is where I am working now. Five years ago, I never would have dared to dream of this. Things went badly at first, but then it all came together. I recovered, and I have made a new beginning. A flying start, by any standard. After all I have been through, all the years of torment, I have become a healthy, energetic, happy, slim and once again successful version of myself. I am back on the right track, and I feel years younger. Professionally, I now work in the marketing department of the VUB technology transfer interface department, helping to valorize its applied research. A perfect position for me to hold, because, when you get right down to it, I have research to thank for making me the healthy person I am today.

For a moment, he doesn't know what he sees. Dizzy Me no longer exists. Today he meets a storm named Tania. 'He' is Floris Wuyts, the man who helped to cure me and who has become my co-author. After all this time, we sit together again, discussing strategy for the new edition of our book. We feel sure of our ground, since the first edition of *Dizzy Me* completely sold out. Our approach caught on and seems to have been groundbreaking. So why not a new edition? Who knows, maybe we will even try to crack the international market! And this will not just be a new printing - we are going to prepare a new and improved *edition*. That's the conclusion we reach as we finish our first pint.

This time, it will really be *our* book. Floris will be responsible for the scientific section, which he will populate with all the latest insights. And I will work on my diary. Because, by the time *Dizzy Me II* comes out, there wi'll be a six-year gap to fill. There is an amused expression on Floris' face, and he jokes - half seriously - that I have become a bit of a MILF. Maybe I have, but I have worked damned hard to get here!

The depths. I tell him about the pit I have clawed my way out of. The mental and physical crash you could see coming if you read between the lines of my blog - if, that is, you were a perceptive reader. But I don't want to go into detail about that period. I'd rather focus on the trajectory I took to work my way back to the surface. Those eighteen bad months were, in retrospect, a gift. But still: my husband Thomas thinks I should at least sum them up in a brief paragraph. Otherwise, he worries, I might leave people with the impression that everything works out all by itself, which could do more harm than good.

Imagine that from one day to the next you find yourself diagnosed with chronic-fatigue syndrome, just at the point when - thanks to your wonderful surgery - everything's supposed to be copacetic. I had all the symptoms of CFS, my doctor said. What led up to this? For fifteen years, I had amassed a collection of balance disorders, difficult pregnancies, miscarriages and delicate deliveries. The trigger? Those cursed mycoplasmatrons, which had been rattling around inside me for six months without my knowledge. Inside a body which, by the way, was still recovering from surgery. I was a working mom, wrestling for half a year with a mysterious illness that umpteen doctors couldn't seem to pinpoint. Put all that together, and it was enough to throw my thyroid out of whack.

When you get right down to it, I was nothing but a bag. A bag dumped on a padded table in a doctor's examining room. A bag who worried she wouldn't be strong enough to make it through another day. Where once before I had been given a snow globe to help me visualize my drifting crystals, now I was asked to imagine a rubber band stretched hopelessly out of its original shape. What did that mean in practical terms? I was ordered to put just about all my normal activity on hold. To admit that I simply wasn't capable of living the life I had only just recovered. To give up my job and mope around the house. To rest my arm after the strenuous effort it took to turn down the radio's volume. It meant that my road to recovery was suddenly strewn with potholes. It was about as pleasant as being hit in the head with a mallet.

More than once, I wondered if I wouldn't have been better off going on as Dizzy Me. I had boasted to my friends, to my employer, that I felt fine, but in fact I felt worse than ever. And the explanation was really quite simple: after years of combat, my resilience was gone. On doctor's orders, I had to rearrange my life, to reconcile myself to slowing down to a crawl, to begin to apply the twenty-minute rule: absolutely no physical movement was permitted for more than twenty minutes at a time. For the rest of my life. The fact that this wasn't in my character was just too bad.

Time and patience - and sport. It took me six months to process this news. I was so ashamed that all I wanted to do was hide. But finally I began to accept it. Only then was I able to truly rest, and to begin to enjoy myself while recharging my batteries. And at last my motivation began to re-establish itself. I started making plans, got ready to re-engage in my life. One such plan came under the heading 'sport.' That one word turns out in my opinion to be the key to my recovery.

I had to do *something*, being gifted with an elevated hematocrit level. For twenty years, I had had a Peugeot racing bike in storage. I put it in the shop for a major tune-up, and then I hit the road. Extremely carefully, at first. Three twenty-minute rides in a row, separated by three-minute 'mindfulness' rest periods. This was already more than the rules technically permitted. But it was clearly helping me. I was pedaling twelve to fifteen miles a week - and then, by sheer coincidence, I got invited to go for a ride with the local bike club. I accepted. And that was my turning point.

At first, I rode about thirty miles. Today, I can do one hundred and twenty-five. I am on my third level of altitude training, and on my new Trek Madone I can sometimes hit an average speed of seventeen miles an hour. I also began jogging, although I don't really have either the feet or the body for that. Jogging goes against my nature, although part of me loves it, whether it's because of the mist that floats so beautifully over the fields or the cows I stop to chat with along the way.

It's different for everyone, but, for *me*, sport was a step back in the direction of my 'real' life after a long stretch of illness. It took time, patience, and perseverance, but it helped me regain my health and function more effectively, both personally and professionally. Although the professional piece was harder to see. When you have been absent for a while, some employers may be understanding, but others may not. I knew that marketing was my thing, and I believed that my struggles simply added one more tool to my toolbox, but it was hard to find anyone at work who shared that opinion. So, with twenty years experience behind me, I found myself starting all over again, from Ground Zero. Really? Puh-*leeze*.

Well, I found something. Pretty quickly, in fact. Underpaid, sure: you get taken advantage of when they know you're hungry. And it was contract work: eighteen

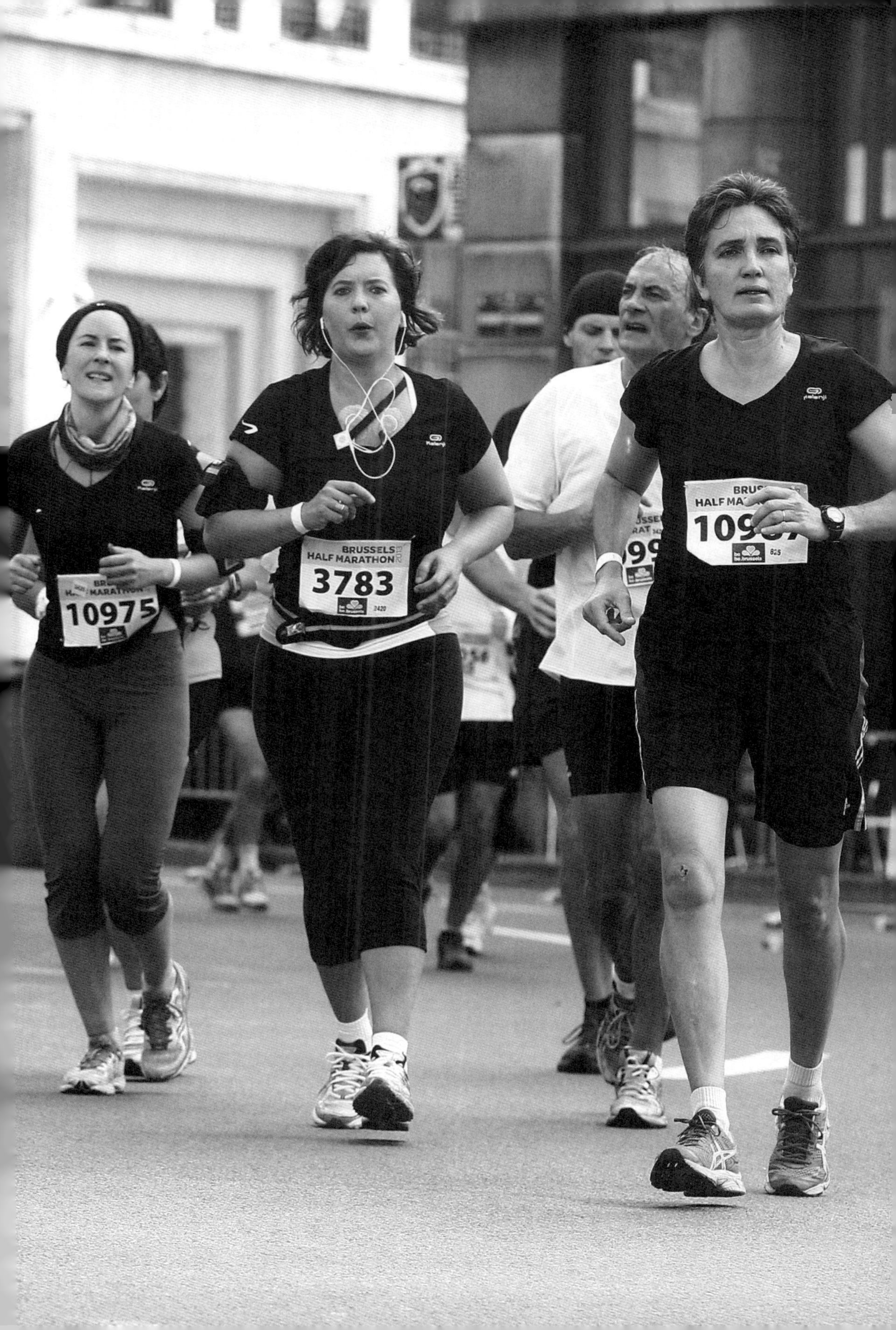
BRUSSELS
HALF MARATHON 2013
3783
2420
10975

months, and then back out on the street again. But marketing often involves short-term contracts; I had been down that road before. So I threw myself into the assignment, and it was a great first test of my readiness. My mission was to pull farmers and the producers of local food products together beneath one umbrella brand, and guide them into the establishment of a cooperative, *Lekkers uit het Pajottenland* ('Treats from the Pajottenland'). It sounds simple enough, and in the media and to the general public I became known as Madame Pajottenland, the woman who ran around tasting every local delicacy and licking her fingers with relish. Behind the scenes, though, it was a different story.

In some ways, this was the biggest chance of my career to play Wonder Woman. If I could get this project off the ground, I would be on my way. My task was to develop a blueprint - including online store - which the rest of Flanders would be eager to copy, a working model that looked big but was scaled down to our regional needs. I took care of the trademark application, the business plan, the policies and procedures, the product catalog, the pricing, the general and specific marketing plans, local events and press releases. I raised the capital needed to launch the co-op and coordinated the efforts of a group of small-business owners who were used to working at their own speeds, in the face of opposition from the major players in the food-production industry. The province, the Farmers' Union, even the local mayors - not counting mine! - were all against us…

But now my farmers have their own distribution network, independent of the old-school channels. I am confident that this lovely group of local producers - and their selection of products - will continue to grow. The only problem was that, at the end of my eighteen-month contract, I was out of a job again. But now I had something unique on my resume, and I found a new job almost immediately at the Vrije Universiteit Brussel.

'Steeds beter'. So, my last name is Stadsbader, which sounds sort of like '*steeds beter,*' which translated from Dutch to English means 'ever better'. In other words, since her surgery and her battle against the mycoplasmazonians, Stadsbader is steeds beter - or, as the Beatles would have put it, 'I have got to admit it's getting better, a little better all the time.'

Get it?

Anyway, when it comes to sport I have certainly been doing *steeds beter*. This was something I needed to build, one step at a time, but looking back I see that my growth during the first two or three years was enormous. My first biathlon was a joke. But I finished it. And then came a second competition - in which I placed first in the 'older women' category! - and a third and a fourth, and even two triathlons and two half marathons. In 2013 I biked my first Pajottenland 200 (that's two hundred kilometers, about one hundred and twenty-five miles), and I did it again in 2014 and 2015. Of course it's discouraging to start out as the one fatty surrounded by a mass of hardbodies. But after four years of training, *my* body has taken a definite turn for the better. And my spirit likes the improvement a lot!

My idealism has helped me to go beyond what I thought were my limits: I have organized such events as 'Biking for the Trees' and participated in 'Running for Plankton.' (Seriously. That was a real thing!) To be honest, though, my motivation has been to better myself. I can do things today I never could have dreamed of, years ago, things that *three* years ago I could perhaps have dreamed but could never have accomplished. And now I find myself making some - for me, anyway - pretty crazy plans for the future. I am determined to learn how to swim in the ocean, so I can compete in a *serious* triathlon. I promised myself that, by the time I turned forty-five, I would ride in one of the classic European bike races - such as the Paris-Roubaix (one hundred and five miles, including thirty-two miles on cobblestones!) or Milan-San Remo (one hundred and eighty-five miles in one day and over a mile of elevation change) - and I *did* it, riding Paris-Roubaix in 2015 as part of the crowd funding campaign which raised the money to get this book translated into English! What an amazing experience that was - I will never forget it.

Sport has become my second life. Once I threw myself into it, everything else followed. I feel more comfortable in my skin, and you can *see* that I am my true self again and not just an example of a rare illness no one really understands. Even my thyroid has settled down and stopped giving me trouble. Without pills! Doctors are far too eager to write prescriptions, in my opinion. Looking back, I am proud of what I have accomplished - and I have done it basically on my own. Like the Little English That Could, I told myself 'I think I can, I think I can'... until, lo and behold, I *did*!

Perseverance has been my second key word. It takes time and patience to persevere, but I *had* time, and I *had* patience, and I invested them both in myself. Today I wear a biking jersey that has the legend *Steeds Beter* printed on it, partly a joke and partly a proud nod to my family heritage.

The doctor, the researcher, and the patient. I am sure there must be a lot of really good doctors out there somewhere. But I don't even have a regular family doctor any more. I see one when I need one, but I don't blindly accept their diagnoses or follow their advice. I am sorry I have to be so blunt about this – actually, I am sorry that I feel this way – but it's the plain and simple truth. Doctors are people, just like you and me – and that means they're capable of making mistakes. Which is why I find I can no longer trust them. In my experience, they don't *listen* often enough, and when they *do* listen they don't always listen *closely* enough. They miss things. They do *not* take their patients seriously.

Doctors are afraid because patients have gotten smarter. They forget that we often know the ins and outs of our bodies better than they do, and they often ignore the signals we ourselves can recognize, signals that may be integral to seeing the full picture of a patient's condition, establishing a proper diagnosis and arriving at an appropriate course of treatment. Time and again I have had to find my own way through the maze of available information. And then they have the nerve to accuse me of 'doctor shopping'.

When you have finally found your way to a cure, and you write a book about your experience and – after fourteen years of mistaken diagnoses – reach out to the three ENTs who failed to help you in all that time, the doctors surprise you yet again. They roll their wagons in a circle and go all 'don't you dare challenge my position' and 'why should we read a book written by a layman and a researcher?' Such a pity. What I find extra staggering is that, according to my fellow sufferers, today's doctors are still making the same mistakes. That's *really* a shame.

Honestly, I am not angry at doctors in general. But I hope that, despite their precious status, they can learn to change their perspective and share their knowledge. As I have discovered, though, that's a difficult balancing act for them to perform.

Doctors, please set aside your pride. I hope you'll realize that it's possible even *you* can potentially learn something of value from others. Do it for the sake of your patients. Take for example the researchers, who doctors owe so much. Researchers – as Floris wrote in his foreword to the first edition of *Dizzy Me* – have an unquenchable urge to continue learning, and a desire to *use* what they've learned for the benefit of humanity. That's the fundamental force that motivates them. As Floris says, 'Research is anything but boring. Sometimes, though, it's challenging, when you feel that you are approaching an answer but just can't find it, or when an experiment fails or your 'working' model doesn't work, or the results come out differently than you expected. But it's wonderful when you can see from your interactions with patients that what you've done might perhaps have helped. It's the patients who keep me grounded as I continue to search for answers.'

It's that ongoing search, that attitude, which has made it possible for me to become a new and improved Tania.

Doing dumb deeds daily. Dizzy Me has indeed evolved into Happy Me. Of course, that's easy for me to say. In retrospect, it all seems to have happened so effortlessly. I no longer have to ask myself whether or not I am capable of doing something I want to do. I can roll around in bed, climb a ladder to pick fruit from an orchard, look left and right before crossing the street, hunt for bargains at the store without risking an attack. I can get my hair shampooed at the beauty parlor, bounce on a trampoline in the summer, and lean back in my beach chair without fear. Most important of all: my children no longer have to worry about their safety when mama's at the wheel!

Daily dumb deeds: I can do it all, now. And most *pleasant* of all is that the kids have almost forgotten the days when their mother was unwell.

The woman who wanted to fly. I have lost weight. I walk on high heels every day. I may not have become the housewife Thomas wanted, but he's happy to acknowledge that I have become a lot sexier. And even though in the difficult days we came up with some creative bedroom workarounds, the sex today is better than ever before.

Speaking of sex, I still get e-mails from fellow sufferers on a regular basis asking me - among all their other questions - about balance disorders and sex. Seriously, who asks their *doctor* about such intimate matters? Pretty much nobody, right? We need to get past that taboo, I think. So Floris and I agree to change our book's cover photo to one of me in my highest heels.

Floris and I round off our conversation with a ride in his convertible, and I volunteer to take a parabolic flight so he can measure my reactions. I figure he couldn't ask for a more suitable subject than me - and if I don't ask the question, I can't possibly get a yes for an answer. 'Great idea, Tania,' he says. 'It's a date: we'll take that flight together.'

I am ready for this next challenge. I mean, I have earned it, haven't I?

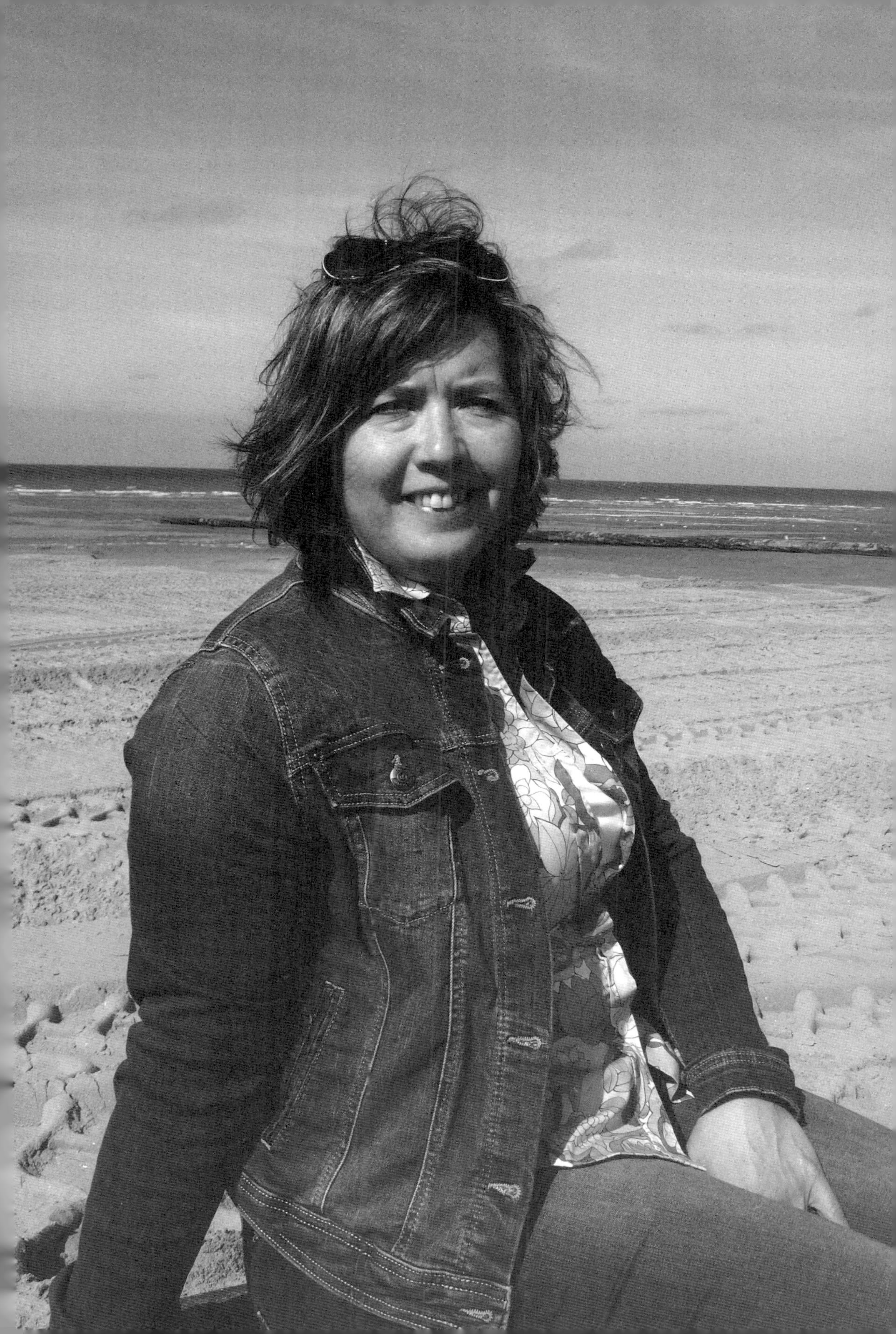

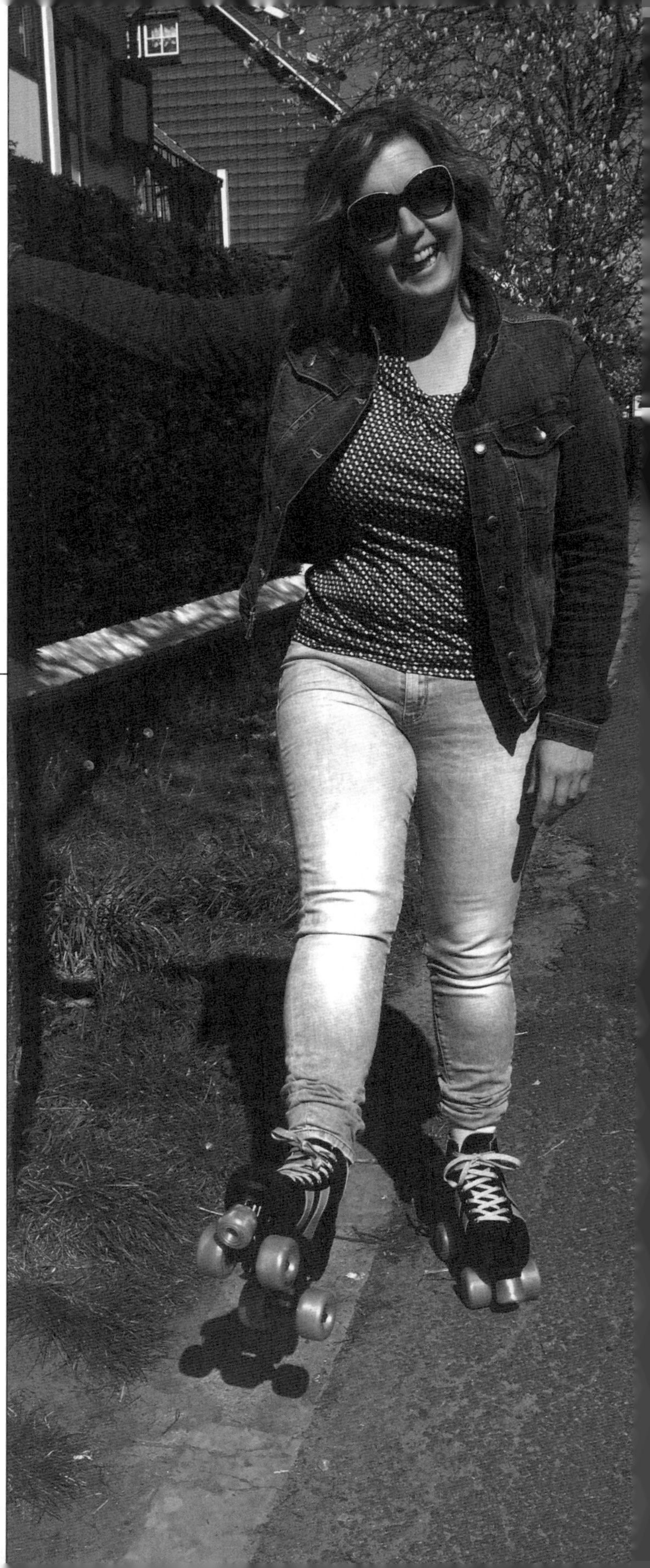

Chapter 4

The Dizzy Me Solution

2017. We did it. What you now hold in your hands isn't merely a book. It's a tool of immeasurable value, a tool that can make doctors smarter and patients healthier. That's also the bottom-line purpose of all the personal stories people sent me for the last chapter of this book. But to reach that goal, we need more and I have got to say a few challenging things at this point. Unless we all pound the table together and demand that this knowledge be widely disseminated, as long as we continue to scurry along beneath the world's radar, nothing important will ever change. Despite our work.

Lurking accomplishes nothing. Are you familiar with the Internet's onepercent rule? It suggests that, in any online community, only one percent of the members - the 'creators and contributors' - actually generate new content, while the other ninetynine percent - the 'lurkers' - observe without participating. Lurkers read the postings to an Internet forum or chatroom but never - or, at most, rarely - contribute. They are the online equivalent of a voyeur.
There is no law against lurking. But I want you to know that, if you have been one of the lurkers online, you are making the work of Dizzy Me harder than it needs to be. As it is, I have to divide my time between my family, my job, and the volunteer work I do for Dizzy Me. But lurkers seem to think that they are entitled to the lion's share of my every day's hours. Please, it doesn't help dizzies forward if everyone bombards me via chat or my personal e-mail account. Most of your questions are answered in this book and online. And we rather need this stolen time to bring change for all.

The Dizzy Me solution: shared responsibility. Will we achieve our goals? That truly depends on you. I believe in the principle of shared responsibility. Let me encourage you right here, right now, to think about it and change attitude, for the sake of all the dizzies of the future. And stop believing that I can somehow bring off a miracle and educate the rest of the world all by myself. Sticking to this passive expectation guarantees you'll need to wait a whole lot longer before anything really changes. Unless you're prepared to raise your voice, the medical community - and, yes, even your own personal community - will minimalize the importance of the problems with which you wrestle. Only greater involvement - in public instead of in hidden facebook groups - will produce the results we need.

Great Expectations. I have been asked if there will be a French edition. A German edition. Even an Italian one. What am I supposed to say to the people who have made that request? How can we help them and give these people access to this information? It starts with visibility. You can help again. Like my personal friends do and that one percent contributors of my Internet community. Even though they may themselves be suffering, they have rolled up their sleeves and helped with the work of spreading the Dizzy Me message around the world. They are my ambassadors and they give me the energy to go on. But it's been a challenging row to hoe!

Good rules make better friends. To take better care of myself, I have created a new set of rules. Oneway engagement has been the death knell for many worthy projects. And what we have achieved yet is far too valuable to sacrifice. So as of today, here is my new rule: I will continue to help you, but from now on I expect you to think of those who will come after you. That means no more chat, no more private emails. This way, something I take the time to write in response to one person's question might possibly help hundreds or even thousands of others with the same question. This will give me some peace, and allow me to focus my time and energy on furthering our cause. Opening up our dialogue will generate more visibility and help us to achieve our goals.

Don't throw out the baby with the bathwater. I also have something to say about the official organizations and quasi-official social-media forums that concern themselves with one or more of the many types of balance disorder. Dizzy Me has allowed me to build up a gigantic network of contacts. I belonged to many groups, and I followed many Facebook and Twitter accounts across the globe. Something I have noticed is that quite a lot of them seem primarily concerned with their own narrow interest. Their own posts, their own statistics. Their individual blinders prevent them from seeing the potential value of seeing the complete picture of all vestibular disorders, from working with others, from understanding the value of a more general scientific resource such as Dizzy Me. They mostly publish posts in which their members empathize with each other's troubles. Empathy is fine, but if we don't include the latest knowledge, honestly, what larger good does that do? Please don't throw out the baby with the bathwater. Remember: it's the baby we're supposed to be taking care of. We dizzies - whether we have got Ménière's disease or Mal de Debarquement Syndrome, Vestibular Migraine or BPPV... Cultures may well differ, but we Dizzy Deans and Donnas are one big family, sharing common needs wherever we call home... United, we'll progress. Divided, we'll fail.

Stardom. You know how you will sometimes see a public figure become a spokesperson for this or that disease? Once they open their mouths, the world gets interested, and the medical profession finally begins to pay attention. Well, there are international stars who suffer from dizziness, and for years I have been trying to get one of them to come forward and speak for the rest of us. But all I heard from most of them is either a no or radio silence. Dear stars, you could have made a real difference. But you have chosen not to. I guess you were too busy just being celebrities. Some of you have benefited from the help of others, but your ongoing silence denies us ordinary mortals a chance to get the same kind of assistance you've gotten. If you were only willing to pitch in, you international luminaries, we could have accomplished so much more by now. What's held you back? Maybe someday you'll decide to use your fame for the general good. . Being a celebrity too, it was Mark Cuban who finally gave me a go to share his story. Thank you for your courage and open mind, Mark.

If you meet a guru on the road, watch out! Shadowy figures who try to lure you into their inner circle with private web pages. They exist. Even here in Dizzyland. You know the type. Within the first five minutes of meeting you, they are trying to sell you their book and promising to heal you with their miracle diet. They present themselves as if they were scientists. I have checked many of them out, incognito, a spy. And once they know who I really am, it takes them about three minutes to suggest we write a book together and rake in the profits. When I tell them our agendas don't correspond, poof! They kick me out.
Good Readers, please don't fall for their schemes. No one can guarantee you a cure. All we can do is help you along your path and hope for the best.

King Kash. The corporations that earn money from our suffering? I have approached them all, those big names you are all talking about, invited them to contribute. But they are not interested. I expect they are playing by the basic rule of commerce: the more people know, the harder it is to make money off their illness.

Them's the brakes. The lurkers, the associations, the stars, the gurus, the corporations: those are the entities which brake the Dizzy Me movement. They may brake us, but they will never break us. And if we can find a way to break through their resistance, then nothing can stop us, and we will surely reach our destination. In the next section of this book, you'll find a treasure chest filled with information, greatly needed scientific knowledge that my co-author Floris Wuyts is eager to share with the world. This knowledge - together with my story and the stories of my fellow sufferers - can help turn the tide for dizzies.

Will you help them to do so: that is the Dizzy Me Solution. Or will this all be nothing but another volume taking up space on your bookshelves? That's up to you.

Tania
Leave your comment on *Dizzyme.eu* and social media pages.

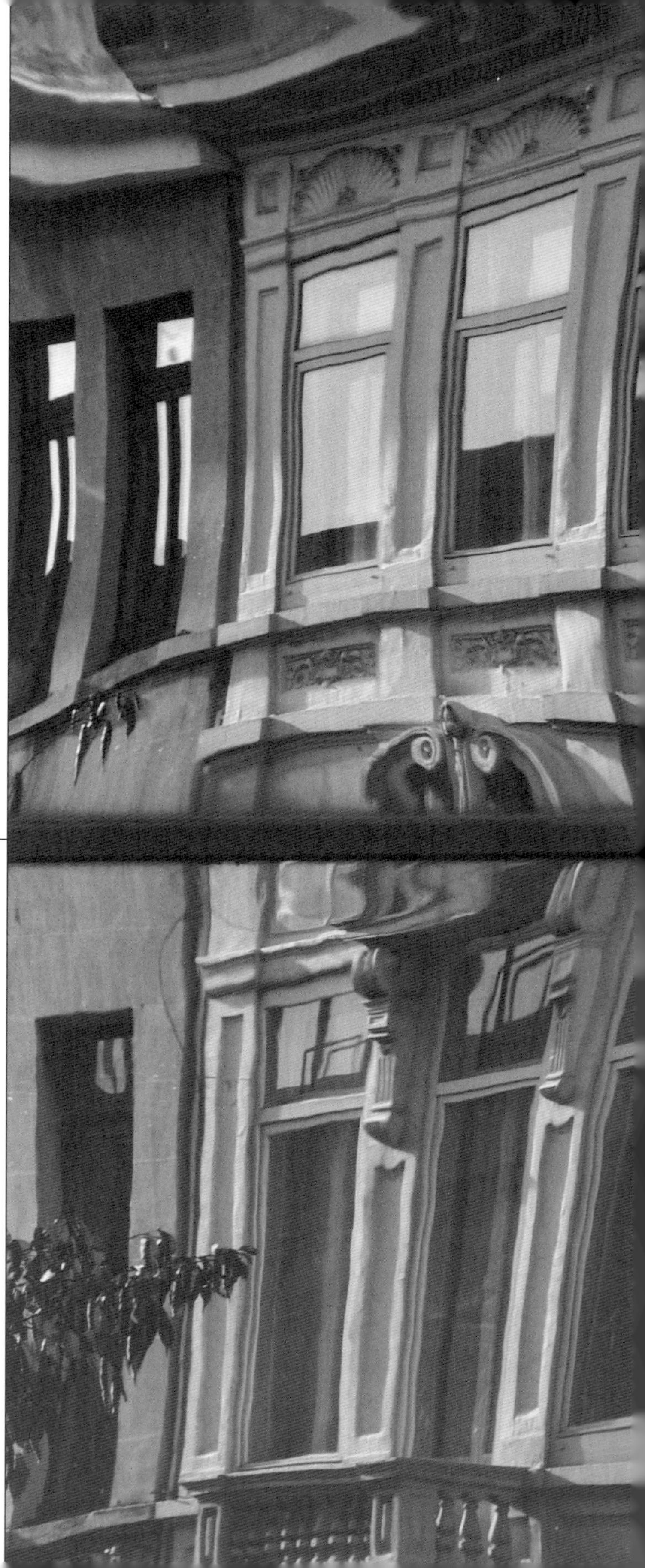

The brain continously tries to make sense of visual, vestibular and proprioceptive information, so that we can interpret "where we are in the surrounding space". This can be jeopardized by distorted vision, like during a vestibular migraine attack.

Chapter 5

Anatomy and Physiology of the Equilibrium

Peer review

All medical information in this work is derived from scientific publications. The difference between the texts you find on the Internet and the scientific literature lies in the key term 'peer review'. Anybody can put almost anything on Internet. When researchers, however, discover something, for example, 'corticosteroids help with the treatment of Ménière's disease', then they do not just write it down and publish it in a scientific journal. The process is much more complicated than that since the scientists have to go through a whole series of steps before their discovery can be made public. First, they have to set up a study protocol which has to be approved by a university ethics committee or an institutional review board. After approval, the scientists will do accurate research running tests on a large number of people or laboratory animals. The results will be statistically analyzed and the conclusions need to be explained and clarified. All the results and analyses will be noted in a manuscript by the researchers. This manuscript is sent to the publisher of a scientific journal. The publisher will send it to two to five international domain experts who are asked to study this manuscript thoroughly and verify whether or not there are mistakes, whether there are errors in reasoning (hypotheses that are not entirely correct), or methodological errors (wrong analysis techniques or statistical methods), or interpretation errors (e.g., too few cases examined in order to generalize), etc. Subsequently, the experts send their usually long list with remarks and criticism back to the publisher who sends it to the investigators. This way the reviewers remain anonymous for the investigators. The investigators in their turn will adapt the manuscript, clarify if necessary, re-run some experiments if necessary, re-analyze the data and so on, until they have accurately resolved the proposed changes to the manuscript. The improved version will be once again sent to the publisher who sends it to the experts. This will be done several times – it can take up to several months – until the reviewers eventually approve the manuscript for publication. The system of peer review is probably the only way of narrowing down inaccuracy in scientific publications. Published scientific research is at the basis of further research and if it is incorrect, it would lead to a downward spiral of knowledge. Information on the Internet is not subject of peer review and incorrect information is hardly intercepted. If all statements and allegations are acknowledged by the source of scientific publications the information is more likely to be reliable. Peer review, may not be perfect, but there is no alternative and it is still the best guarantee of quality research.

Balance is not only literally, but also figuratively between the ears, it relies on a system. Because gravity pulls our body down every moment of the day, we are unconsciously constantly working to ensure that we do not topple. One of the most important organs that deals with this, is the balance organ in the inner ear: the peripheral vestibular system with its labyrinths. Although balance is regarded as our sixth sense, we are completely unaware of it. We even ignore in most cases where the labyrinths are, until they fail or something goes wrong further down the line.

The vestibular system

Humans have a vestibular system for each ear, located in the inner ears, as shown in Figure 1. It measures the head position relative to gravity, just as a spirit level works, and also registers the speed and direction of movement. It measures how you turn your head from side to side or how you nod your head. In fact, it registers every movement one makes with the head. Further on in the book is explained how this exactly works.

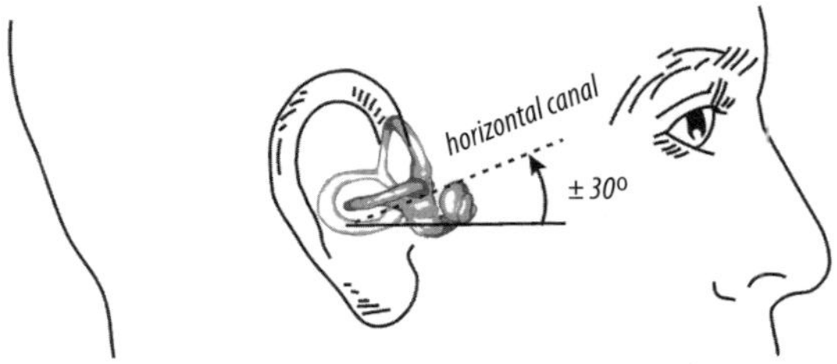

Fig. 1a — The balance system is part of the inner ear.

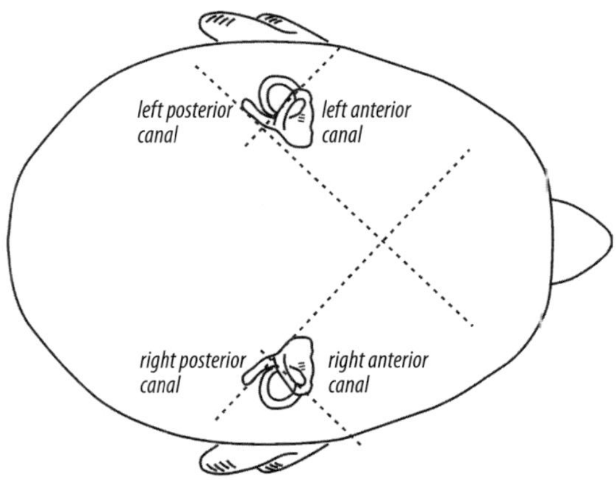

Fig. 1b — Location of the two organs of balance in the head. The left anterior semicircular canal is practically parallel with the right posterior canal, and vice versa. The horizontal canals are orientated at approximately 30 degrees above the horizontal plane, when looking straight ahead.

The ingenious vestibular apparatus is essentially part of a much more complex balance system. This balance system provides a number of essential reflexes. These arose during millions of years of evolution and are so critical to survival that almost all mammals have virtually the same balance system.

Structure of the balance system.

The entire balance system consists of different parts, located peripherally and centrally. The peripheral part constitutes the balance organs in both inner ears that transmit their signals through the eighth cranial nerve (Vestibulocohlear nerve or N.VIII) to the vestibular nuclei in the brainstem. From there on, there are projections to several locations. The first projection leads to the oculomotor nuclei a bit higher up in the brainstem, that drive the eye muscles to generate the vestibulo-ocular reflex (VOR). This VOR ensures gaze stabilization upon head movement. The second projection goes to the spinal cord through the vestibulo-spinal tracts, to ensure posture and balance. A third projection goes to the cerebellum to allow for motor coordination of movement and balance control. A fourth projection from the brainstem leads to the autonomic medullary centers to generate the vestibulo-autonomic reflex that controls breathing and blood pressure. And finally, there are projections from the vestibular nuclei to the thalamo-cortical structures, to enable the cognitive perception of motion — 'where am I in the surrounding space' —, spatial orientation and navigation.

In specific cortical brain centers, visual information and proprioceptive information coming from muscles and tendons is merged with vestibular information to generate a congruent internal representation of orientation, as well as the appropriate reflexes. The is schematically represented in Figure 2.

An experiment with the VOR

The following experiment, that you can try yourself, illustrates how complementary the different senses work. Stretch your arm in front of you, put your index finger up and shake it quickly. Your finger looks blurry. Now hold your finger steady and shake your head quickly while looking at your finger. Normally, you should see your finger sharp and clear. In both cases, your finger and eyes move identical with respect of each other but in the first case there was no clear image as opposed to the second case. This is because of the vestibulo-ocular reflex (VOR). The balance system measures precisely which head movements is made, and this information is used by the brain to control the eyes to make perfectly compensating eye movements. The eyes, in their eye sockets, move in the opposite direction than the head. Your eyes can voluntary follow slower movements by fixating and following an object, but that mechanism takes up to approximately one hundred milliseconds and is too slow for fast movements. At that moment your balance system takes over. The result of the VOR is gaze stabilization. This reflex ensures, for example, that one can read inscriptions such as street names while walking or running, or that you can read the words in this book even if you shake your head while reading. If this doesn't work out for you, then you should keep on reading to know why it goes wrong and what you can do about it.

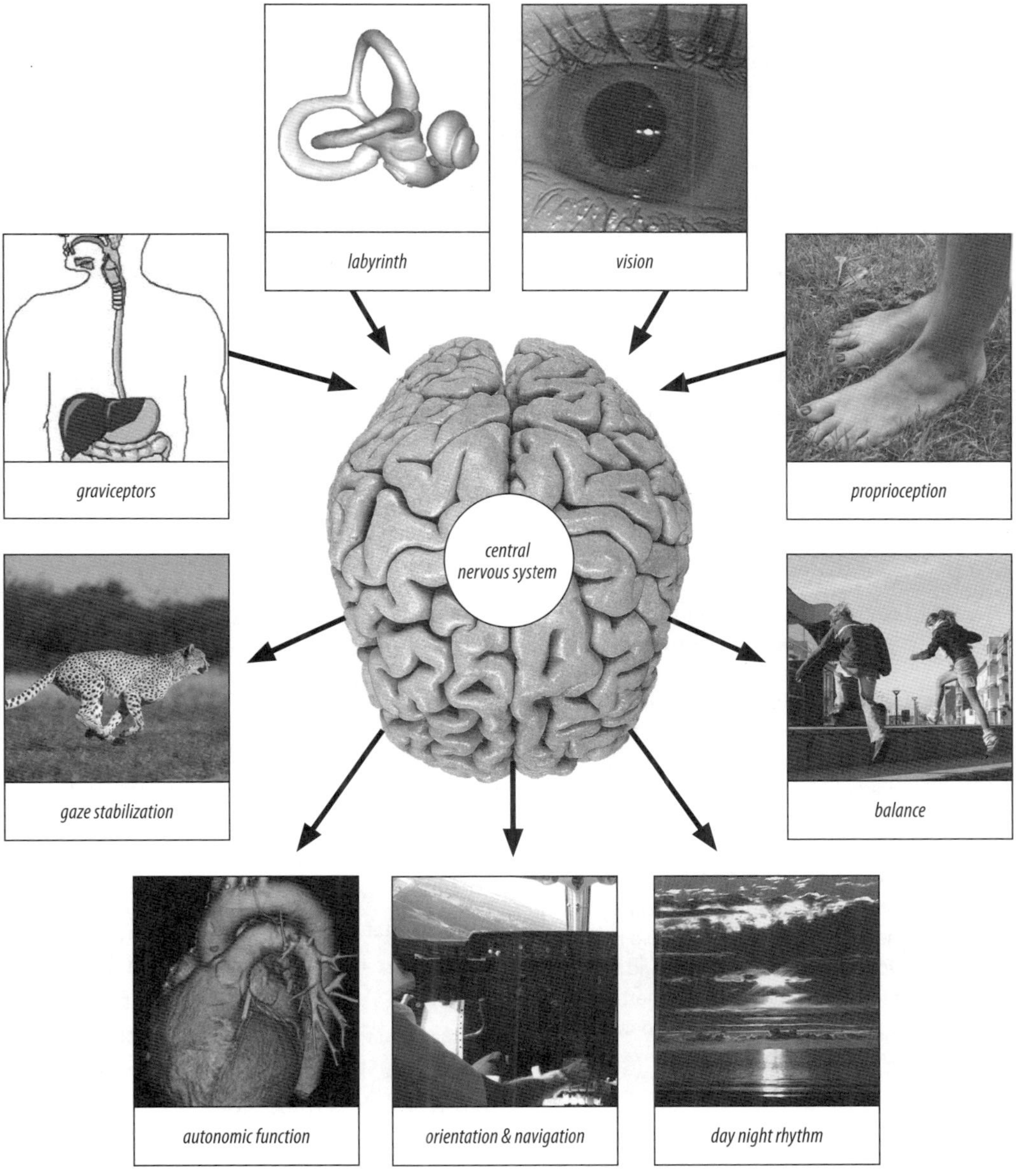

Fig. 2 — An overview of the balance system. The eyes, organs of balance, muscles and graviceptors give information to the brain about how we walk or stand. The brain integrates this information and makes sure we have a stable view, that we can navigate and orientate ourselves, that we can move in a balanced way, that our heart rate is adjusted when needed and even that our circadian rhythm is not disrupted.

Postural reflexes. If you are leaning a bit too much sideways or bend over, your muscles and joints feel that your body is changing its posture. Based on the balance organ in the inner ear which tracks the direction of gravity, and information provided by the muscles and joints about the body position, the vestibular system in the brain generates reflexes so that the legs take the necessary steps sideways or forward so one does not fall. The reflexes that keep the body from falling, are called postural (or vestibulospinal) reflexes and have two parts, the lateral and medial tracts. The lateral vestibulospinal tracts instruct the muscles of the trunk and the lower part of the body how to move and react on perturbations so that we always have a 'balanced' walk and especially so we always maintain a stable posture. The medial vestibulo-spinal tracts serve to adjust neck and shoulder muscles in order to keep the head upright by means of the vestibulo-collic reflex.

THE VOR

Go stand in front of a mirror, look yourself straight in the eyes and nod violently yes or no. Your eyes stay focused on yourself because they go the opposite way than your head. But even in the dark, when your eyes cannot see anything, the eye reflex works. You can test this by closing your eyes and putting your fingers on your closed eyelids to feel your eyeballs. Move your head left and right like when nodding. Your fingers should feel that your eyeballs move right and left. This shows that the VOR is generated by the vestibular system, and it does not rely on visual information.

Heart. The balance system also regulates the heart rate so it beats faster when one gets up. When you lie down in bed the balance system measures the direction of gravity and 'knows' where the ground is. You also feel it by the pressure of the mattress or the ground on your body. When you get up the balance system detects almost immediately (within a few thousandths of a second) that the direction changed and that you got up. This change of posture entails that your blood flows in a different way through your veins and that quite a lot of blood 'stays behind' in the compliant blood vessels in your legs since they expand because of their elasticity. It is possible that because of that, the brain does not get enough oxygenated blood, and one experiences a syncope or a pre-syncope (feeling like you are going to faint) especially when one gets up too fast. This is called orthostatic intolerance. The balance organs try to prevent that by sending the necessary position signals to the brain which regulate your heart rate. The brain also relies on the blood pressure sensors (baro receptors) in the blood vessels but this feed-back signal has a delay of approximately one second compared to the balance organ signal. This phenomenon hampers astronauts in their daily activities and functioning in the first few days after they return from space, partly because the organ of balance becomes unsettled due to their prolonged stay in weightlessness in space.[1]

Integration. A good collaboration of all our senses ensures that we know if the room moves or if we are moving. It is through the integration of this information that we know if we occupy an unusual position in the surrounding space. On the following pages we will explore this further.

Essential visual information

The eyes give, by means of processing visual information from the environment, important information on the position of your body. Visual information is very dominant for humans and a very large part of our brain is constantly occupied with pattern recognition. It takes about one hundred milliseconds for the visual mechanism to make the necessary conclusions. Hence, the visual system alone is too slow for the fast gaze stabilization, which takes about ten milliseconds. Nevertheless, visual information in the context of a broader understanding of 'where you are in a room or the surrounding space in general' is essential. One of those visual clues that are essential in this context, is the horizon. There are also centers in the brain that are specifically concerned with the processing of moving images on your retina and your own movement. This is called optic flow. When a disturbance occurs, particularly, when the brain pays too much attention to optic flow, it can cause visually induced dizziness.[2] This syndrome was only recently unveiled and will be further discussed in this book.

Proprioception

One of the other essential senses that keep the body balanced is proprioception. In all the muscles and joints are miniscule sensors that are called proprioceptors. These proprioceptors are continuously measuring the tension and position of the muscles and the position of the joints. The sensors in the neck for example are important for giving the brain additional information about the position of the head on the torso and about the movements the head makes, such as shaking the head from left to right.

Cervicogenic vertigo, still not proved

According to some, vertigo is caused by neck problems. But until now there is little to no scientific proof of that hypothesis. Except for very rare cases of rotational vertebral arterial syndrome, and cases after neck trauma, proprioceptive cervicogenic vertigo is still very controversial. Until today there does not exist a clinical test that objectifies cervical vertigo. In addition, in the majority of cases the cause of vertigo lies somewhere else, such as for example vestibular migraine.[3] The famous German neurologist Thomas Brandt wrote a scientific article in 1996 on this subject with the remarkable title 'Cervical vertigo – reality or fiction?'[4] Even now, more than twenty years later, there is still no clarity about it. Recently, it was well-demonstrated in scientific studies in monkeys by professor Kathleen Cullen's team from Canada, that when both systems of balance are not functioning any more, *i.e.* turned off , signals from the neck are used as replacement for the signal that normally comes from the organs of balance.[5] But this mechanism of replacement only happens when both balance organs do not work, which rarely occurs.

So, when we take everything into account, it seems that until today there is no cogent proof that neck problems are the cause of dizziness, although there are a few individual cases where neck problems are caused by for instance a vascular problem. One has to be very critical and extremely cautious in claiming that the problem of vertigo is caused by neck problems. Consequently, no scientific evidence has proven the beneficial effect of manual neck therapy for balance disorders. On the contrary, there are several case reports where stroke was shown to be caused by neck manipulation. Thus, chiropractic manipulation (cracking) of the neck is discouraged because it can damage the inner layer in blood vessels of the neck, *i.e.* dissection of the cervical arteries. This in turn can induce stroke, caused by loosened particles of the inside of the arteries that are carried along in the blood stream and block the blood supply to certain brain area, hence cause stroke.[6]

Not only sensors in your neck but also those in your ankle-joint play a crucial role. They indicate how your foot is standing with respect of the lower leg. If this angle differs from an angle of ninety degrees, then it can be considered as an 'unbalanced position'. Also, there are sensors which mark pressure such as those on your soles, thighs or back, which also give information about your position to your brain.

Auditory system

We can orientate ourselves in a room by determining the direction from which the sound came. Other receptors, such as receptors of blood pressure and gravito-receptors, give information from which we can tell if we move, if the environment moves or if we are standing in an unusual way.

Vestibular organ

The organ of balance in each inner ear registers head movements and the orientation according to gravity. This will be further explained in detail later on in the book.

Assessment

Each of these systems – vestibular, proprioceptive and visual – use references on which they rely. The vestibular system relies on inertia and gravity. The proprioceptive system uses the surface on which we stand or that we touch. And the visual system relies on the visual environment. In general, these three systems constantly work together to form a coherent image of the position in which we find ourselves in the room. The relative importance of each source of information will be dependent of the environmental factors. For example, if there is too little light to be able to see accurately, the other systems become more sensitive. If the surface is unstable, such as when walking on the sandy beach or on a driveway with gravel, then the visual and vestibular systems take over. If we find ourselves in a moving environment, the visual system is challenged and the other systems should take over. When there are unusual movements, such as in a rollercoaster, the balance system gets into more trouble. We know how to deal with 'abnormal' situations, but it requires more effort, and usually training. You can test this yourself: stand on one leg and try to keep balance. If you manage this, it is fine, but once you close your eyes it becomes a lot more difficult to keep your balance. You have to correct yourself a lot more with the muscles in the leg you are standing on and you probably cannot manage it as long as when you were doing it with your eyes open.

Pirouettes

Training is important, especially for the vestibular system. Look at the following example. You know from experience that it is not simple to spin around a couple of times and to stand stable on your feet afterwards. In the case of ballet dancers and figure skaters, it is completely different: they can spin around several times without being dizzy and moreover, they are steady on their feet! But how do they do that?

Ballet dancers and figure skaters use a specific technique called spotting: before undertaking the pirouettes they look at one specific point in the distance, usually in the back of the room. While spinning they look as long as possible at that point and turn their head at once, so they can focus again on that point in the distance. Through training, ballet dancers and figure skaters learned to interpret multisensory input correctly and also to optimize their postural balance.

They also use a second trick: after spinning around they nod vigorously. In that way they use a very peculiar quality of the balance system. They would normally stagger a bit after spinning around, but by nodding, they apply a physiological trick: they suddenly stimulate another part of the equilibrium (the otoliths) by placing their head in a new position. That 'new' signal ensures that the previous signal coming from the semicircular canals, as a result of the spinning around, is being erased (otolith dump).

Conflict

Based on all inputs from the different vestibular, proprioceptive and visual sensors, our brain makes an internal construct, or representation, of how we are situated in space. This internal image tells wether we are sitting behind a desk, lying on a bed, driving a car, walking, running, and so on. This construct is constantly stimulated by several sensors in the body which adjust and update the internal image if necessary. But if there is a conflict and the internal image deviates from reality, one becomes dizzy or disorientated. In other words, the internal image is a sort of predictor of what you will feel or experience the next moments.[7] If the prediction diverts too much or for too long from the actual experienced motion, several alarm signals will be generated, *i.e.*, neurovegetative reactions will come into play, with the result of becoming pale, start sweating and eventually vomiting. This is motion sickness. But also other disorders such as Mal de Débarquement Syndrome (see later) could be explained by this model of a conflict between the expected movement and the real movement. Other causes for a conflict can be faulty sensors (visual, proprioceptive or vestibular) due to specific diseases that affect for example the vestibular organ. A simple example is vestibular neuritis that causes the same nausea and vomiting as during severe motion sickness. Unnatural movements with strong visual stimulations, like in flight simulators can likewise generate problems of nausea and dizziness, called simulator sickness. But also specific movies projected on large screens can make people nauseated. Virtual reality goggles can also generate similar conflicts that make healthy people nauseous, particularly when the visual scenery lags too much behind the motion of the head, for example during looking around.

Motion sickness

The best-known example of a conflict between the different senses is motion sickness (also: travel sickness). Motion sickness is actually not a disease but in fact completely normal and a sign of a healthy vestibular system. Take for example a cruise ship. When you are walking on the lower deck your eyes give information to the brain that you are walking in a stable environment. At the same time your organ of balance detects that the whole ship is swaying, as well as that you are walking, supported by the proprioceptors that confirm this state. If your internal image is mainly based on the dominant visual information that tells you that you are in a stable environment (when not looking outside), your expected motion will not be the same as the observed one. The sensed motion will be based also upon your vestibular organs and proprioceptors that tell you that much more is happening than only walking. This is especially true when the ship is swaying a lot, which may lead to sea sickness being a special case of the more general motion sickness or kinetosis. The internal image of yourself in a seemingly stable environment is not confirmed by the other sensors in your body. This conflict is the reason why you are nauseous, start to sweat, become pale and may eventually vomit. This conflict can be partially solved by going outside and watching the horizon, especially lengthwise of the ship. It is also better to be in the center of the ship than to stand at the ship's rail, because the waves passing the ship's hull provide a visually strong impression of the ship's speed while the balance system does not experience this movement. This is because the balance organ is designed to mainly measure speed changes and not constant speeds. Adding to that is also the visual stimulus of the passing waves that generate 'vection', being the sensation of moving while this is not the case. In other words, this all creates conflicts since visual, proprioceptive and vestibular inputs just don't match, causing sea sickness. The link between nausea and seasickness is apparently old news because the word 'nausea' is derived from 'naus', which is Greek for 'ship'.

Sea legs

As soon as you go ashore, it is possible you still experience the swaying of the ship even though you are walking through the streets or sitting behind your desk or on the couch. This has something to do with the plasticity of your brain. When you were sailing, your brain has tried to adjust to your 'new' situation on the ship where you were on a moving platform. Because the ship's

The ingenious organ of balance is one of the oldest sense organs. There are indications that the organ of balance was developed very early in the evolution of life on earth. The very first fish had a simple organ with only a few direction-sensitive hair cells. With the emergence of moveable eyes, such as the eyes of later fish species and mammals, the organ of balance has developed into the complex three-dimensional structure we know today. The current form of the organ of balance is apparently developed in a very effective way. This is demonstrated by the fact that the structure of the apparatus of balance as we know it now even existed in dinosaurs.

The eye reflex, which comes about thanks to the organ of balance, is probably not designed to read books or fly in airplanes but to go hunting. If you want to go hunting you have to be able to move, run, jump and so on. If, just at the moment you want to catch your prey, you do not have a stable image of your prey then you will fail to catch it and go away empty-handed. Most likely you eventually will die of hunger. Gaze stabilisation is crucial for survival, and thus optimized throughout evolution for perfomance during hunting, and that applies to all mammals. People are, therefore, designed to hunt, rather than going to the supermarket and pick a half-prepared chicken from the shelves. We cannot change thousands or even million years of evolution just because in the last few centuries there has been a change in our 'hunting' behavior. Quite a few stimuli from the daily life of today are essentially very unnatural, and it is therefore normal that some people experience problems. Travel sickness is a good example.

movement is relatively monotonous and predictable, the brain learned quickly to integrate that movement in the internal representation of how you move in the environment. Even though this learning was 'on short notice' there is a delay on plasticity. When you are ashore, it takes a while before your brain adjusts back to the old, familiar 'land situation'. This gives you the feeling that you are still swaying. If you are still staggering because of that, this is called sea legs. This feeling normally goes away after a couple of hours or days after the cruise. But when this feeling stays after weeks or even months then we are speaking of the Mal de Débarquement Syndrome, which is a real 'disease', contrary to seasickness. Mal de Débarquement Syndrome will be described later in the section called 'diseases abc'.

Car sickness

Car sickness can typically occur when you are, for example, reading on the iPad or text messaging on a smart Phone while sitting in a moving car, bus or train. Similar to the sea sickness, a conflict arises between the senses, where the eyes suggest a head-stable environment, while the vestibular organs and the proprioceptive input confirm the movement of the car. The driver of the car never suffers from travel sickness because he or she can anticipate every movement. He or she 'sees' how the car 'moves' and can estimate how it is going to feel in the next turn. Hence, the driver is already leaning his or her head in the direction of the turn before making that turn. This refers again to the crucial role of prediction of the next movement by this internal model.[7]

Children and travel sickness

Children are prone to travel sickness, partly because they cannot see sufficiently outside of the car and thus they cannot know what motion is coming, neither can they match what they feel with what they see. Moreover, they are sometimes bouncing up and down; those movements make it more difficult for the balance system to know what is happening. Given that they also lack driving experience, they are not able to anticipate the movements of the car.

The chance of seasickness is fifty percent higher in girls than in boys. A scientific study shows that girls at the age of eleven years are most prone to seasickness, whereas boys are most sensitive to seasickness at the age of twenty-one years. The sensitivity for seasickness decreases with age and at about thirty years there is no difference between men and women in terms of sensitivity for seasickness.[8]

Pilots

Pilots are a special case. Because the organ of balance is not sensitive to slow movements or sustained rotations, it occasionally occurs that pilots do not experience how the plane is orientated, in particular they can have difficulties to know if the plane is turning or flying horizontally. This is an example of 'spatial disorientation' and it should be taken very seriously. Yet, again, it is perfectly understandable and normal that it can happen. Humans are not designed to fly airplanes. It is because of the specific design of the vestibular system - not optimized for flying — that pilots are trained to believe their instruments and not their balance system. Nevertheless, occasionally accidents do happen, especially with fighter jets that fly very fast with a very short response time for the pilot to correct a misinterpreted position. Colleagues from the research institute TNO Soesterberg in the Netherlands have estimated that world wide, one commercial airline plane per year crashes due to spatial disorientation of the pilot.

By continuous exercise and habituation, the brain can eventually adapt to the most challenging situations, such as astronauts floating in a condition of weightlessness in space, or ballet dancers doing dizzying pirouettes, or dervish dancers from Turkey who spin endlessly in a very special way with their head turned over. Apparently, the brain is able to make a coherent and accurate sense of the multisensory input.

Seeing, hearing, feeling...

Even though the eyes are important, visual detection of movements has its limits. Our visual system alone cannot make a difference between a head movement and a movement of the total environment.

If you only rely on the input of your eyes, you can be fooled by illusion

You have probably been through this before... you are in a train at the station, with another train next to you. You look at the passengers on the other train. You wait. Your train leaves. That is what you think! The moving image of the leaving train fills your entire retina and thus gives the illusion of self-motion. A split second later you know that you have been tricked by your eyes. All the signals of the other senses that could confirm the self-motion are lacking: the balance organ does not detect movement, there is no sound of the engines, nor any feeling of the vibrations of the engines or of the train moving, and neither is there a sensation of pressure of the seat indicating acceleration. At that moment, you realize that the train next to you is leaving and your train is standing still. This is called optokinetically induced vection.

Another good example of how visual environment in a certain context can be dominant and deceiving is the so-called 'broken escalator' phenomenon, described by Professor Adolfo Bronstein from London. When you step onto an escalator that you know does not work, you still feel your body kind of wobbling. Your muscles adjust the posture as if the escalator is moving, even though you obviously see that the escalator is stationary. This is a result of a kind of rugged conditioning in your brain for gait patterns, and possibly a built-in reflex from prehistoric times to walk on moving logs of wood on a river.

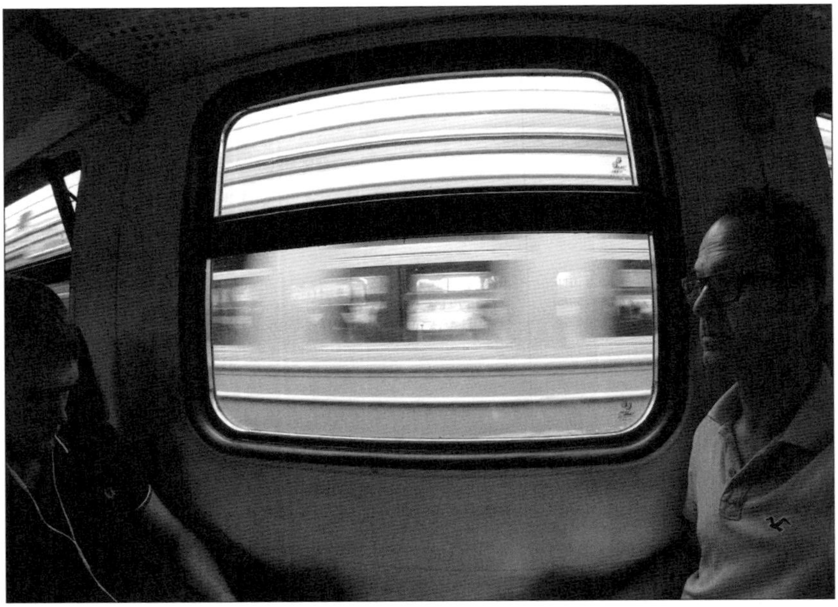

Hardware and software of our vestibular system

Why does one person want to go on a rollercoaster ten times while the other becomes nauseous after the first ride? Or why can a gymnast walk seemingly effortlessly on a balance beam while in other situations people are so dizzy they cannot even stand up straight? In all such cases, the vestibular system plays an important role. Irronically, the rollercoaster person that doesn't become sick after ten times may have a very weak vestibular system. Normally, the complex vestibular, visual and proprioceptive sensations during a roller coaster ride cause at least some sort of sensory conflict, similar to the ones that can cause motion sickness. People with a very weak or no vestibular end organ will therefore hardly encounter any form of neuro-sensory conflict. On the contrary, the person who gets sick after one ride in a rollercoaster may have a very sensitive vestibular system in combination with not being used to acrobatic or complex movements. Surely the gymnast has a very good and well-trained balance system

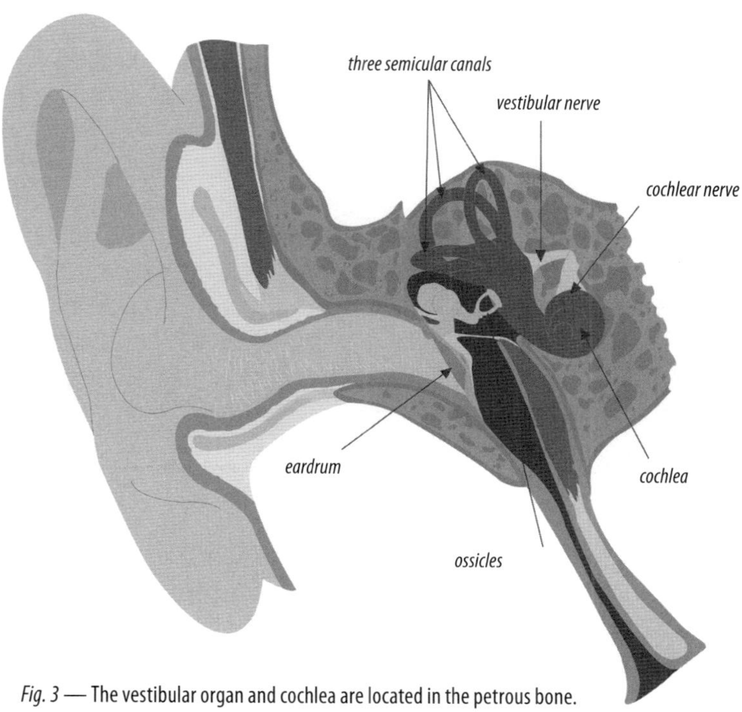

Fig. 3 — The vestibular organ and cochlea are located in the petrous bone.

that functions optimally and cooperates well with the visual and proprioceptive system to maintain the posture of the body. In the case of sudden dizziness, there is a disturbance in functioning of the vestibular system, either peripherally, centrally or both. In this section we explain how the vestibular organ perceives movement, at the cellular level, how signals are generated proportionally with the head or body movement and how they are integrated in the brain. Finally, we explain how balance disorders can occur.

Anatomy. In humans and most other mammals, the vestibular organ is part of the inner ear and is tightly packed together with the auditory organ in the petrous portion of the temporal bone in the skull. If you tap on your skull right behind your ear, then you are tapping the temporal bone.

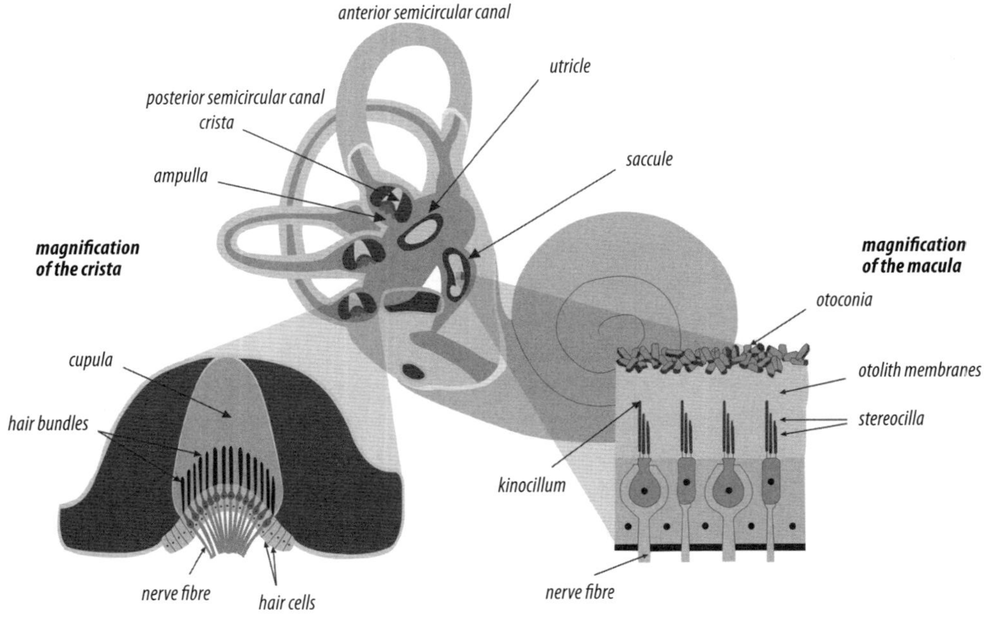

Fig. 4 — Overview of the vestibular organ.

The organ of balance is built as a relatively complex system of cavities and passages, which is presumably why it is called 'labyrinth'. Inside the cavities and passages, there is a closed membrane that has the same shape as the bony shell. That membrane is filled with a fluid which is called 'endolymph'. Around this membrane there is another fluid, called perilymph. Endolymph is rich in potassium (K+) ions and low in Sodium (Na+) ions, whereas the reverse holds for perilymph which is rich in Na+ and has low K+ concentrations.

Inside the organ of balance there are two separate systems to determine the position of the head and the head movements: on the one hand, the semicircular canals detect turning motions and angular accelerations, and on the other hand, the utricle and saccule are sensitive to linear accelerations, including gravity.

Angular accelerations characterize the rate of change of angular velocity, for example while suddenly turning the head around to look behind. Then there is both acceleration and deceleration of the head rotation. The rotation speed is expressed in degrees per second. Linear accelerations are experienced in, for example, a car that accelerates or brakes. Any object undergoes a linear acceleration even during rotations. Centripetal forces are required to make sure that an object does not slip out of its circular orbit. That is why a passenger in a car will move sideways when the driver takes a brisk turn. The inside of the car pushes the passenger in the new direction. The 'anticipating' driver, however, will lean in the direction of the turn and tilt his head in that direction even before the turn. Passengers on the other hand, who do not see the movement coming, will experience the opposite: leaning outwards. This difference in anticipation – predicting the next move – is one of the most important reasons why a driver is never carsick. Or (with reference to the previous comments on the internal representation of 'what is your position in the surrounding space' and on possible conflicts between expected and sensed motion) the driver updates his internal model optimally by using his anticipation to predict the coming motion.

Hair cells function as detectors of movement. Here we describe how 'movement' of the head and body is converted into an electric signal that is transmitted to the brain via nerve bundles. This is achieved by the hair cell which is the actual motion detector for both angular and linear accelerations.

A hair cell looks like this up close:

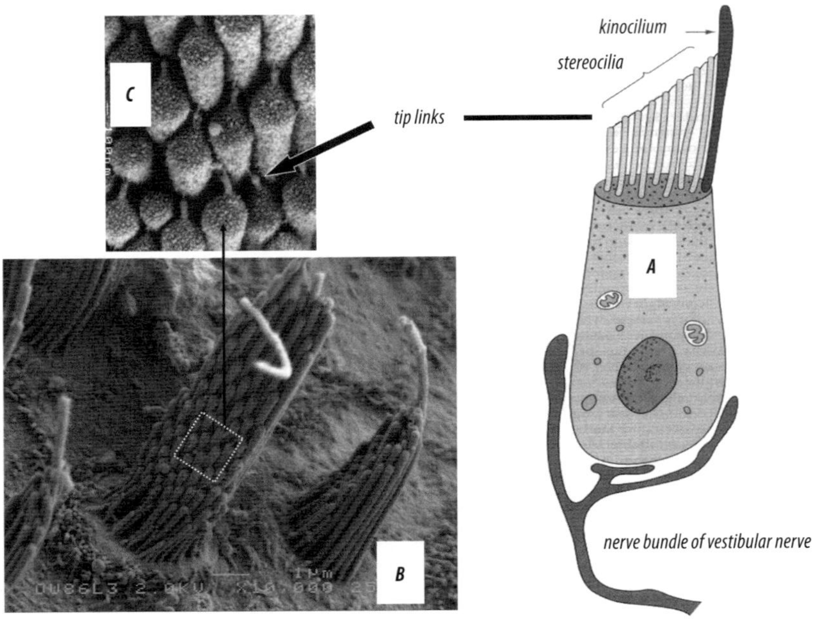

Fig. 5 — The hair cell as motion detector.
A. Schematic representation of the hair cell — B. Figure of a few hair cells —
C. Figure of the 'tip links' which connects the tips of the hair cells with each other.

Every hair cell has thirty to two hundred cilia. When you look at the stereocilia from the side, they look like a staircase. They become gradually longer in the direction of the longest cilium, the kinocilium; this corresponds with the polarization direction of the hair cell. The stereocilia are connected to each other at the top by elastic connections or tip links. The cilia are in fact channels through which ions such as potassium ions pass from the top to the bottom, *i.e.*, from the endolymph to the perilymph. The positive K^+ ions are attracted to the inner of the hair cell because the electric potential inside the hair cell is negative (typically -70 to -80 mV for Type-I hair cells and -50 to -60 mV for Type-II hair cells). Close to the tops are small gates that open and close depending on the tension in the tip links. This tension is determined by the position of the cilia. The cilia are embedded in a gelatinous mass. Every head movement results in some kind of deflection of the cilia. If the cilia bend in the direction of the longest cilium, then the tip links are being stretched. This open the gates of the channels, whereby K^+ ions start to enter the channels and flow down, right to the nucleus of the hair cell. If the cilia move away from the kinocilium, the tip links shorten. This closes the gates and little to no ions pass to the hair cell (Fig. 6).

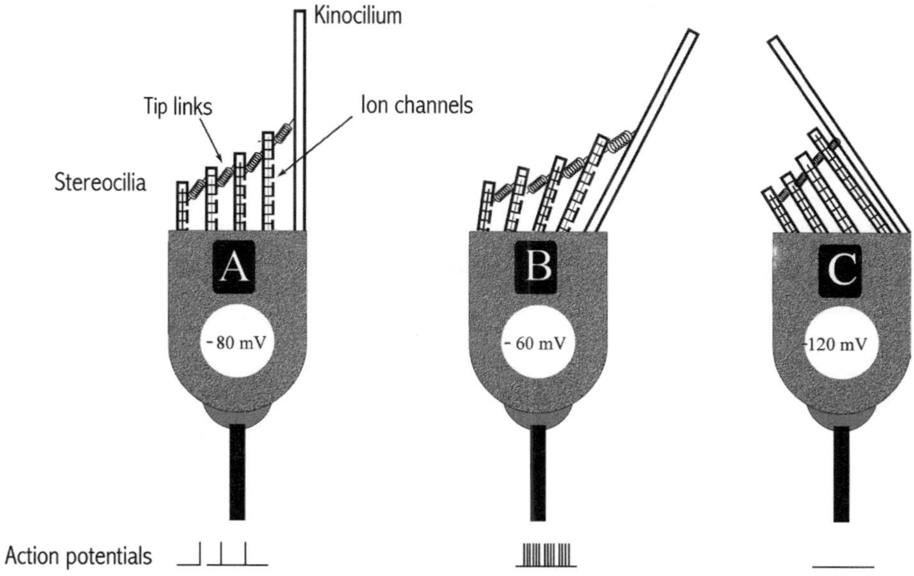

Fig. 6 — Hair cells and how they cause action potentials by moving:
A. At rest (± 100 action potentials/s) with normal tension on the tip links and partially open ion channels — B. Upon stimulation (*e.g.*, 200 action potentials/s) with great tension on the tip links and more open ion channels. — C. Upon inhibition (0 action potentials/s) with little tension on the tip links and consequently closed ion channels.

Every time K^+ ions enter the hair cell, they provoke a chain reaction, resulting in the release of neurotransmitters between the basal plate of the hair cell and the nerve endings. This creates an electrical discharge of the hair cell, so that a short electrical pulse or action potential is transmitted through the vestibular nerve to the brain. There are various specialized brain centres or nuclei that receive a kind of Morse code signal of different short electrical pulses. The frequency of those pulses increases or decreases depending on how the cilia are being bent. The brain decodes those changes of frequency as signals of how the vestibular organ is being stimulated, and this information is then further processed in order to operate the eye and body muscles. In a resting state (or at constant speed), the cilia stand straight up and only ten to twenty percent of the ion channels are opened, so that a spontaneous frequency discharge of about one hundred pulses per second are sent to the brain. Although accelerations trigger the movement of the hair cells, the system evolved in such a way during evolution that the angle of deflection of the hairs is proportional to the speed of the head movement. A higher speed of the head results in a larger deflection of the hairs and a higher frequency discharge is passed on to the central vestibular nuclei in the brainstem. The information is decoded there and sent higher up to different other nuclei in the brain that provoke the necessary reflexes for correction of eye movements, *i.e.*, gaze stabilization and for the correction and maintenance of the body position.

The hair cells are an asymmetric sensor with a higher sensitivity for the detection of movements of the cilia towards the kinocilium rather than away from the kinocilium. The asymmetry is larger with high accelerations than with small accelerations. The specific sensitivity for angular or linear accelerations is caused by the way in which hair cells are embedded in the semicircular canals and in the utricle and the saccule. There is a preference in each ear, but if you look at the whole balance system in both ears then it seems that there are just as many hair cells orientated in all possible directions.

If the cilia move toward the kinocilium or away from it, then this frequency can go up to several hundred pulses per second or decrease to zero. This activity makes it possible that the vestibular system is virtually not limited by a threshold. Even the smallest head movement has the capability to change the spontaneous activity and is detected and processed by the brain. The sensitivity of the system can be attributed to the stereocilia's sensitivity which ensures that even the smallest deflection of the stereocilium (only a few Ångstrøms; 1 Ångstrøm = 0,0000001 mm) can be detected.

The otolith organs. The membranous labyrinth has two otolith organs: the utricle and the saccule (Fig. 7). Because of the horizontal orientation in the head, the utricle is especially sensitive to forward, backward and lateral accelerations in the horizontal plane. Because of its vertical orientation, the saccule is especially sensitive to vertical accelerations. But since both organs show an obvious curvature, the otoliths detect just about every head movement. The utricle and the saccule are characterized by a gelatinous layer with crystals on top. These otoconia are calcium carbonate crystals with a higher relative density than the surrounding liquid or structures. A comparison from the world of pastries is a 'nougatine cake', a cake with nuts on top.

The otoconia play an essential role in the story of benign paroxysmal positional vertigo (BPPV), but this will be more extensively discussed later. While the top of the utricle contains the otoconia embedded on the gelatinous layer, the bottom of the gel is permeated with cilia that stick into the gelatinous layer. The gel is located on the structure of the hair cells that, as explained above, consist the ultimate detection sensors of movement. This whole system of hair cells, gelatinous mass and crystals is called macula (Latin for 'spot').

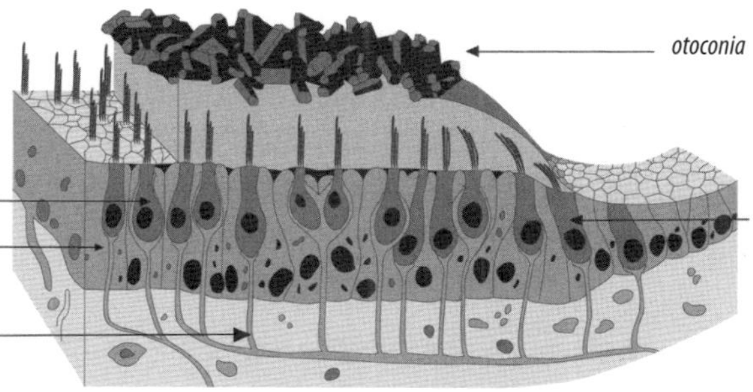

Fig. 7a — The macula of the utricle with the calcite crystals or otoconia.

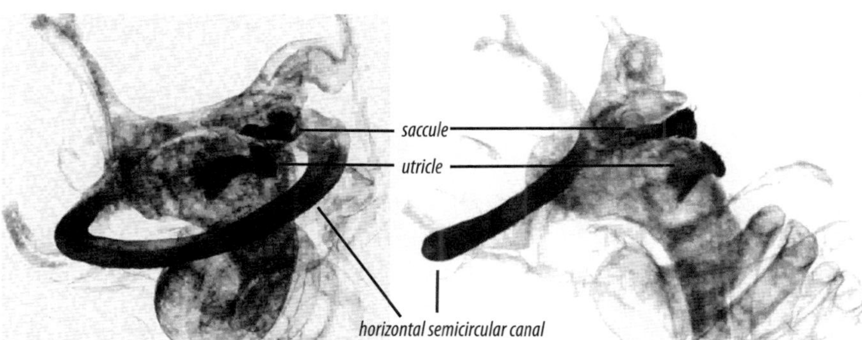

Fig. 7b — Picture of the utricle, saccule and lateral canal with a micro-CT scan of the organ of balance of a gerbil. The utricle can be imagined as a kind of tongue that is sticking in a cavity of the vestibule while the saccule is a curved surface that is orientated vertically – somewhat similar to a curved right hand with thumb up. The famous Australian scientist Professor Ian Curthoys who made the CT-scans, compares the saccule with the inside of a sugar pot: the crystals that stick to the side of the sugar pot represent the otoconia. The utricle is mainly horizontally orientated and the saccule vertically. (*Courtesy of Prof. Ian Curthoys, University of Sydney, Australia*)

The working of the otolith organs is based upon the principle of inertia. Any movement of the head (getting out of bed, bending over, standing, walking and so on) generates linear accelerations. The underside of the macula in the utricle follows that kind of movements immediately, because the underside sticks to the bony labyrinth, which is part of the skull. The otoconia on the upper side of the macula stay behind when the movement changes direction because of the principle of inertia. This fact can be easily illustrated by the next example. Imagine putting an orange on the top of a car's antenna. The moment the car starts moving, the orange will stay behind relative to the car and the antenna will thus bend backwards because of the inertia. The bending backwards is indicating that there is a forward acceleration. The greater the bending backwards, the greater the forward acceleration. At a constant speed, and when we neglect the friction of the orange with the air, the antenna's resilience or elastic restoring forces will ensure that the antenna returns to its straight-up position. When the car slows down, the antenna will bend forward because of the inertia of the orange, and the angle of the antenna is an indicator for the amount of deceleration. The hair cells in the maculae of the otoliths play the same role as the antenna and the otoconia play the role of the orange. The bending of the hair cells causes the opening and closure of the ion channels on the vestibular hair cells with the necessary increase or decrease of discharge frequencies which are passed on through the nerves to the brain as described above.

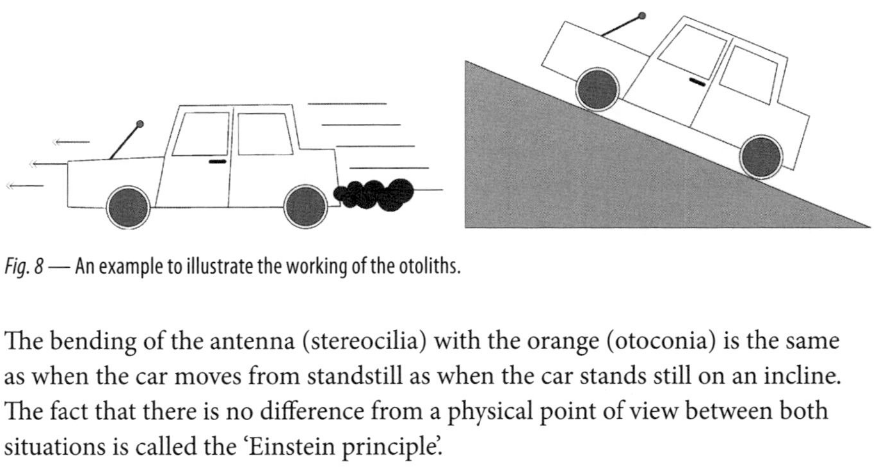

Fig. 8 — An example to illustrate the working of the otoliths.

The bending of the antenna (stereocilia) with the orange (otoconia) is the same as when the car moves from standstill as when the car stands still on an incline. The fact that there is no difference from a physical point of view between both situations is called the 'Einstein principle'.

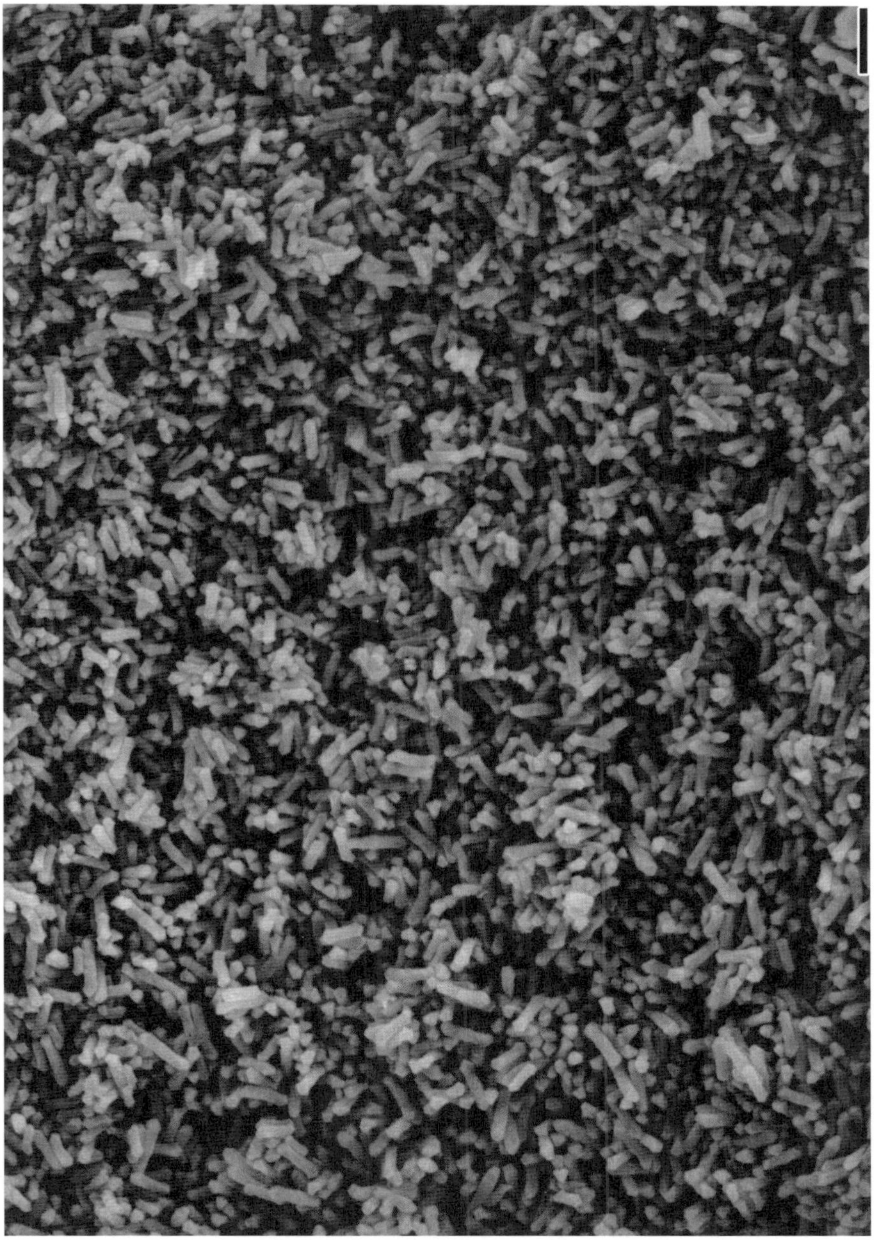

Fig. 9 — Detail of the otoconia which are located on the utricle or the saccule. Picture taken by an electron microscope. The line represents ten micro meter. (*Courtesy of Prof. Anna Lysakowski, University of Illinois, Chicago, USA*)

The vestibular system is particularly sensitive because accelerations of 2 cm/s^2 can already be sensed. This is five hundred times smaller than the force of gravity.

However, only changes in speed can be detected, not constant speed. If the speed is constant, the otoconial membrane bounces back because of its elastic restoring forces, within a couple of seconds until it is back in its neutral position. The otolith system measures no stimulus at that time, independent of the current speed: it is impossible to distinguish stand-still and constant speed, in other words: only accelerations can be detected.

The otolith system also detects the position of our head in regards to gravity. If the head is tilted out of the vertical plane, gravity exerts a shearing force on the otoconial membrane, causing the cilia to bend. The size of the shift and bend is a measurement for the position of our head in regards to this force of gravity. We can conclude from Figure 8 that the otolith system, for physical reasons, cannot make a difference between linear accelerations (moving) and inclinations with regard to the vertical. Thus, the vestibular system reacts the same way to a forward acceleration as to a backward tilt of the head. This can create problems of disorientation, *e.g.*, in pilots flying airplanes. Flight simulators and amusement park attractions, on the contrary, make use of these otolith limitations. Subtle tilts of the simulator cabin combined with visual images that suggest movement, can stimulate a quite realistic take off or landing with its concommittant linear accelerations.

Lessons from space. In weightless conditions, the linear accelerations are being detected by the otolith organs, and the principle of inertia still applies. The otolith system, however, is not capable of detecting the orientation of the head relative to the vertical, since there is no 'vertical' in space. It is a misconception that there is no gravity in the International Space Station (ISS), since it flies only four hundred kilometres above the earth's surface, so there is virtually the same gravity field as on the earth's surface. But the space crew does not experience gravity because they are constantly falling, together with the ISS, just next to the earth.

Either way, this constant falling creates a quite difficult situation because gravity is not a reference any longer and this can lead to space sickness with nausea and vomiting as a result, among other things. Nearly sixty to eighty percent of the astronauts experience space motion sickness. In the last couple of years, our team of investigators at AUREA (Antwerp University Research center for Equilibrium

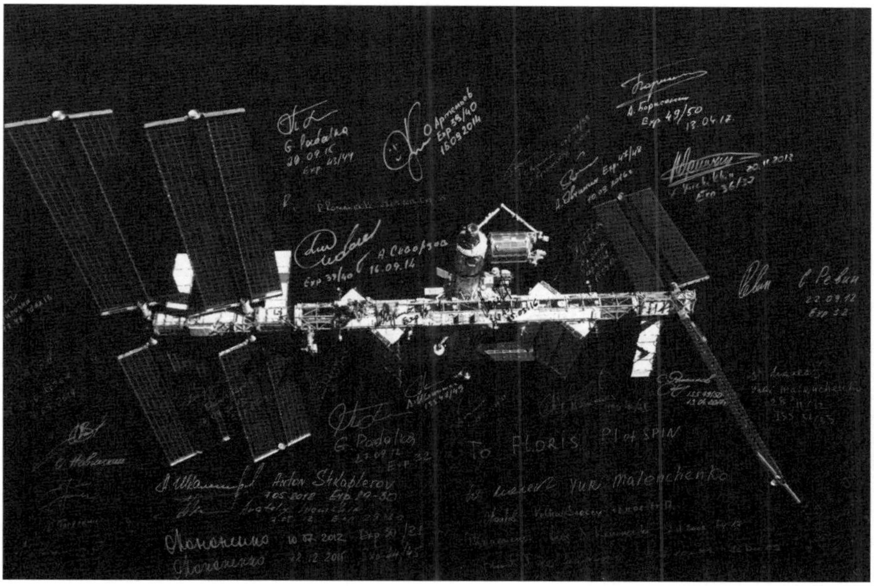

Fig. 10 — Poster of the ISS with the autographs of 35 cosmonauts who spent 6 months in the ISS and who participated since 2007 up to the finishing of this book in ESA experiments SPIN and GAZE-SPIN (in collaboration with Roscosmos) in our laboratory in Star City near Moscow. In these research projects, we have shown the link between the otolith system and the regulation of the blood pressure.[1,9].

and Aerospace) has had the privilege to investigate cosmonauts before and after their six-month spaceflight in a project commissioned by the European Space Agency (ESA). At the moment of writing this edition of the book, we have tested 35 cosmonauts. From this research, we have unraveled a connection between a disordered function of the otolith system and a reduced function of the vestibulo-autonomic reflex.[1] The latter allows for regulation of blood pressure when we go from a lying position to standing up. This research, which shows the link between the system of balance and the autonomic system, cannot be done quite so easily on earth because it is impossible to deregulate the otolith system selectively and temporarily in humans in order to investigate the blood pressure regulation.

This shows the undeniable value of the ISS as an immense laboratory. Through this research, new theories can now be elaborated about the working of the human body, which then need to be further verified. Thus, knowledge and science are still advancing.

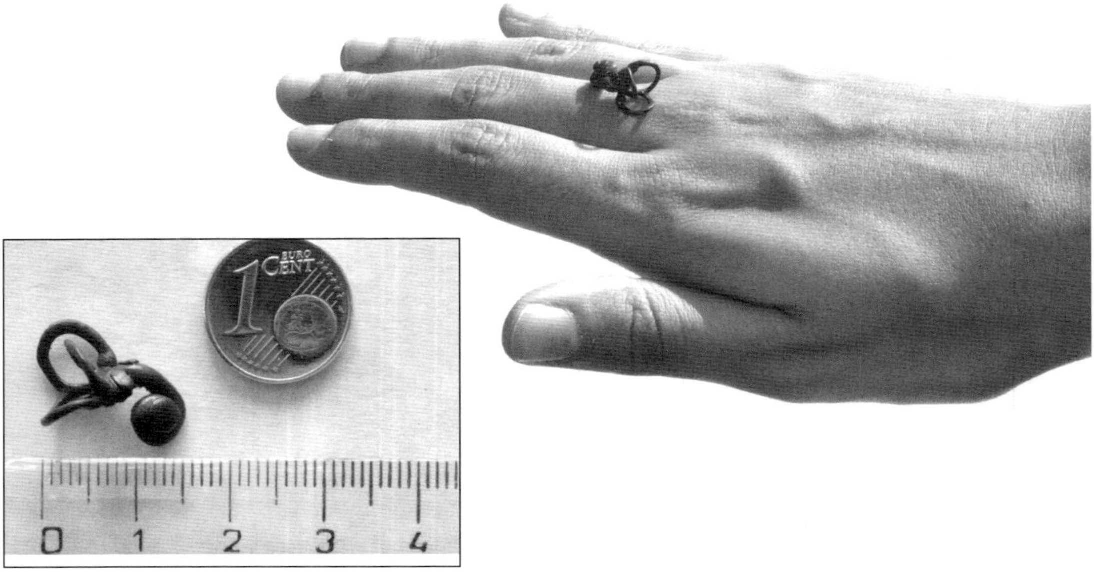

Fig. 11a en 11b — The human organ of balance.
Photo above: The organ of balance in its actual size.

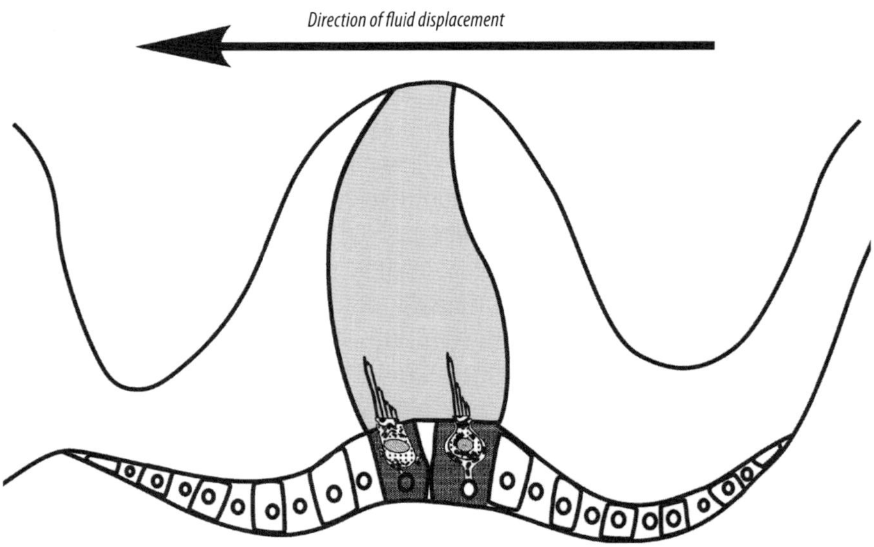

Fig. 12 — Cupula that bends during a movement because the endolymph fluid pushes against it due to inertia.

Semicircular canals

Anatomy. Both labyrinths contain three semicircular canals (also called ducts), intersecting each other at right angles (Fig. 1b): the horizontal, the anterior (or superior) and the posterior canal. In humans, each canal has a total diameter of approximately seven millimetres. The diameter of the 'tube' of the membranous canal is approximately 0.6 mm. When we bend our head twenty to thirty degrees forward when standing up, the lateral canals are approximately in the horizontal plane. The vertical canals are almost straight up, and form an angle of ninety degrees with each other. In all semicircular canals, we find ampullae near the location where one end of the canals merges into the central cavity, called the utricle. The ampulla consists of a dilation containing the crista (Fig. 12). On the crista are the hair cells that stick in a gelatinous mass with their cilia and with that they form an elastic structure called the cupula. The cupula closes the connection of the canals to the utricle on one side and is, assumingly, loosely attached to the wall of the canal. The other side of the canal has an open connection to the utricle. In all hair cells within each cupula, the orientation of the stereocilia with regard to the kinocilia is the same.

Inertia. When turning the head, the semicircular canals undergo an angular acceleration and the endolymph stays behind due to inertia. The endolymph thereby exerts force on the cupula, causing the cilia of the haircells to bend (Fig. 12). This deflection is limited to only a few thousandths of a millimeter, but the system is extremely sensitive. As an example of the range of sensitity, consider the following. The detection threshold for rotation corresponds with a deflection of the stereocilia of approximately 2 nm. A typical head rotation on the contrary yields 400 deg/s which corresponds with a hair-bundle displacement of 0.6 µm, which is 300 times larger.

Due to the friction with the membranous labyrinth and the resilience of the cupula, the endolymph comes to a halt within approximately ten milliseconds. The gain of the hair bundle deflection is calculated as 0.003 degree per angular rate of the head expressed in degrees per second. This implies that the cupula only has a limited movement, but the consequent deflection of the cilia leads to the opening and closing of the ion channels and thus to the change in the discharge frequency which is sent to the brain through the vestibulocochlear nerve. The discharge frequency is proportional to the deflection of the cupula, which is in turn proportional to the speed of the head, so the vestibular nuclei can decode almost immediately how fast the head movement is.

With a constant speed of turning on the other hand, the cupula bounces back to its original position within around ten seconds because of its elasticity, and the stereocilia go back to 'resting position'. The canal system cannot make a difference between constant speed and standstill. You can check this, for example, when you are in an airplane while it is making a long turn. If you do not look outside, after about twenty seconds it seems as if the airplane is flying horizontally. Only until the pilot commands the airplane to fly horizontally again, you feel the rotation. As mentioned before, pilots are being trained to 'not trust' their balance system, but to rely on their electronics. Experts from the TNO Soesterberg research facility in The Netherlands analyzed that world wide, one fatal plane crash occurs each year in commercial airlines due to spatial disorientation, which is directly linked to the discrepancy between the perceived flight path by the pilots and the actual flight path of the airplane.

Suppose a person starts turning around on a rotation chair with a constant speed. Even though the cupula bounces back to its original position within ten seconds, rotation will be experienced during about twenty to thirty seconds. The accompanying eye reflexes last that long. This is due to a system in the brain called the *velocity storage mechanism*, which saves the movement in its memory. The real function is not completely understood by science, but we know that the system increases the sensitivity of the balance system for very slow movements, and it may also guarantee to make a difference between acceleration and incline (tilt), since the otoliths are not capable to do that.

The canal system functions best for fast head movements: when you nod or shake your head very fast, the cupula move in the exact opposite direction and indicate in which direction the head is turning. Typical head movements when walking and running are situated around 1 and 2 hertz (if we walk normally, our feet touch the ground two times per second) and that is largely in the middle of the frequency domain of 0.5 to 5 hertz in which the semicircular canals function optimally.

Direction sensitivity. It is logical that the only movements in the plane of the respective semicircular canals stimulate those canals. Because we have three canals which are perpendicular, we can detect angular accelerations in three dimensions (Fig. 1). The canals act antagonistically when considered in pairs. The left horizontal canal is, because of polarisation of the hair cells in the cupula, the most sensitive to a rotation to the left; the right horizontal canal is the most sensitive to a rotation to the right. But both are, albeit to a lesser extent, also sensitive to the opposite rotation. In the brain, the difference in activity between both labyrinths is used to state which direction the head is moving and with what speed. On the basis of this information, postural balance and gaze stabilisation are optimized.

Gaze stabilization and VOR. The system of push-pull – on one hand an increase of activity, and on the other hand a decrease – is at the origin of an effective balance system, but can also explain sudden dizziness.

The hair cells are active all the time in the left and right vestibular organs. Even at rest, when not moving, the hair cells 'fire' with about a hundred action potentials or spikes per second. The hair cells on the left and right side in resting position fire with the same rate and in the brain both signals are constantly compared with each other. Upon a gentle turn of the head to the right, the cilia in the right horizontal canal are deflected towards the kinocilium (K in Fig. 13) and the hair cells increase their firing rate, from around 100 to 150 spikes per second. Additionally, the cilia in the hair cells of the contralateral horizontal canal at the left are also being bent, but because of the mirrored orientation they are deflected away from the kinocilium and the number of action potentials decreases, say from 100 to 50. The right and left vestibular nuclei in the brainstem receive frequency-modulated signals from respectively both sides: 150 per second from the right and 50 per second from the left. On the right side, where the spike frequency increases, signals are relayed from the vestibular nuclei to the oculomotor (III) and abducens nuclei (VI) further on in the brain stem. These motor plants coordinate and drive the appropriate eye muscles (medial rectus of the right eye and lateral rectus of the left eye respectively) that control eye movements. On the left side, where the discharge frequency decreases, the vestibular nucleus will send antagonistic signals to the respective motor plants to relax the antagonistic eye muscles (respectively the medial rectus of the left eye and the lateral rectus of the right eye - this is not schematically shown in Fig. 13). The result is that the eyes move in the opposite direction of the head so that they compensate for the head movement. That is why one can continue reading this text, despite movements of the head from one side to the other, or why one can still read street names or recognize faces while walking on the street.

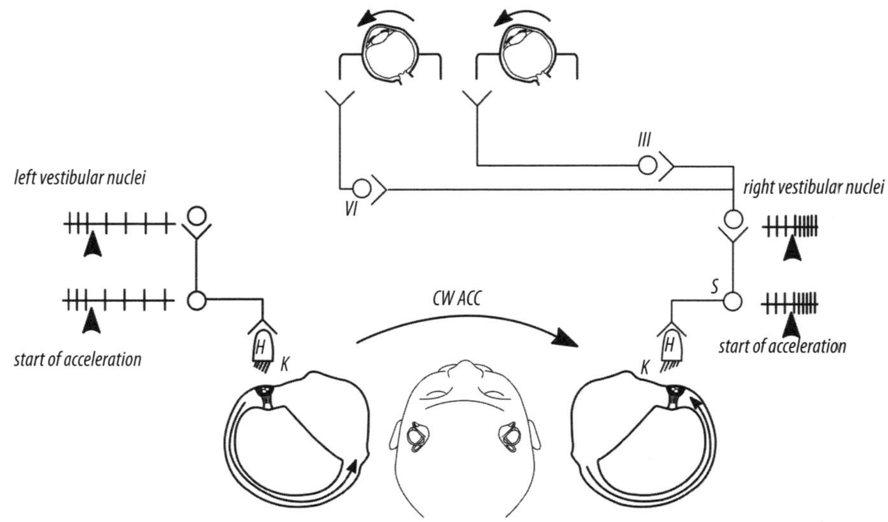

Fig. 13 — The VOR generates as a 'simple' three-neuron reflex compensating eye movements, via a push-pull mechanism of the left and right vestibular organs during the turning of the head. The oculomotor nerve (III) and the abducens nerve (VI) are the cranial nerves that operate the eye muscles to make a corrective eye movement to the left when the head turns to the right. The symbol K indicates the side of the kinocilium on the hair cells (H) on each side. The first circle (S) is the Scarpa's ganglion that serves as a relay station where approximately 18000 afferent nerve fibers enter. From there, the signals travel further down to the vestibular nuclei in the brain stem (second circle), and to the respective nuclei that dirive the eye movements.

This eye reflex is called the vestibulo ocular reflex or VOR. The study of this reflex is the basis of a lot of research on equilibrium. If something is wrong with the balance system, it can be noticed by a poorly functioning VOR.

Nystagmus. The VOR generates compensatory eye movements. Because the eyes are limited in their movement by the eye sockets, they move according to a certain pattern of movement called 'nystagmus': the eye moves slowly in a certain direction and when it comes near the edge of the eye socket, it makes a fast reset movement to the opposite direction and starts again with the original slow movement. The slow phase is dictated by the vestibular system, while the fast eye movement is a 'resetting phase'. It is impossible to see your own nystagmus, but it can be easily spotted in a fellow traveller in the train when he or she is watching the passing landscape. The observed nystagmus is actually driven by vision since the train traveler is looking outside and is, in this case, called optokinetic nystagmus, but it is quite similar to the VOR nystagmus.

When the VOR mechanism fails, complaints of dizziness can occur. Some complaints are a result of signals that suddenly break down on one side, which results in the firing rate of the vestibular hair cells being disrupted. This will be further explained in the section about vestibular neuritis, one of the vestibular diseases. A failing VOR can occur when both vestibular systems are hampered like after a serious bacterial infection for example of the heart. When high doses of antibiotics have been given to cure the infection, the side effect is that the hair cells in both vestibular end organs may have been damaged. Consequently, when turning the head, only limited compensatory eye movements will be generated, with a blurred vision as a consequence during movements. Also this will be further elaborated in the section Diseases-ABC.

Vestibular nerve. The nerve that leaves from the organ of balance to the brain is called the equilibrium nerve or vestibular nerve. We distinguish a lower (inferior) and upper (superior) branch of the nerve. The nerve fibres that come from the horizontal semicircular canal, anterior semicircular canal and the utricle constitute the superior branch of the vestibular nerve. The nerve fibres that come from the posterior semicircular canal and saccule form the inferior branch. It is useful to know this because some diseases typically affect the superior branch of the vestibular nerve and others the inferior nerve branch. A handy mnemonic trick to know which nerve branch (superior or inferior) innervates which vestibular part, is 'HAUSSPI': Horizontal canal, Anterior canal and Utricle go to the Superior branch; Saccule and Posterior canal go to the Inferior branch.

The human vestibular nerve contains approximately 10.000 to 20.000 afferent nerve fibres, and 500 to 1000 efferent axons. The efferent fibers branch more extensively than the afferent ones.

Misinterpretation. For years, clinicians have generalized the results of 'standard' balance tests to the whole vestibular apparatus while the standard balance tests evaluate only certain parts of the vestibular end organ. And there are considerable differences troughout the world regarding the applied vestibular tests. In Belgium, the 'standard' balance test includes the caloric test and rotatory chair testing. In the caloric test (see the section on 'balance tests'), clinicians investigate the function of both horizontal semicircular canals separately. If this test indicates

Inertia

As an example, to make clear in which way the stereocilia bend in angular acceleration, thereby causing stimulation of the hair cell, let's consider a cup of coffee. Imagine that you are swivelling a cup of coffee on a dish by pushing the handle with your finger. In the beginning the coffee will stay behind because of the inertia. After a while the coffee will begin moving because of the friction and everything will rotate at the same time. When you stop swivelling the cup of coffee, the coffee will still be swiveling.

In analogy to this example, the endolymph (coffee) will be moved in an angular acceleration of the head over a small angle in regards to the membranous labyrinth (the cup). The rate of displacement of the endolymph moving in the semicircular canal, is strongly limited by the presence of the cupula which completely closes the canal and only bends a little bit by its elasticity. The angle of deflection of the ciliae of the hair cells determines directly how much the ion channels open or close. This again leads to signals to the brain, where they are decoded in different brain centers to generate the appropriate reflexes.
This model explains why after turning on a rotating chair or just turning on your own axis, as children like to do, and then suddenly stop, one still feels dizzy, since the endolymphe continues moving in the canals. Close observation of eye movements would reveal a nystagmus.

that there is no response on one side, it can, at the most, be concluded that either the horizontal canal is shut down at that side, or the superior nerve branch of the vestibular nerve is disrupted. However, a statement cannot be made about the inferior branch. New tests such as the cervical vestibular-evoked myogenic potential (cVEMP; see the section on 'balance tests') partly solve this problem.

Vestibular nuclei. Both of the superior and inferior vestibular nerves project on the vestibular brain centres via a transitional stage, Scarpa's ganglion. The vestibular nuclei in the brain stem project multisensory information on the cerebellum, from which this information is sent on to the cortical regions in the cerebral cortex that is responsible for the 'perception' or the awareness of movement, position and orientation in the surrounding environment. The vestibular nuclei send parallel information to the neck muscles and to the leg muscles through the medial and lateral vestibulo-spinal tracts respectively, to maintain postural balance through the vestibulo-spinal reflex (VSR). Finally, the vestibular nuclei sends image stabilization signals to the oculomotor nuclei: the nucleus oculomotorius, the nucleus abducens and the nucleus trochlearis, which operate the six extraocular muscles, the muscles that can move the eyeball in almost every direction. The neural network that takes care of this VOR is a three-neuron reflex arc (Scarpa's ganglion, vestibular neuron, oculomotor neuron; Fig. 13).

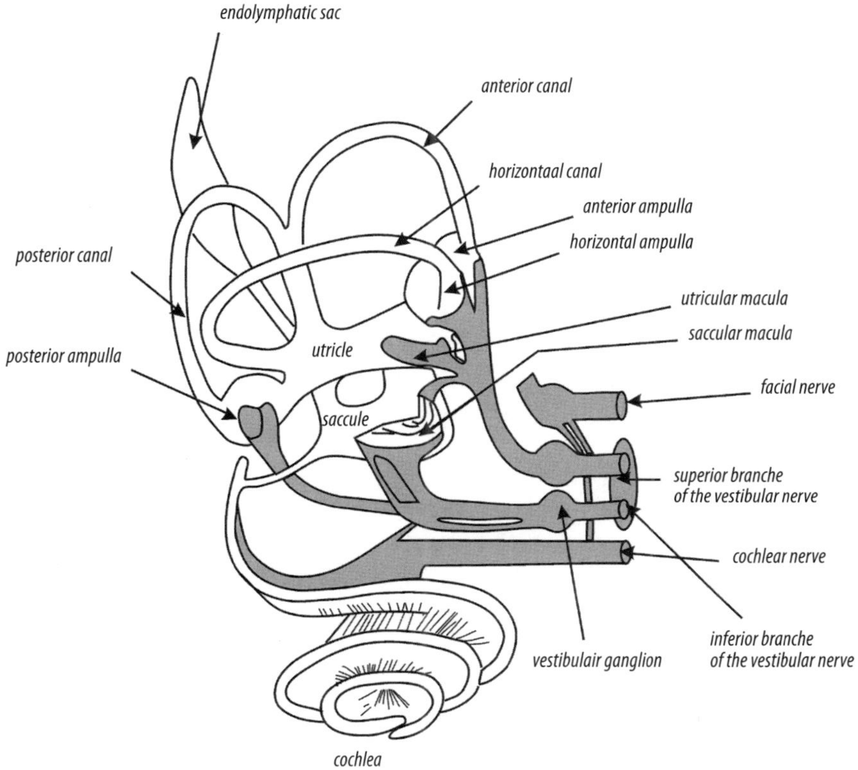

Fig. 14 — Overview of the membranous labyrinth with the nerves.

The primary action of the extraocular muscles is located in the same plane as where the horizontal, anterior and posterior canals are located. The result of that is, despite the plane of head rotation, that there is always an opposite eye movement in the same plane so that the gaze direction of the eyes stays stabilised. The establishment of the VOR is a lot more complicated than the three-neuron reflex. The left and right vestibular nuclei in the brain stem are constantly communicating through commissural fibers or connecting tracts to compensate, adjust and optimise the VOR and the VSR. In addition, there are many built-in parallel circuits to make these reflexes as robust as possible.

From ingenious hardware to sophisticated software

Internal model. The information from the vestibular organ is constantly compared with other sources of information, such as the visual and proprioceptive (originating from the muscles, joints, pressure receptors in the skin, and so on) and the brain constructs an internal model of where are we in the surrounding space and how are we moving, standing, sitting, lying and so on. This internal model is constantly being adjusted to have a representation as correctly as possible of this position in space. If something goes wrong somewhere, the model gets adjusted on the basis of the information that is reliable. But if there is a sustained conflict of different sensory information, one become nauseous and dizzy. It is as if some kind of alarm goes off. This is how one becomes travel sick.

The cerebellum is to a large extent involved in this processing and integration of vestibular, proprioceptive and visual input to take care of image stabilisation and equilibrium. It is also called the vestibulo-cerebellum and is the 'adaptation centre' of the vestibular system. The Purkinje cells in that part of the brain are capable of tempering or adjusting quite some processes of the balance system. They can, for example, suppress the whole VOR or even invert it. The retinal-slip mechanism is an impressive result of the vestibulo cerebellar control mechanism, responsible for fixation suppression.

Zebra stripes. One of the possible hypotheses as to why zebras have stripes is that the pattern of stripes disturbs the gaze stabilization and the retinal slip mechanism of, for example, the cheetah that wants to capture them. This is especially the case when the stripes fill up the entire field of vision of the cheetah, or, in other words, when the cheetah is nearly about to attack the zebra. At that moment, the spatial orientation is being disturbed so that the cheetah misses and the zebra can escape.

Why does a normal person not whirl and spin? A short recap: the central vestibular system in the brain takes different sources of information into account: the eyes, the muscles and joints and the vestibular organs in both ears. The eyes tell the brain how the body is situated with regard to its environment. The tension in muscles and joints gives information about how the body moves or is positioned. The vestibular organ in the inner ear provides information about head velocity and orientation relative to earth's gravity. Without a vestibular system, the image on the retina would jump at every step, every heartbeat or whenever the head slightly moves. Moreover, there is no means to react in time when getting out of balance or almost fall. If the information of the eyes, muscles, joints and the vestibular organ is processed properly, a stable gaze and posture is guaranteed, even when moving. The gaze stabilisation is achieved by the vestibulo ocular reflex (VOR) and the postural balance by the vestibulo spinal reflex (VSR). If something goes wrong, the eyes do not make the expected compensating eye movements, vision is blurred, the risk of falling increases and ususally dizziness emerges.

But what is dizziness? Dizziness is the illusion of movement, or in other words, undergoing a pattern of movements while they do not exist in reality. It is an undervalued problem and reduces the patient's quality of life considerably.

Living a dizzy life

Dizzy, giddy, spinning, swaying, lightheaded, rocking, bobbing, tipsy, unstable, groggy, wobbly, heavy head, nauseous, queasy, sea sick, vertigo… These and many more are terms patients use to describe their complaints. And these words can refer to different causes or etiologies. Vertigo is a special case of dizziness, referring to a sensation of rotation (vertere in Latin means to turn). Vertigo is different from instability. The words sometimes refer to the part where the problem could be. For example, the word 'vertigo' suggests that the problem can have something to do with the semicircular canals, while lightheadedness doesn't quite point to a disturbed part of the vestibular organ. Vertigo is usually associated with heights, like

Retinal-slip mechanism

Look at your thumb while holding it at arm's length. Then move the upper part of your torso along with your head and arm from left to right, with your thumb at arm's length while continuously fixating your eyes on your thumb. Normally, you can manage that and you can clearly see your thumb. Put your thumb down, move your head from side to side and then look at an object in the distance. Again, you can see the object perfectly. Those movements (moving your head from side to side whether or not while looking at your thumb at the same time), are identical for your vestibular organ. But the eyes behave completely opposite. In the first case, they move along in the eye sockets while fixating the thumb, whereas in the latter case, they just move from side to side in their eye sockets while fixating the object in the distance. This is caused by the retinal-slip mechanism which is controlled from the vestibulo-cerebellum with the Purkinje cells. In case of cerebellar lesions or atrophy, this fixation suppression mechanism is hampered. In that case, a nystagmus will be present, corresponding with the rotation, despite the fixation of a target that like the thumb moves together with the subject. Consequently, during the caloric irrigation test the ability to overrule the nystagmus by fixation is typically investigated to identify possible cerebellar lesions.

in the Alfred Hitchcock's film of the same name. In scientific literature, however, vertigo refers to a sensation of whirling and loss of balance caused by a disease affecting the inner ear or the vestibular nerve. To make it easier, we will use the word 'vertigo' from now on. Vertigo is an illusion of movement. In a recent consensus publication,[10] a group of experts suggested the preferred terminology to use from now on in scientific research. Their definition is: 'Vertigo is the sensation of self-motion when no self-motion is occurring, or the sensation of distorted self-motion during an otherwise normal head movement.' All terms such as 'giddy', 'dizziness', 'sea sick' and 'lightheaded' refer to different kinds of vertigo. That same scientific publication describes the term dizziness as 'the sensation of disturbed or impaired spatial orientation without a false or distorted sense of motion'.

The term 'unsteadiness' indicates a wobbly and unstable feeling, whether you sit, stand or walk, in which you do not have a clear preference of direction.

Now that we have described the different terms that are linked with 'vertigo', the next step is the anamnesis, the determination of the medical history, acquired through an interview with the patient in which the clinician asks the patient about his or her complaints to form a first impression leading to a possible diagnosis.

SO STONED - anamnesis of the dizzy patient

The anamnesis of a dizzy patient is of utmost importance to differentiate the possible causes or etiologies of vertigo. The key factors that allow a first approximation of diagnosis identification are based on the time profile, symptom profile and trigger profile of the disease. The here proposed mnemonic 'SO STONED' comprises eight different dimensions that characterize the vertigo-related complaints of the patient and guide the clinician in his or her decision scheme.[11] 'SO STONED' refers to Symptoms, Often (frequency of occurrence), Since, Trigger, Otology, Neurology, Evolution, Duration. Since the most common vestibular diseases have different fingerprints when all dimensions are considered, this tool can facilitate the identification of the appropriate vestibular diagnosis.

For patients presenting with acute vertigo symptoms at the emergency unit, a two-minute, three-item bedside oculomotor examination (HINTS) has been proposed by Kattah and colleagues[12] to differentiate between acute peripheral vestibular lesions or central pathologies, like cerebellopontine angle infarctions. HI stands for head impulse test, N for nystagmus during the gaze-evoked test, TS for test of skew during a cover test where alternating each eye is covered. When the head impulse test is normal, an alternating gaze-evoked nystagmus appears at eccentric gaze, and the eye makes a vertical realignment upon uncovering it after the cover test, then a very high likelihood exists for an infarction in the region of the PICA or the AICA, being the posterior inferior cerebellar artery and the anterior inferior cerebellar artery. This simple bedside test has a 100% sensitivity and a 96% specificity which is much higher than imaging scans can provide in the early stage of the symptoms. In 17% of the PICA infarctions, the only symptoms are vestibular. Yet, it is a very important to identify the true etiology and not to think the patient has a 'trivial' vestibular disorder like a neuritis because in a considerable group (approximately one third) an oedema will develop that is severe enough to cause potentially lethal compression of the fossa posterior structures. Infarctions of other brain regions are more easily identifiable as stroke since they present with speech problems, disarthria, ataxia and other neurologic symptoms.

Once stroke is excluded, it remains a challenge to identify the etiology of the vertigo. To this purpose, clinicians need a quick and comprehensive assessment tool, comprising a structured overview of all the indispensable history information. Based on literature and our own experience, we made an inventory of how the most common vestibular disorders manifest themselves. This revealed a set of eight independent, but closely related dimensions necessary to discriminate between several diagnoses. The acronym 'SO STONED' is a useful tool to memorize these eight questions. Recently, Brandt and his co-workers[13] as well as Roland *et al.*[14] proposed a similar concept, without, however, putting it in an 'aide memoire' tool, and without covering all our proposed dimensions. The SO STONED tool increases the likelihood of a proper differential diagnosis, which obviously needs to be confirmed by clinical, laboratory and imaging examinations.

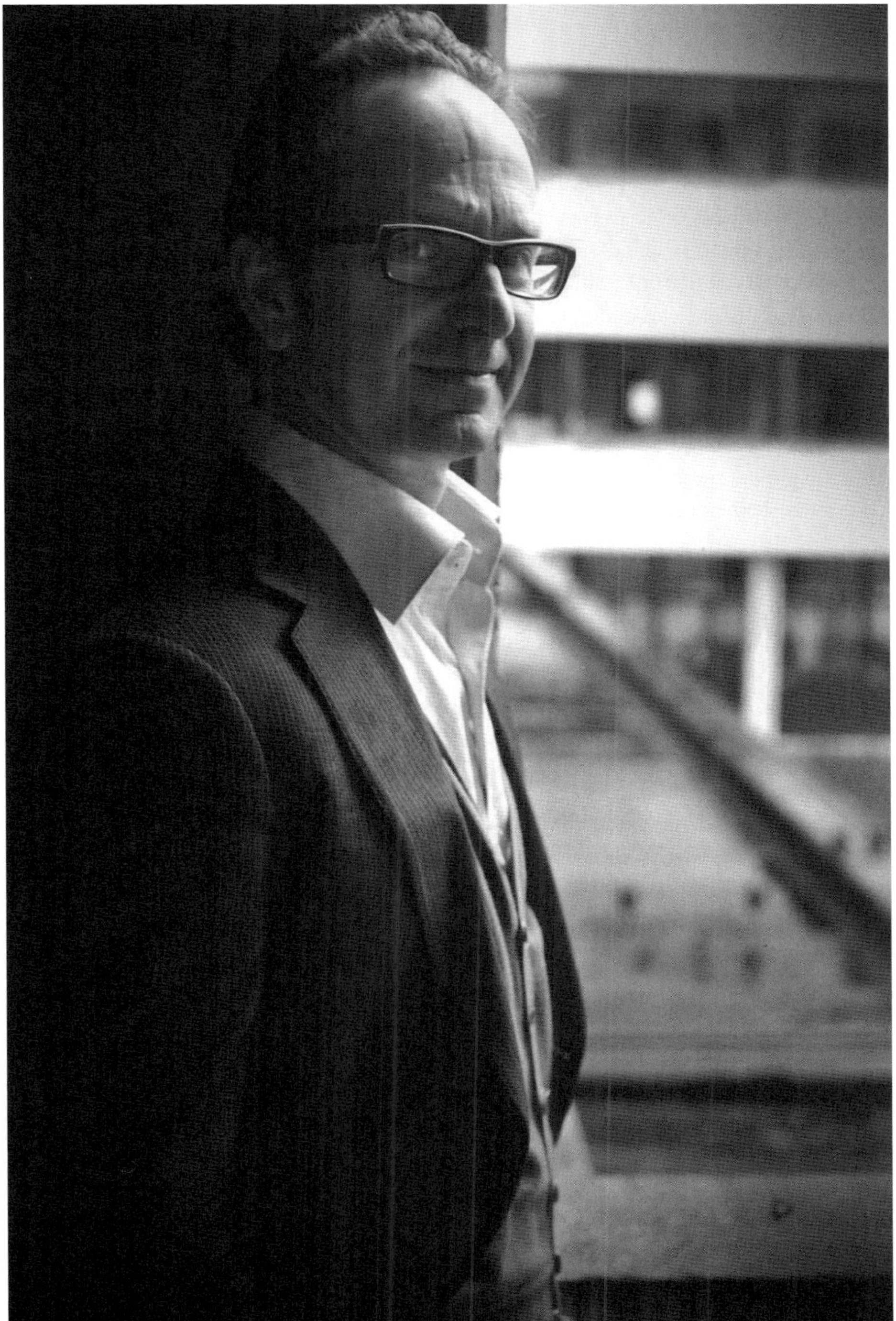

EIGHT DIMENSIONS

The letters of the acronym 'SO STONED' represent: Symptoms, Often (frequency), Since, Trigger, Otology, Neurology, Evolution and Duration. Table 1 provides an overview of the different questions that should be asked to the dizzy patient. The table on the inside of the back cover presents typical characteristics of different diseases according to the SO STONED history. Classification of the vestibular diseases was based on the ICD-11 beta version of the WHO classification, which divides vertigo in three different categories, namely acute, episodic and chronic. Since posterior fossa stroke can manifest itself as acute vertigo, stroke was added to the table of diagnoses.

The SO STONED tool proposes a systematic approach to the vertigo patient by using the complementary information provided by the different dimensions. Besides the frequent diagnoses presented in Table 2, other less common diagnoses should be taken into account when appropriate. In the following, we provide the rationale of the different dimensions.

Symptoms

Characterization of the symptoms helps to locate the problem. Vertigo or spinning, *the illusionary sensation of rotation is primarily referring to semicircular canal-related problems such as vestibular neuritis, benign paroxysmal positional vertigo (BPPV), superior semicircular canal dehiscence (SSCD), Ménière's disease (MD), etc. However, vertigo is also a common symptom in stroke.* Postural instability *is mainly typical for bilateral vestibulopathy or neurologic disorders such as polyneuropathy or cerebellar ataxia, although it can occur in other pathologies (see Table 2).* Lightheadedness *and or* dizziness *can be caused by panic attacks, agoraphobia and phobic postural vertigo, examples of persistent postural perceptual dizziness (PPPD). Dizziness is also reported in vestibular migraine, vestibular paroxysmia, bilateral vestibulopathy and in stroke. Some medications can also produce vertigo or lightheadedness.* Linear sensations *or a* tilt of the perceived vertical *are more suggestive for otolith dysfunction. Drop attacks or a sensation of being pushed to the ground or in another direction are signs of Tumarkin's otolithic crisis in MD, but beware of vestibular paroxysmia.* Lateropulsion *as well as* oscillopsia *occur in general when the labyrinth is affected, but may also occur with central lesions.*

O ften

A single attack of acute vertigo is a hallmark of vestibular neuritis or labyrinthitis, as well as stroke. Attacks that occur almost daily are typical for BPPV, but also for vestibular migraine, perilymphatic fistulas, SSCD and vestibular paroxysmia. When primarily spontaneous attacks occur several times per day, the likelihood for vestibular migraine decreases compared to vestibular paroxysmia. MD triggers vertigo attacks more than once, but the symptom-free intervals are rather weeks to months. Chronic vertigo can also be episodic, where the symptoms severity fluctuates in such a way that some complaints are always present as typical for PPPD. Bilateral vestibulopathy has a more continuous character.

S ince

This item focuses on possible causes for the vertigo. A head trauma occurring some weeks or days before the first symptoms is suggestive for BPPV, but also SSCD or perilymphatic fistula can be triggered by such an event. A viral illness might be the cause of vestibular neuritis, which in turn may induce delayed BPPV. Acute periods of stress may cause MD. Prolonged sleep disturbances can precipitate vestibular migraine. Inefficient compensation after an earlier period of vertigo can lead to chronic subjective dizziness, part of PPPD. Ototoxic medication or autoimmune disorders can lead to bilateral vestibulopathy.

T rigger

Bending over, lying down, rolling over in bed, looking up may all trigger short vertigo attacks, typical for BPPV. It is of great importance to discriminate if the symptoms occur during or just after the lying down or after rising up. Vestibular problems due to BPPV should cause vertigo in particular upon lying down, and often also during the sitting-up movement. If problems only occur during the erecting phase, think of cardiovascular etiologies and orthostatic hypotension. Rapid head movements causing instability or dizziness are rather hallmarks for a unilateral or bilateral labyrinth dysfunction, but are also aggravating factors for vestibular migraine and PPPD. Vestibular paroxysmia are sensitive to gravity changes, because the irritative blood vessel/vestibulocochlear nerve contact may elicit concomitant vertigo spells lasting several seconds, similar to BPPV. Therefore, when position changes in which the orientation of the head relative to the vertical position cause the symptoms, vestibular paroxysmia should be differentiated from BPPV based on the other dimensions of SO STONED.

Besides movement triggers there are also other types of triggers that can elicit or aggravate vertigo attacks. Valsalva manoeuvre, coughing or loud sounds that cause vertigo can be attributed to perilymphatic fistulas or a third mobile window lesion, e.g. the superior semicircular canal dehiscence. Attacks of vestibular migraine may be provoked by stress, lack of sleep, alcohol or exertion. If visual surroundings cause problems, visual vertigo should be considered. Open squares, shopping malls, crowded spaces can cause panic attacks that may present with concomitant dizziness, typical for PPPD. Some vertigo attacks occur completely spontaneously such as those caused by MD, but also vestibular migraine, vestibular paroxysmia and stroke. Vestibular neuritis usually starts without a trigger, but during the subsequent days each head movement will aggravate the vertigo symptoms. When postural instability is increased in darkness or with an unsteady underground, bilateral hypofunction or areflexia could be a differential diagnosis.

O tology

Sudden hearing loss accompanied by a single attack of vertigo may suggest labyrinthine deficiency. A combination of tinnitus, hearing loss and pressure in the ears or aural fullness, is suggestive for MD, although other pathologies, such as vestibular migraine, vestibular paroxysmia and third mobile window lesions may occur with some of the above otological complaints. When autophonia or hyperacusis of bodily sounds (hearing eye ball movements or pulsatile tinnitus) are present, third mobile window lesions should be excluded by means of temporal bone imaging.

N eurology

This dimension serves to rule out lesions of the central nervous system, such as posterior fossa ischemia, which could be screened by the HINTS tool.[12] *Additionally, this dimension aims to identify vestibular migraine with its typical characteristics such as headaches, current or past migraine, photophobia, scotoma, phonophobia, paresthesia, diplopia, etc. The absence of specific neurologic items serves to rule out other diseases that present with episodic vertigo attacks, such as MD, BPPV, third mobile window lesions, etc.*

E volution

Vestibular neuritis is typically very disturbing in the early stage with gradual improvement over days, whereas MD is characterized by sudden attacks, with periods of little to no vertigo in between. All other forms of vertigo typically have a stable course of intensity or are characterized by progressive or fluctuating severity of symptoms. One of the rare vestibular disorders that may worsen over time is PPPD.

Duration

The duration dimension has a very discriminative power to exclude specific disorders. For instance, MD cannot last seconds to a few minutes, whereas BPPV cannot last hours. Moreover, the dimensions 'duration' and 'frequency' are closely linked to each other. A single attack, lasting days, can point to labyrinthitis or vestibular neuritis, while short but frequent attacks in the order of seconds suggest rather BPPV, vestibular migraine, vestibular paroxysmia, perilymphatic fistula or third mobile window lesions. To discriminate between these diagnoses, the combination with the dimension 'trigger' and concomitant 'neurological' and 'otological' signs is crucial. Less frequent attacks that last hours are likely to represent MD or vestibular migraine. It should be noted that vestibular migraine can last from seconds (accumulated per day to a total of five minutes) to 72 hours.[15]

The combination of all dimensions is the key factor using the SO STONED acronym and provides a fingerprint of specific diseases. Clinical examinations, auditory and vestibular tests, and imaging obviously should be done.

To conclude, the acronym 'SO STONED' covers eight different dimensions while taking the systematic history in a vertigo patient. Since the most common vestibular diseases have different fingerprints when all dimensions are considered, this tool can facilitate the identification of the appropriate diagnosis.

It is nothing more than a guideline and additional questions are necessary, but this mnemonic contains the minimum of questions which are necessary to initiate a diagnosis.

If the patient gives a clear answer to these eight questions, and complementary information on which medication he or she takes, family history, what his or her medical history is, and so on, the doctor immediately gets a first impression of what the cause could be, and especially, which diagnosis it is not. In addition to that, the anamnesis is ideal to identify combined diseases.

A good example of this is a patient who is known to have Ménière's disease (MD). If he then comes back for a consultation and talks about a recent attack of dizziness, the doctor would quickly think that the MD is flaring up again. If the patient answers the Trigger-question ('what triggers the complaints?') with the answer 'especially when I lie down on my bed' and also 'bending over', the doctor should know what is going on, because in that case the answers do not fit the story of Ménière. When the doctor asks the Duration-question ('how long are you dizzy?') and the patient answers 'about twenty seconds', it strongly indicates a position-bound dizziness such as benign proximal positional vertigo (BPPV). It is strongly advised to complete the investigation with additional clinical tests and, when appropriate laboratory test and/or medical imaging. In this specific example, the Dix-Hallpike test will confirm the initial 'differential diagnosis', of BPPV in addition to the existing MD. The additional therapy will then be based on this new diagnosis.

Once the anamnesis is done, there need to be some extra tests to confirm the supposed diagnosis. These can be relatively simple tests, such as the head impulse test, or the more complicated tests, such as vestibular function tests. Hearing-screening tests need to be done to come to an accurate diagnosis. MRI or CT scans can also be part of additional evaluation, but this depends on the presumed pathology. The following chapter elaborates on the different vestibular function test.

Table 1. SO STONED questions asked to the patient for a structured history taking.

Dimensions	Questions	Targeted additional questions
Symptoms	What are the symptoms?	Vertigo, dizziness, nausea, postural instability, falls without syncope, falls with syncope, lightheadedness, rotatory or linear sensations, tilt of the vertical, oscillopsia, drunken feeling, lateropulsion, to-and-fro rocking…
Often	How often does 'it' happen?	Daily (once or several times a day), weekly, monthly, irregularly, continuously, only once, only during the trigger
Since	Since when do you suffer from this problem? Related to both time and circumstances	A day, week, month, year, decade ago. After a viral illness, a head trauma, a medical/surgical intervention, a journey on a boat, train or plane, without any clear cause
Trigger	What triggers the complaints/symptoms and what makes them worse, *i.e.*, aggravating factors?	General head movements, walking, rolling over in bed, bending over, looking up, being a passenger in a car or plane, walking in supermarket aisles, walking in semi-darkness, coughing, noise, visual stimuli, or … completely spontaneous
Otology	Do you experience any concomitant otological symptoms and when do these occur?	Hearing loss (fluctuating), tinnitus, aural fullness, hyperacusis, autophonia, draining ear, otalgia. Before, during or after the attacks, in between, long-lasting, *i.e.*, independent of the symptoms
Neurology	Do you experience any concomitant neurological symptoms?	Headache, migraine (current and in the past), face or limb paraesthesia, scotoma, phonophobia, photophobia, numbness, palpitations, hyperventilation, speech problems, diplopia, cervical problems
Evolution	What is the evolution of the symptoms?	Persistent, improving, worsening, ups and downs
Duration	What is the duration of the symptoms?	Seconds, minutes, hours, days, continuously

In the following chapter,

different equilibrium tests will be explained so that an insight can be acquired in the information that is gained from different tests. Especially, what the tests do not tell is not unimportant.

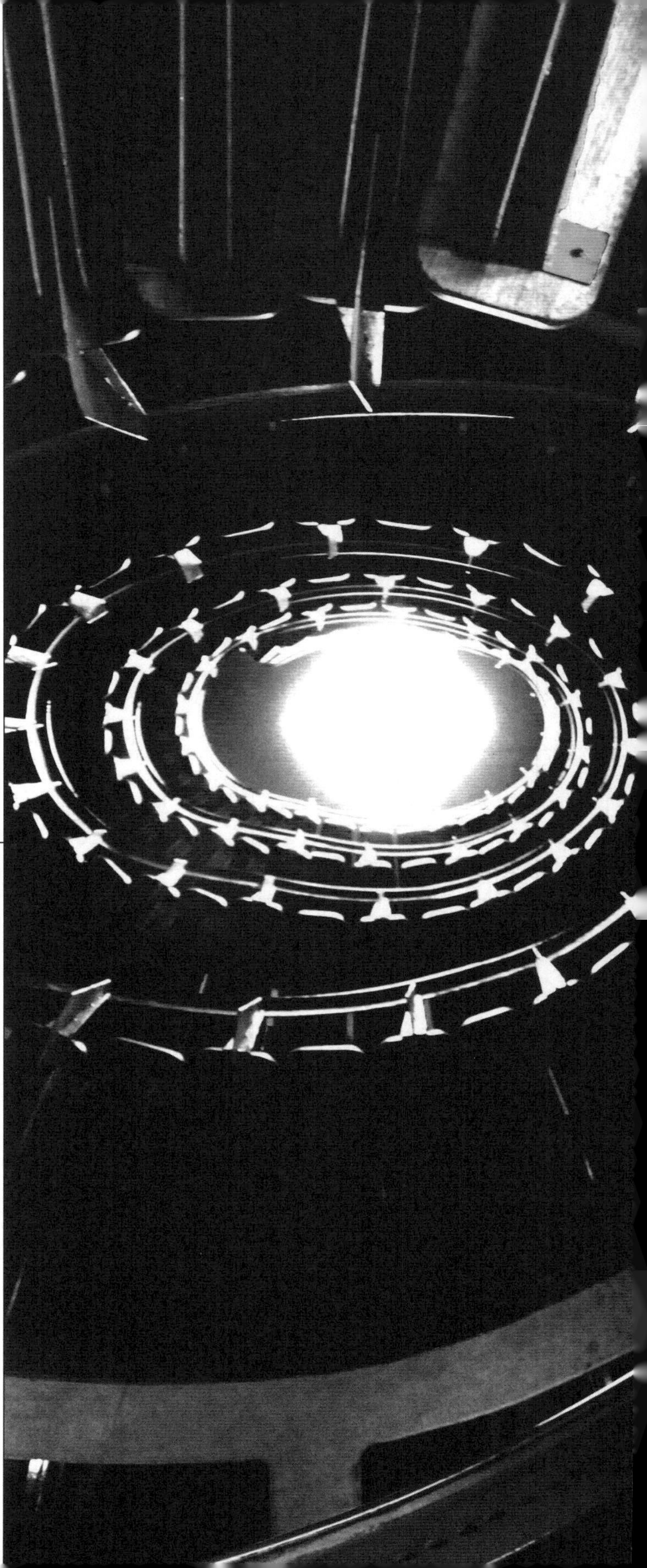

Chapter 6

Equilibrium Tests

In the inner ear is an organ of balance which consists of five parts: the three semicircular canals and two otoliths, saccule and utricle. In equilibrium tests we try to evaluate and quantify the working of the different parts of the organ of balance. This has two reasons: on the one hand to confirm or adjust the proposed diagnosis of the clinician, and on the other hand to map the evolution of the vestibular function, within the scope of a treatment, or the progress of an illness. For about a hundred years, equilibrium tests were limited to evaluating the working of the horizontal semicircular canals. But that has changed in the last twenty-five years, mainly because of newer research methods and faster computers. This in turn, provided better insights, although different tests are still under debate of what they really tell us.

Table 3 is a survey of different tests to examine different parts of the peripheral vestibular organ. Some tests examine the vestibular system as a whole, others examine the working of each side separately.

Table 3. Clinical examination and laboratory tests for different parts of the vestibular end organ

Part of the organ of balance	***Method***	***Left/right separately***
Horizontal semicircular canal (SCC)	Electronystagmography or videonystagmography with rotatory chair testing caloric test Videoscopy (v)HIT	no yes yes yes
Posterior (SCC)	Videoscopy (v)HIT	yes yes
Anterior (SCC)	Videoscopy (v)HIT	yes yes
Utricle	Unilateral centrifugation Lateroflexion oVEMP	yes no yes
Saccule	cVEMP	yes
Global evaluation	Subjective visual vertical Galvanic stimulation	no yes

Electronystagmography (ENG) or videonystagmography (VNG),
used for testing the horizontal semicircular canals

An important function of the balance system is to generate the VOR, which is the compensating eye movement in relation to head movement. A lot of vestibular research is done by examining and quantifying this eye reflex. The most widely used methods to register eye movements are electronystagmography (ENG), videonystagmography (VNG) and the closely related video head impulse test (vHIT). ENG involves placing electrodes around the eyes of the patient (Fig. 15). VNG involves placing a kind of diving goggles on the patient, with inside the goggles video cameras that observe the eye movements closely. These images are analyzed by computer image processing techniques (Fig. 16). ENG and VNG are considered basic methods to evaluate the VOR.

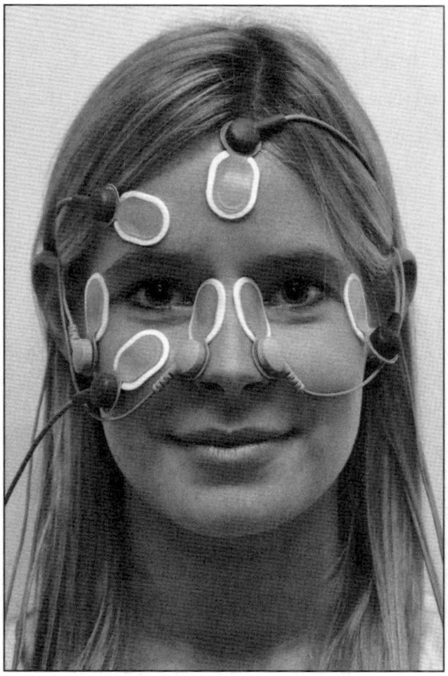

Fig. 15 — Electronystagmography (ENG), with electrodes around the eyes.

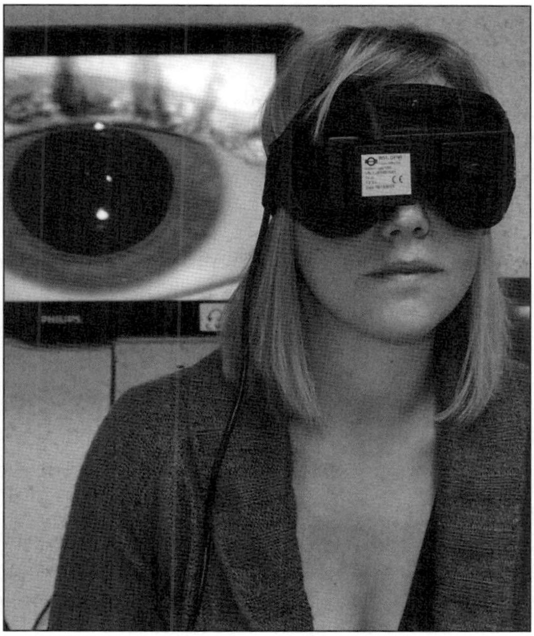

Fig. 16 — Videonystagmography (VNG). By way of a kind of diving goggles with cameras, an image of the patients' eye movements is obtained.

ENG relies on the fact that the eyeball can be considered as an electric dipole, *i.e.*, it is positively electrically charged on the front (cornea), compared with the back of the eye, where the retina is negatively charged because of all the electrically negative ions in the blood that flows through the retina. This cornea-retina potential difference is only a few millionths of a volt; however, by placing the electrodes correctly and amplifying the signal appropriately, one can achieve clear signals (Fig 18). These are proportional to the eye movements in the horizontal plane, since the electrodes are placed on the left and right of the eyes (Fig. 15). The electrodes can also be placed above and below the eyes, but these signals predominantly represent the eye blinking of the patient. Unfortunately, vertical eye movements cannot be trusted and torsional eye movements cannot even be measured with ENG-techniques. Horizontal eye movements, on the other hand, can be measured reliably, under the strict condition that calibrations are done consistently and multiple times, and especially prior to each caloric irrigation.

ENG has been used for decades, and this method is still used in many places worldwide. The great advantage is that the patient can close his or her eyes during this test. There are several publications with normal limits[16-19] for the use of this method and it is a proven method that is almost always applicable, both with very young as well as very old patients.

Videonystagmography or VNG (Fig. 16) has the advantage that it only needs to be calibrated once per patient and it can quantify both horizontal and vertical eye movements. The most important disadvantage of video techniques is that the patient must keep their eyes sufficiently open. When the patient blinks repeatedly, when the eyes are not completely open, or when the eyelids cover the eyes too much, the video technique measurements are not reliable. This is especially true when a patient has nystagmus, which causes frequent blinking.

Some video systems are also able to quantify torsional eye movements but they are more expensive (Fig. 17). Most VNG systems work at speeds of 30 to 60 or 100 images per second, depending on the video camara technology which is usually slower than ENG (typically 100 to 200 Hz). For saccades – looking from one point to the other very quickly – some video systems can be too slow to register movement in a reliable manner. But technology evolves quickly and more and more video systems can be delivered with fast cameras (at an additional cost).

VNG is growing, but for the time being ENG and VNG will both be used because each system has its advantages and disadvantages.

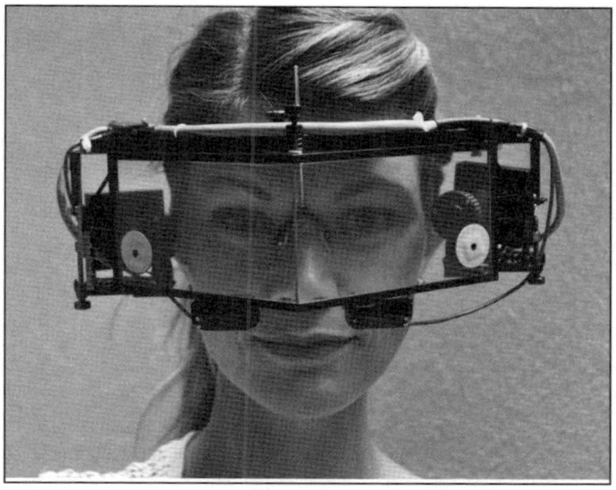
Fig. 17 — More complex system for videonystagmography (VNG).

Standard parts of the basic balance test

In general, the next tests are part of the ENG or VNG-test battery:

- Gaze-evoked test
- Spontaneous-nystagmus test
- Test of the eye movements comprising saccades, optokinetic and smooth pursuit tests
- Rotating-chair test
- Positional test
- Caloric test

Gaze-evoked test

Some patients have trouble to focus on an object, regardless of the emmetropia or vision status of the patient. When fixating on a target itself leads to nystagmus, it suggests a neurological problem. This is tested by having a patient fixate on objects which are projected at different locations on the screen. In normal circumstances, one has to be able to maintain the gaze at any central or lateral position, without deviations or nystagmus. Abnormalities suggest central nervous system problems, unless the patient also has a spontaneous nystagmus.

Nystagmus test

In normal conditions, one should not have a nystagmus when the head is held still and there is no visual input. If a nystagmus is present, without specific stimulus, it is called a spontaneous nystagmus. The typical characteristics of a 'spontaneous' nystagmus are that this eye movement appears when there is no visual input, and disappears by focusing on an object. This rather suggests a problem of one of the labyrinths, but can also indicate a disturbance in the central nervous system. In any case, the nystagmus, observed in this first part of the test battery, will manifest itself in all the subsequent test items, and this needs to be taken into account when interpreting the results.

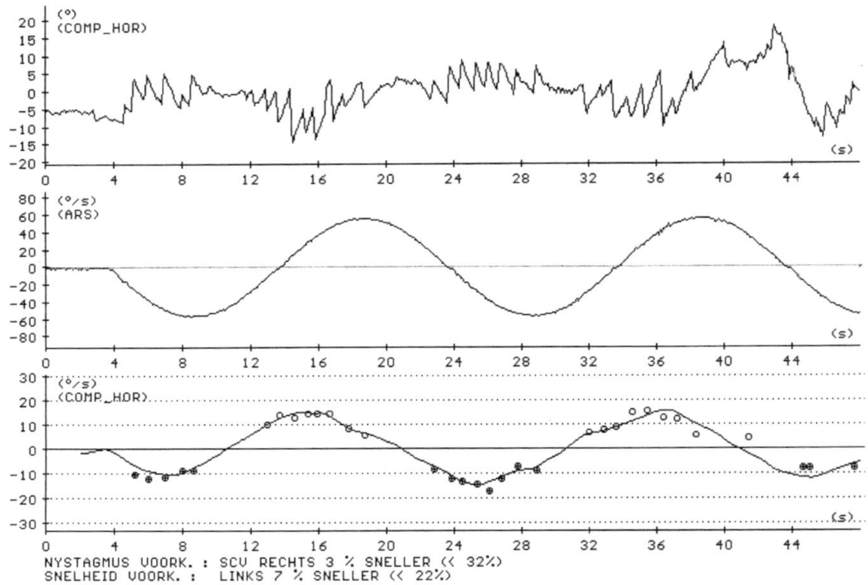

Fig. 18 — Result of ENG during a rotating test.
The first graph: The vertical axis shows the size of the eye movements. By convention, an eye movement to the right is depicted as a deflection upwards on the graph. The horizontal axis shows the time in seconds. Nystagmus can be recognized as a sawtooth pattern. Successive nystagmi to the right and left are generated by rotation of the subject to the right and left on the rotating chair, of which the speed is shown in the graph in the middle. The chair moves in a sinusoidal pattern, first to the right at a maximum speed of 50 degrees per second, and then to the left. The bottom graph shows the velocity of the eye movements. Each dot represents the velocity of the slow component of a nystagmus which is shown on the first graph. The eye velocity follows also a sinusoidal pattern as a reaction on the movement of the chair. For this patient, the VOR is symmetrical, because the nystagmus speed of the movements on the rotating chair to the left are as fast as the movements to the right. But the maximum speed of the nystagmi is too slow and consequently the VOR gain is too low as a result (in this case 17%, whereas it should be above 30%). Additionally, the phase is abnormal high. The tops of the sine waves on the bottom two graphs do not match. This suggests a large delay in the processing of the VOR. If only the (a)symmetry is considered, then this patient can be regarded as normal. If also gain and phase are considered, then abnormalities can be found.

Oculomotor tests

It needs to be verified that the vertigo or dizziness does not originate from a central neurological problem. Neurological conditions often result in abnormal eye movements that can be observed when patients perform specific tasks to be carried out with the eyes. The patient for example, needs to look at lights that jump back and forth on a screen (saccade test). Adequately following an object that sways back and forth is also part of the test (smooth pursuit eye movement test). The optokinetic test evaluates the ability to follow a pattern of stripes that move to the left and to the right at different speeds. The stimulus field (with stripes or dots) in this test should be as large as possible. These are tests that only examine eye movements, and in which the vestibular organ is not stimulated. Normally, patients needs to be able to execute these tasks without problems, provided they are adequately concentrated.

Rotating-chair test

As described earlier, one of the essential outcomes of an appropriate working vestibular system is the generation of a VOR during head rotation. Thus, measuring the VOR is an efficient method to quantify the function of the vestibular system. This is especially beneficial since no method exists to test the vestibular organ directly, such as a hearing test or a vision test. These senses, compared to balance, are very simple to assess, because it is sufficient to present a stimulus (sound, optotypes) and to ask the patient if he or she hears or sees the stimuli.

To test the VOR, the patient needs to undergo movement. The stimulus should be as specific as possible, so that it can be repeated. This can be achieved by, among other things, rotating the patient on a special rotating chair (Fig. 19). The most widely-used manner is moving from one side to the other, according to a sinusoid, with a maximum speed of 50 to 60 degrees per second and a duration of 20 seconds per sway, which equates to a frequency of 0.05 Hz. This is called the sinusoidal harmonic acceleration test (SHAT). One can move faster back and forth, or slower, but the results differ little compared to the 0.05 Hz-stimulus. It has been shown that 0.01 Hz has a slightly greater sensitivity to identify certain conditions, being 73% instead of 70% for 0.05Hz.[20]

To quantify the VOR properly, two signals need to be measured. On one hand, the speed of the movement, preferably of the patient's head, and on the other

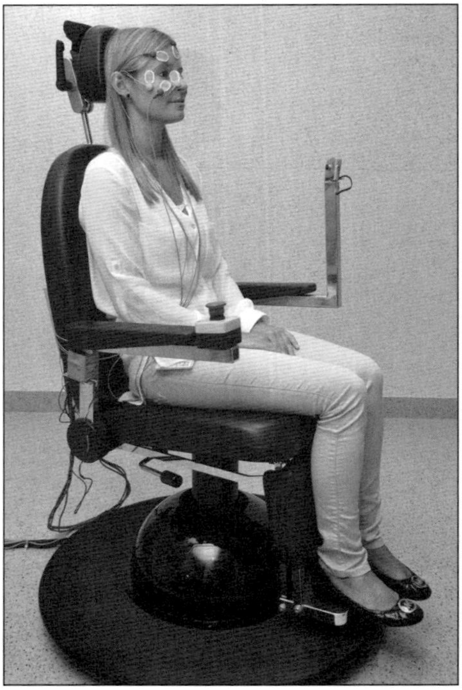
Fig. 19 — Rotating-chair test

hand, the speed of the eye movements. By comparing these two signals with each other, we can characterize the VOR by measurements of 'gain', 'phase' and 'asymmetry'. The gain, or efficiency, is the proportion between eye speed and head speed. When the lights are switched on in the room, the gain is equal to one, so your eyes move as fast to the left as when your head moves to the right when shaking your head. If not, your gaze stabilization would not be optimal, and you would have a blurry vision with every head movement. At slow rotation speeds, the VOR is assisted with the visual system (smooth pursuit, OKN and saccades) thus the gain equals one. With faster head movements, the gain is still one, but the reflex is mainly due to the vestibular system because the visual system is too slow to generate compensatory eye movements (approximately 90 ms delay). Because the rotating-chair test is rather slow, the test needs to be done in complete darkness. This can be done by letting the patient close the eyes in an already dark room (ENG), or by closing the video glasses with a lightproof lid (VNG). If the rotating chair test is done while the patient can vaguely see his or her environment, the results of the VOR test are incorrect and will not make much sense.

A patient whose vestibular organs failed to function on both sides will still generate completely normal test results in semi-dark conditions, since the eyes provide sufficient information to generate a VOR, while in complete darkness no VOR would be measured by the ENG or VNG test, indicating abnormal results. This shows how important methodological details of test protocols are for making a diagnosis.

The gain, or efficiency, of the VOR in the dark lies between 30% and 90%. Unfortunately, the gain is strongly influenced by the alertness of the patient. That is for example why patients are always asked to count down out loud from two hundred to zero by threes while rotating in the dark. The phase is also calculated, which is a measurement for the 'delay' in the vestibular system. Because it is not only sufficient that the eyes move as fast as the head and in the opposite direction, it also needs to be approximately at the same time. If the VOR happens too slowly, then the patient is dizzy. Lastly, there is asymmetry. Does the vestibular system convert head movements to the left as easily as those to the right in compensating eye movements? Asymmetry levels of more than 20% to 25% are usually considered as abnormal.

In a nutshell, to have a proper VOR, the response needs to be sufficiently large, instantaneous and symmetrical. It regularly occurs that only one of the three complementary parameters - gain, phase and asymmetry - is abnormal. However, each component is essential because it can be just that one part that explains why the patient complains of dizziness. It is also important to have the normal limits from each parameter so that abnormal values can be identified. For example, just as determining a cholesterol level is too high when a value is above the limit, we can determine a too high phase or a too high asymmetry of the VOR. It is unfortunately a fact that the methods in vestibular tests differ a lot more than the methods for blood checks. Every equilibrium laboratory should establish its own standards, measured for example in about forty healthy volunteers, and preferably published.

Is 'sophisticated' really useful?

Why is it relevant to measure also phase, and not only gain and asymmetry as in most 'simple' rotation tests? Imagine a patient who has a symmetrical VOR, with normal gain, but an abnormal phase. This means that the patient's VOR is compensated properly in terms of speed and symmetry, so movements to one side and the other side are converted into equivalent compensatory eye movements. The eye speed is also sufficiently high, but the phase is abnormal which indicates there is a delay of time in the eye reflex. This can indicate a delay in the processing of the signals in the brainstem, or typically a reduced function of one peripheral labyrinths (so that the other labyrinth has to take over at the cost of extra processing time). This kind of delay can partially impact the other systems, especially vision and proprioception which demands extra energy and effort to maintain continuous balance and gaze stabilization. If the patient is tired, has had too little or insufficient sleep, the complaints of vertigo may worsen. The patient will report his problems as 'not being on top of things' – or cheap drunk – since the VOR-driven compensatory eye movements arrive just a bit too late. If the phase is not measured during the balance tests, this aspect will be missed, and the VOR will seem normal. So, despite the fact that the patient has complaints, and the phase is abnormal, the 'simple' test will be negative, and thus not in agreement with the disease. The calculations of gain, phase and asymmetry are based on physical and mathematical principles (such as Fourier calculations).

Almost every patient can tolerate this test because the chair moves slowly back and forth, the test takes place in total darkness and it usually takes no longer than two minutes.

Finally, the head of the patient in the rotating chair needs to be positioned upright, and not bent forward. In the past, some clinicians assumed that the optimal VOR reaction could only be obtained for the horizontal canal if it lies in the plane of the rotating movement, such as when the head is bent forward 30 degrees. But scientific research has proven that it is better to position the head straight up because the variability of the gain is smaller, and thus, abnormalities can be observed more easily in patients.[21] Moreover, humans walk with their head straight up, rather than looking down at the ground in daily life.

Positional tests

Positional tests are performed to search for positional nystagmus, *i.e.*, a nystagmus that appears when a certain position is taken, for example, laying down. Nystagmus can appear when a patient goes to lay down or after they are in the laying-down position. It is important to observe and to record the nystagmus when someone is dizzy. During this test, the patient is laid down, like during the Dix-Hallpike manoeuver, first, with the head hanging and leaning to the left, and then to the right. Investigate whether there is a persistent nystagmus or a transient nystagmus and in which direction it goes. There is a preference to use VNG instead of ENG because the vertical and/or torsional component can be measured with VNG.

Caloric test

The Austrian surgeon Robert Bárány won the Nobel Prize for Medicine in 1914 because of the caloric tests. It is still used every day and performed almost all over the world. The essence of this test is to inject in the auditory canal water that is seven degrees warmer or colder than the average body temperature. When the patient is positioned in the supine position, with his or her head at a 30-degree angle, this caloric test stimulates the horizontal semicircular canal in the inner ear. Indeed, this positioning of the patient makes that the horizontal canal is actually orientated vertically. The effect of the temperature of the warm or cold irrigated water causes a convection current of the endolymph in the canal. This causes the warm endolymph in the part of the semicircular canal that is relatively close to the ear canal to rise, since it is lighter than the cold endolymph on the other side of the canal at body temperature. Due to this, the cupula bends slightly in one direction or another (depending on whether it is cold or warm water). This bending causes movement of the cilia in the hair cells that are embedded in the cupula, which results in a signal of excitation (more stimulation) or inhibition (less stimulation) to be sent to vestibular nuclei in the brainstem. The endolymph moves, just as when there is head movement, causing the VOR to be evoked. A warm stimulus provokes nystagmus that beats toward the side of the irrigation, and a cold stimulus generates a nystagmus that beats towards the opposite side. A simple mnemonic helps to remember this: COWS, *i.e.*, 'Cold Opposite, Warm Same'.

The special thing about this test is that it allows each horizontal canal to be tested individually, because there is only a reaction on the side where the water is irrigated in the auditory canal. The reaction occurs specifically in the horizontal semicircular canal because it is the nearest to the auditory canal (Fig. 20a). Typically, 200 ml of water of 44 and 30 degrees Celsius is injected for 30 seconds, in each ear. One often begins with the warm water on the right and then wait five minutes, in which one registers the eye movements during the first two minutes. Then the same is done on the left side and the reaction is measured again. After five minutes, the procedure is repeated with cold water on the right, to end with cold water on the left.

When using ENG, it is crucial to calibrate each time before every 'irrigation'. If this is not done, the results of the test are not reliable. The eye potential, which is measured with electrodes, is very sensitive to perspiration as well as other factors that, for example, have to do with alertness (linked to pupil diameter).

The patient lies in the dark, and after the start of the irrigation, he or she soon feels a sensation of movement. This sensation has a typical crescendo-diminuendo-sequence. It comes and goes. After about two minutes, the sensation ceases. The patients are always asked to count, typically from a hundred to zero, in twos. Some patients feel like they are really spinning, while others barely notice it. The feeling of dizziness is caused by the brain having a sensory conflict, because the stimulus only comes from the irrigated ear and not the other ear. The brain is also not receiving any additional information from the other senses, such as vision, since the eyes are closed, or proprioception. This conflict only takes place for a short period of time. When we inform the patient that these

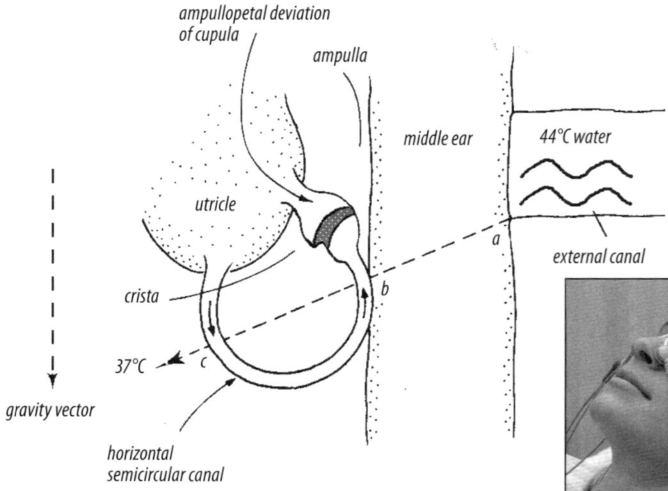

Fig. 20a — Schematic overview of the working of a caloric test. The ossicles are not drawn in this figure.

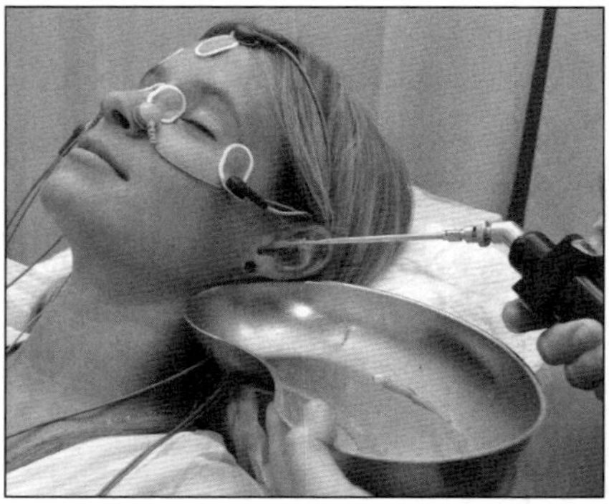

Fig. 20b — Warm and cold water are alternately injected into the ear during a caloric test. The patient lies in such a manner that the horizontal canal is orientated vertically.

sensations are completely normal, many patients are reassured, causing them to feel less dizzy, or they can tolerate the dizziness better. Nevertheless, this test can lead to vomiting with patients who are very sensitive. However, in my personal experience, and I have done thousands of vestibular tests, this number can be limited to a very small percentage, mainly by informing and comforting the patient.

The slow component velocity of the nystagmus is the value that is used as measurement for the caloric excitability of the labyrinths. This measurement is taken at the peak of the reaction for each of the four irrigations. The difference between the left and right side is calculated and then it is divided by the sum of all irrigations. This measurement shows the 'asymmetry' between the excitability of the left and the right horizontal semicircular canals (Fig. 20c). Thus asymmetry yields [(right warm + right cold) – (left warm + left cold)]/(all four irrigations). In addition, it can be derived if the nystagmus to the left or the right is being

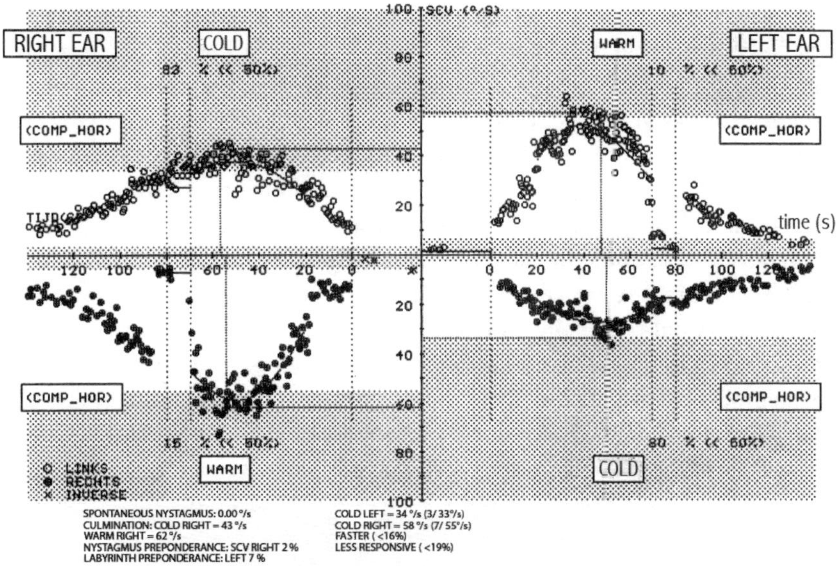

Fig. 20c — Butterfly chart of the four caloric irrigations. From the center of the figure, time runs in seconds, both to the left as to the right on the horizontal axis. The vertical axis shows the slow component velocity of the nystagmus that is generated by each irrigation. The reaction of the right ear is shown on the left side of the figure, and the function of the left ear on the other side of the figure. Each time one can recognize a build-up of the reaction and then a decrease of it. The result for this patient is normal since the labyrinth dominance is 7% which is within the normal range of symmetry (< 19%). So there is no difference between the left and the right horizontal canals. The preference of nystagmus beating to the left is 2% which is also within the normal limits (< 16%). So there is no difference between the sums of the nystagmus to the left and to the right.

systematically facilitated. This is called nystagmus preponderance and obtained as [(right warm + left cold) – (left warm + right cold)]/(all four irrigations).
If the nystagmus preponderance exceeds normal values (> 16%), and in absence of other abnormalities on the ENG or VNG, it is suggestive for central neurological problems and needs to be further investigated.

Complementary with the rotation test. The result of the caloric test is complementary to the rotation test. The caloric test shows to what extent each of both horizontal canals are excitable. The rotation test shows how the integrated vestibular system deals with motion, *i.e.*, how head movements to the left and right convert in an appropriate VOR, despite possible big differences between both organs of balance. Many diagnoses are made or adjusted based on this

test. A typical example is a patient who has complaints that are consistent with vestibular neuritis. It is then presumed that there is an acute failure of one labyrinth. If the vestibular test is conducted shortly after the complaints begin, and the results show that one side barely reacts or at least reacts less to the caloric test than the other side, the clinician can diagnose vestibular neuritis with a high probability, particularly when a spontaneous nystagmus is present and the rotation test is asymmetric too. However, when the caloric test gives a perfect symmetrical result other possibilities need to be considered, such as a brainstem infarction (see the section on HINTS). In that case, several other clinical tests for that patient would normally show signs that are suggestive for a brainstem injury. Imaging (NMR) and further neurological investigations should corroborate the neurological diagnose. Only in some exceptional cases, the rotation test and caloric test provide contradictory information. These cases challenge the knowledge of the clinician dealing with that particular patient.
A complete electronystagmography test takes about one hour.

Head Impulse Test

The head impulse test (HIT) is a fast, effective and simple way to clinically establish if there is a problem with one or both vestibular organs. It is the ideal test to perform at the initial check of a patient who is brought to the emergency room with vertigo and vomiting. Both a brain hemorrhage in the brainstem or something as 'trivial' as vestibular neuritis can be the cause of vertigo and vomiting.

The principle of the HIT. As mentioned before, each vestibular organ at rest sends about one hundred spikes per second to the brain. The discharge frequency increases with a head movement to the ipsilateral side and decreases with a head movement to the contralateral side. If it were a completely symmetrical system, the frequency on the one side would increase as much as it would decrease on the other side. However, since the 'resting state' matches with a hundred spikes per second, there is a non-linearity in the system built in because there can be a lot more spikes sent to the brain than two hundred per second (100 + 100) but not less than zero spikes per second (100 - 100).

For example, imagine suddenly turning the head quickly to the left. The cilia are being bent so strongly in the left horizontal canal that the discharge frequency increases from one hundred to about four hundred spikes per second. The cilia in the vestibular organ on the other side are also being bent but because of their mirrored orientation to the other side, the number of action potentials decreases from one hundred to zero. This non-linear behavior (several hundred spikes per second versus zero) is the basis of the HIT to uncover abnormalities.

How to perform a head impulse test. The clinician stands in front of the patient and asks him or her to look at the investigator's nose or at an object on the wall behind the investigator. Then the investigator takes the head of the patient firmly in his or her hands and turns it slowly back and forth in an angle of about twenty degrees to the right and to the left to loosen up the neck of the patient. This is not essential, but merely to prepare the patient. Then the investigator turns the patient's head unannounced and very fast to the affected side, with a short but abrupt movement. Normally, the vestibular organ on the leading side, *i.e.*, towards where the head was moved, increases its discharge frequency from one hundred to about several hundred spikes per second. But this will not be the case if there is an vestibular failure on that side. The 'healthy' ear on the other side, however, works properly and generates a decrease from one hundred to zero spikes per second on that side. Yet, this decrease contains too little information. The central vestibular system does not know whether the head moved 'fast' or 'very fast' to the affected side because in both cases the contralateral side does not transmit a signal to the brainstem (zero spikes per second). Consequently, the eyes move along with the moving head and they cannot remain their focus on the investigator's nose. The patient soon realizes this and makes a recovery move (a catch-up saccade) with his or her eyes to look at the target – the nose – again. When the investigator moves the head to the 'healthy' side, the patient can maintain his or her gaze on the target because on this side the discharge frequency is sufficiently high to give information to the central vestibular system about how fast the head turned, and consequently how fast the eyes had to compensate. So the side towards which a catch-up saccade is generated upon a head trust is the side that is not functioning properly.

The head impulse test is ideal to find out the side of an affected non-functioning labyrinth, and in general, to see if there is a problem with the gaze stabilization. It is important that the investigator makes sudden and fast movements, otherwise the patient will anticipate and his or her eye movements would be falsely accurate. The movements do not have to be big but should be very rapid in order to saturate (bring it from one hundred to zero) the vestibular organ on the 'healthy' side completely. That is why the investigator needs to take the patient's head firmly into his or her hands. This method is developed for the inspection of the horizontal canals, but it can also be used to verify the integrity of the vertical semicircular canals. When the head is turned from obliquely backwards to obliquely forwards (in the LARP or RALP plane = left anterior canal and right posterior canal or right anterior canal and left posterior canal), the posterior and anterior canal can be tested, although this requires trained hands of the investigator.

The HIT is a so called 'bedside test', which means that this test can be done everywhere, including on the side of the patient's bed. However, it is recommended to perform additional vestibular tests, including a caloric test, to confirm the findings of the HIT, but the HIT is a very quick and easy test for the clinician to evaluate the integrity of each of the labyrinths, without the need for additional equipment.

In the past few years, there has been a development of a digital video version of the HIT which is for sale at different companies. This test is called vHIT or videoHIT. In this version, the patient has to wear a kind of glasses, such as swimming goggles, in which a small camera is integrated to look at the eye movements. The head movement is measured with accelerometers and a computer program on a laptop provides the necessary visualization of the test. Scientific studies show that there is no direct correlation with the caloric test.[22] The high frequencies of the VOR are tested by the vHIT, and the low frequency of the VOR are tested using calorics.

The vHIT is more sensitive than the 'bedside' HIT, according to Mahringer and Rambold but the HIT nor the vHIT can be seen as replacement for the caloric test. A recent review[23] of the vHIT concludes that vHIT is a physiological quick test, testing the VOR of each semicircular canal at high frequency. vHIT is a complementary test for other vestibular tests, especially the caloric test, but not a replacement. As the vHIT is not associated with nausea or vomiting and well tolerated by the patients, it is recommended to perform the vHIT as a first test in each semicircular canal. If the vHIT is normal, then a caloric test is mandatory to rule out a peripheral origin of dizziness. For acoustic neuroma disease, vHIT was not correlated with the tumor size as determined by the MRI being the gold

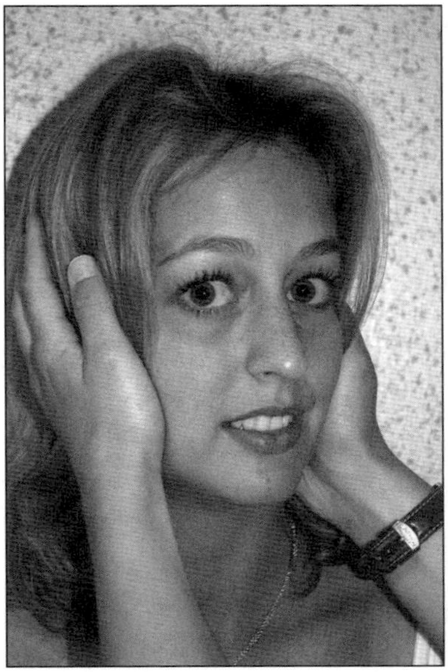

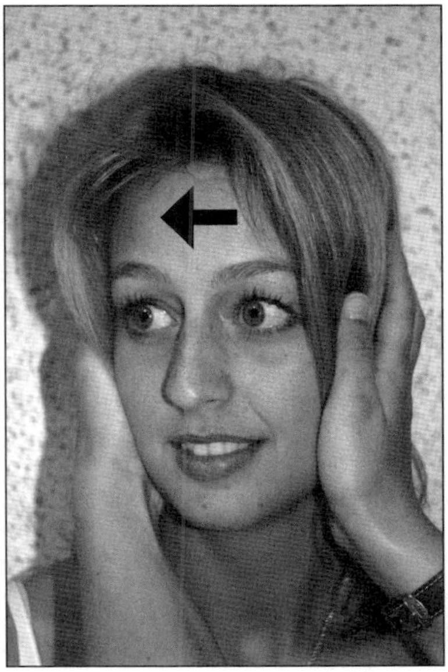

Fig. 21 — Head impulse test. The patient whose head is turned fast from her left side (picture on the top left), to the right (picture on the top right) is not capable of focusing on the nose of the clinician and needs to do a catch-up saccade (black arrow) to regain focus (bottom picture). The patient's right horizontal canal does not work properly in this case.

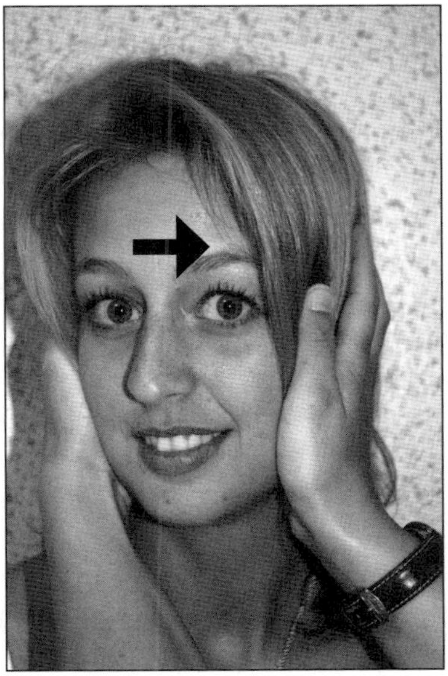

standard, neither with hearing loss, whereas caloric results did correlate with both parameters. The vHIT still needs further study to see the evolution of the VOR gain with the progression of the vestibular disease. So, to conclude, if the vHIT is normal, this does not rule out peripheral lesions!

The cervical Vestibular Evoked Myogenic Potential (cVEMP)

Used for testing the saccular function

The principle. Since 1994, the saccular function has been successfully measured by means of collic or cervical vestibular evoked myogenic potentials (cVEMPs). cVEMPs are inhibitory muscle potentials that are measured by placing an electrode on the contracted neck muscle (sternocleidomastoid muscle) and by subjecting the patient to loud stimuli played through headphones.[24] cVEMPs are the result of these loud sounds (tone bursts of 500 to 1000 kHz) that stimulate the saccule directly through vibrations. This is most likely due to the fact that anatomically, the saccule is located close to the oval window, through which the sound vibrations coming from the eardrum are passed on to the cochlea. The stimulated saccule sends signals to the vestibular nuclei in the brainstem, from which signals are sent to, among others, the neck muscle on the stimulated side. This signal causes the contracted muscles to relax. The EMG (electromyogram) of sternocleidomastoid muscle tension and more particularly the inhibition can be measured through electrodes triggered by short but loud tone bursts presented to the ear of the patient on the ipsilateral side.

The patient needs to contract the neck muscle for this, which can be accomplished, for example, by pushing his or her head against the own hand. It is of great importance to watch the tension of the muscle closely and also to maintain the same level of tension during the approximately thirty seconds that are needed for this part of the test. For this, the patient looks at a monitor on which he or she can see how severely the muscle is tightened (Fig. 22a). This value is also used for further calculations of the signals.[25,26] The peak-to-peak amplitudes (p13-n23) and latencies of these EMG signals (p13 and n23) are interpreted to determine the level of asymmetry between the left and right saccule. Additional measurements that characterize the saccular function are threshold intensities. One starts off with a maximal sound intensity of 95 dB which is lowered until eventually the threshold value is reached. This threshold

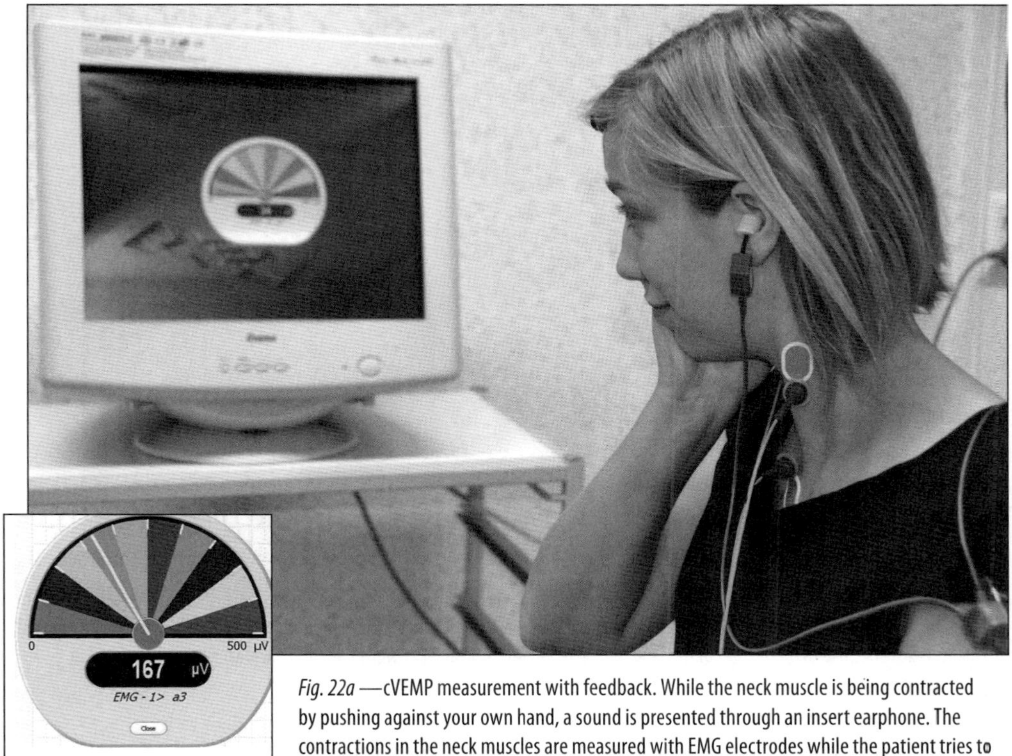

Fig. 22a —cVEMP measurement with feedback. While the neck muscle is being contracted by pushing against your own hand, a sound is presented through an insert earphone. The contractions in the neck muscles are measured with EMG electrodes while the patient tries to keep the tension in the muscle constant through feedback on the monitor.

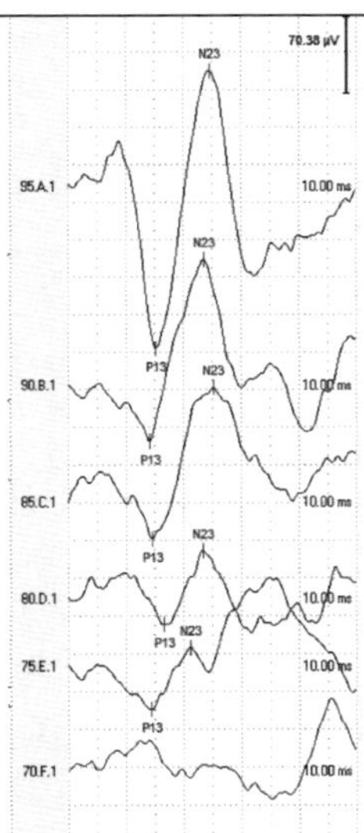

Fig. 22b — cVEMP traces with different sound intensities from 95dB to 70dB. The threshold for this case is at 75dB. Typical for the cVEMP response is the negative peak p13 and the positive peak n23 around respectively 13 and 23 ms after the sound stimulus.

value is defined as the lowest sound intensity that still can evoke a cVEMP response (Fig. 22b). These threshold values seem especially of great importance when identifying the diagnosis of superior semicircular canal dehiscence (SSCD) discussed later in this book. A cVEMP test normally takes about twenty minutes.

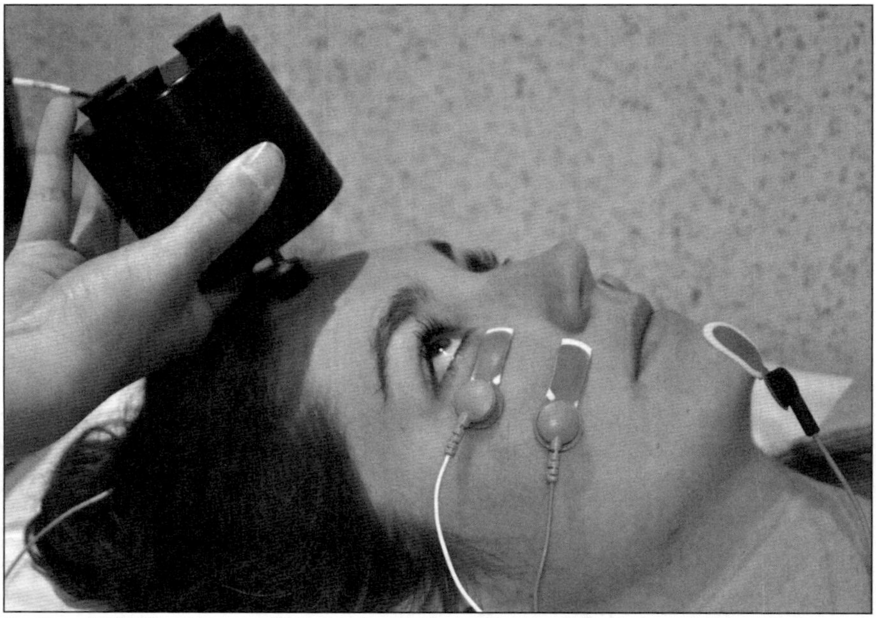

Fig. 24 — oVEMP. Vibrations are applied on the forehead by a mini-shaker while the patient looks up. The lower eye muscles are close to the surface of the skin while looking up. Contractions of the eye muscles are measured with electrodes.

Ocular Vestibular Evoked Myogenic Potential (oVEMP)

Used for utricular function

One of the most recent tests among the vestibular test battery is the ocular vestibular evoked potentials (oVEMPs), in which the eye muscle responses are measured while the patient's forehead is stimulated with a little hammer or a mini-shaker (Fig. 24). A specific part of both utricles is stimulated this way, which results in a signal that goes to the vestibular nuclei in the brainstem, and from there to the inferior oblique eyes muscles. This eye movement is too small to measure with ENG or VNG, but contractions of the eye muscles are measurable with EMG. This test evokes a crossed response: contractions of the right eye muscle originate from a stimulation of the left utricle, and vice versa. Currently, this new test is being investigated thoroughly in several research and clinical centers in the world. The full meaning of this test is still under debate and not entirely clear yet, but it will become unraveled in the next few years.[27]

Unilateral centrifugation (UC)

Used for measurement of the utricular function

The utricular function can also be measured one side at a time with a unilateral centrifugation test.[28,29] More specifically, the sensitivity of the utricle and a possible dominance of the right or left utricle, among other things, can be characterized by means of this test. The centrifugation is executed with a chair rotating around the vertical axis at a relatively fast rotation speed. Patients in the seat must be fastened. The head is firmly stabilized in a head support and is thus prevented from moving forward during the test. Video goggles are then placed on the patient's head (Fig. 25), with which the eyes can be studied in detail and the eye movements analyzed. The chair is rotated with an acceleration of, for example, three degrees per second squared up to a rotation speed of four hundred degrees per second. Then the chair rotates during ninety seconds at this constant speed to fade out the effects of the semicircular canals to a large extent. Next, the chair will, while constantly rotating at the same speed of 400 deg/s, shift alternating 4 cm to the left and right, as in a sinusoidal pattern. After four complete sines, the chair slowes down. The complete duration of the test takes about 13 minutes. During this test, the ocular counter rolling (OCR) of the eyes is measured by means of 3D video oculography. This OCR is a measure of the function of each utricle separately, characterised by gain and preponderance (asymmetry). This test is fully complementary to the other tests of the vestibular test battery.

Video-oculoscopy

for screening of the horizontal, posterior and anterior semicircular canals

The use of video-goggles allows a clinician to carefully investigate nystagmus of any type. Looking in close-up at eye movements may identify subtle abberant eye movements, and in particular transient movements, in different positions that the patient is subjected to, like the Dix Hallpike position or decubitus position. When you can record the eye movements as well as the position of the patients, it allows you to look back at the recording when some special complicated eye movements were seen and better interpret the observations. Obviously, videoscopic investigation of a patient with a suspected BPPV (Benign Paroxysmal Positional Vertigo - see later in this book) is of great use to see the typical eye movements

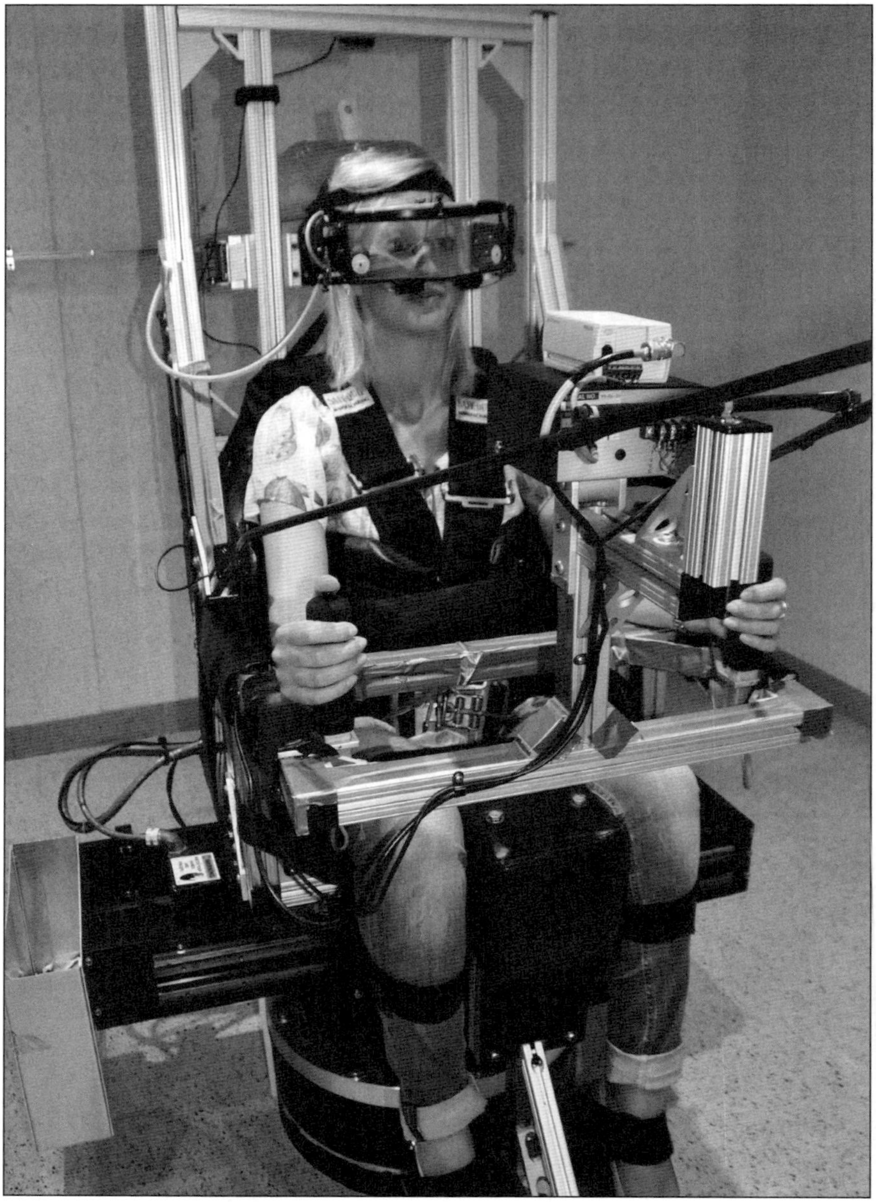

Fig. 25 — Unilateral centrifugation equipment for evaluation of the utricles. During rotation, the chair moves also sideways to align the axis of rotation either with the right or left vestibular organs. The concomitant ocular counter rolling is measured with 3D video goggles.

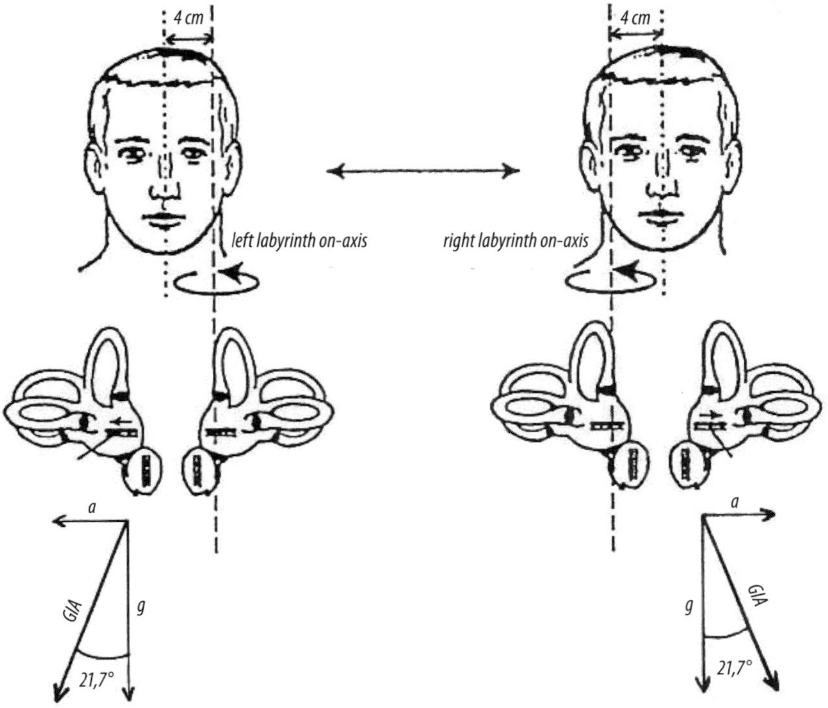

Fig. 26 —The principle of unilateral centrifugation. While the patient is rotating, the axis of the rotating chair is moved, so that it is aligned alternating through the left or right utricle. The other utricle is then being centrifuged. The sum of the gravity (g) and the centrifugal shear force (a) on the otoconia of the utricle results in a tilt of gravito intertial acceleration (GIA), and this produces an opposite counter rolling of the eyes. This is measured with 3D video-oculography.

that are elicited in the Dix-Hallpike position when otoconia are moving in the posterior semi circular canal. Next, during the therapeutic maneuver such as the Epley or the Semont liberatory maneuvers, inspection of the eye movements will allow to verify if the debris of the otoconia are moving in the right direction, or if they are returning back to the initial position. When a patient suffers from horizontal canal BPPV, video-oculoscopy is very useful during the roll test to identify on which side the BPPV is present. Carefully rolling the head from one side to the other while inspecting the horizontal nystagmus direction and particularly the reversing of the direction is a handy tool to lateralize the BPPV. And consequently, that will guide the direction of the liberatory barbeque roll maneuver.

However, video-oculoscopy also allows the clinician to identify possible abnormalities, or unexpected eye movements that cannot be attributed to BPPV. In a study we performed in a group of 36 patients with vestibular paroxysmia (a disorder that will be described in the chapter Disorders ABC), we observed in 80% of the cases a non-BPPV type of nystagmus in the Dix-Hallpike positions. This was presented at the IFOS meeting in Paris in 2017. A non-BPPV type nystagmus is, for example, a pure horizontal nystagmus when the patient is placed in the Dix Hallpike position that triggers the posterior canal and not the horizontal canal (one should see an upbeating and clockwise or counter-clockwise nystagmus with a crescendo-diminuendo time course within a minute). Or when a clockwise or counter-clockwise nystagmus is persistently beating as long as the head-hanging position is taken. Thus, not every positional vertigo needs to be interpreted as loose otoconia floating around in the canal, but it can be due to for example a neurovascular conflict, causing the patient to suffer from vestibular paroxysmia. In case of vestibular migraine, non-BPPV type nystagmi are also frequently observed, as well as when brain tumors or central lesions are present. Finally, when a patient is seated upright after the lying down position, and reports only then vertigo or dizziness while no nystagmus is observed, one should think of a cardiovascular ethiology.

Video-oculography

Video-oculography is the variant of video-oculoscopy referring to the quantification of the eye movements in either two or three dimensions, *i.e.*, horizontal and vertical or with the addition of the torsional component (clockwise or counter clockwise). The latter is quite difficult to achieve and only a limited number of commercial systems are capable of a reliable torsional measurement. This method is essential to measure otolith responses like during unilateral centrifugation testing (Fig. 17, 25). For almost all vestibular tests as well as for specific neurological disorders such as progressive supranuclear palsy, 2D video-oculography is of great use, since it records reliably hampered vertical eye movements.

Subjective Visual Vertical (SVV) test

Used for global perception of verticality

During the SVV test, the patient is seated in a totally darkened room. Then a laser line with a given inclination is projected on a wall. The patient has a hand-held remote control that can rotate the line to the left or to the right. The task for the patient is to put the laser line perfectly vertical. The deviation of the laser line with the true vertical is the outcome measure of this SVV test. This procedure is repeated several times to the left and to the right and the outcomes are averaged. Any object, like a chair or a door, that is seen in the room can serve as a reference and this makes the test fully unreliable, resulting in a false negative outcome. Perfect darkness is crucial to obtain a reliable SVV outcome measure. Neither should the laser line be visible for the patient during the off-setting of it. A healthy subject should not have a deviation from the true vertical of more than 2.0 degrees. In some clinics, the SVV test is made a bit more difficult by asking the patient to tilt his or her head to the left and then to the right, while adjusting the line with the true vertical. This method makes it more sensitive, but on the other hand one should also take proven methodological issues into account.[30] Alternative methods to assess the SVV make use of a simple bucket equipped with a plum line[31] or a commercial available computer program. When measured in acute stages of a vestibular disease, this SVV deviation can be clearly above the normal limit. However, it restores to normal limits within weeks to months. Therefore, the SVV is rather a measure of an acute disorder, and has little specificity for chronic disorders, as well as to which side and which vestibular lesion particularly. In case of an infarction or lesions in the brainstem or cerebellum (*e.g.*, the nodulus), a distinct skew deviation will be present with abnormal SVV results.

Normative data

Data obtained from patients need to be compared with normative data to conclude if a given test is positive or negative. Usually, norms are taken from the scientific literature, but inevitable it is much better to construct proper normative data in the proper setting of the vestibular clinic. Each lab has its own practice, and some methods can slighty alter the outcome. This task of establishing a lab's own normative data is a costly and time consuming, but it has the great advantage that abnormalities are more rapidly detected, because the limits of normality are smaller. Thus, the test methods become more sensitive for aberrant findings when a lab's own norms are measured in a healthy population.

Galvanic stimulation

Used for an overall vestibular reactivity assessment

When small current pulses are provided to the skin by means of electrode patches that are placed behind the ears, one can stimulate the entire vestibular system on either side, depending on the cathode or anode. The effect sensed by the subject is a strong lateropulsion when standing upright. This way, one can evaluate the responsiveness of the entire vestibular system, but it is not very specific. Walking around while galvanic stimulation is activated will provoke a deviant gate, with lateropulsion either to the left or the right, depending on which side is stimulated. This method is mainly adopted in research settings.

Complementarity

In the past two decades, more vestibular tests have been developed than in the entire past century. As specified in Table 3, there are different tests for different parts of the vestibular system. The most reliable investigations so far are the traditional ENG or VNG including rotation testing and caloric testing. These tests have been performed for decades and despite their limitations concerning calibration, as well as the fact that only the horizontal canals are tested, they provide the desired answers to questions such as: is a spontaneous nystagmus present, are the eye movement normal or abnormal, is the VOR symmetric and sufficiently high (gain) and not delayed (phase) during the rotation test; is the caloric response symmetric and do both horizontal canals provide sufficient responses; is there any directional preponderance of nystagmus and is the fixation suppression adequate?

In the recent years, the vHIT (video-head impulse test) has made its entrance in the vestibular clinic and some clinicians claim that it is a replacement of the classic ENG or VNG because it is easier and faster to perform than the caloric test. Other researchers however have shown that the correlation between the caloric test results and the vHIT results is very poor.[22] The vHIT is a high-frequency test of the VOR while the caloric test is a low-frequency test, and as such complementary.[32] Moreover, a very well-trained clinician is needed to perform the vHIT reliably and it can take quite long to record a reliable signal in a patient. However, it has the advantage that it can quantify the VOR of the posterior and anterior canals too, side by side, when appropriately tested. A recent review paper states that when the vHIT is negative, a caloric test is mandatory to rule out peripheral vestibular lesions.[23] In the next decade, more research will reveal the added value of this new test.

The c-VEMP is a test that is mainly relevant to identify the presence of superior semicircular canal dehiscence (SSCD) since it clearly shows abnormalities for that pathology. Ocular VEMP evaluates the utricles, but compared to c-VEMP it is a more complicated test and the scientific literature is not yet fully conclusive about all its aspects. Unilateral centrifugation on the other hand is a more detailed test of the utricles, but much more complicated to perform and sophisticated equipment is needed.

Not every patient needs all these tests. Depending on the anamnesis by the clinician, it will be decided which tests should be performed. Also, different tests can result in different outcomes in the same patient, because the different sub-systems do not necessarily have to be compromised at the same time. And even when all the vestibular function tests are normal, it does not mean that there is no vestibular problem. Indeed, a considerable part of the vestibular problems is situated at a higher level, *i.e.*, in the brain. For these purposes, recent advances in MRI methods offer possibilities to identify problems at the level of the central integration in the brain. Within the next decade, this field of research will shed its light further on the vestibular ethiologies.

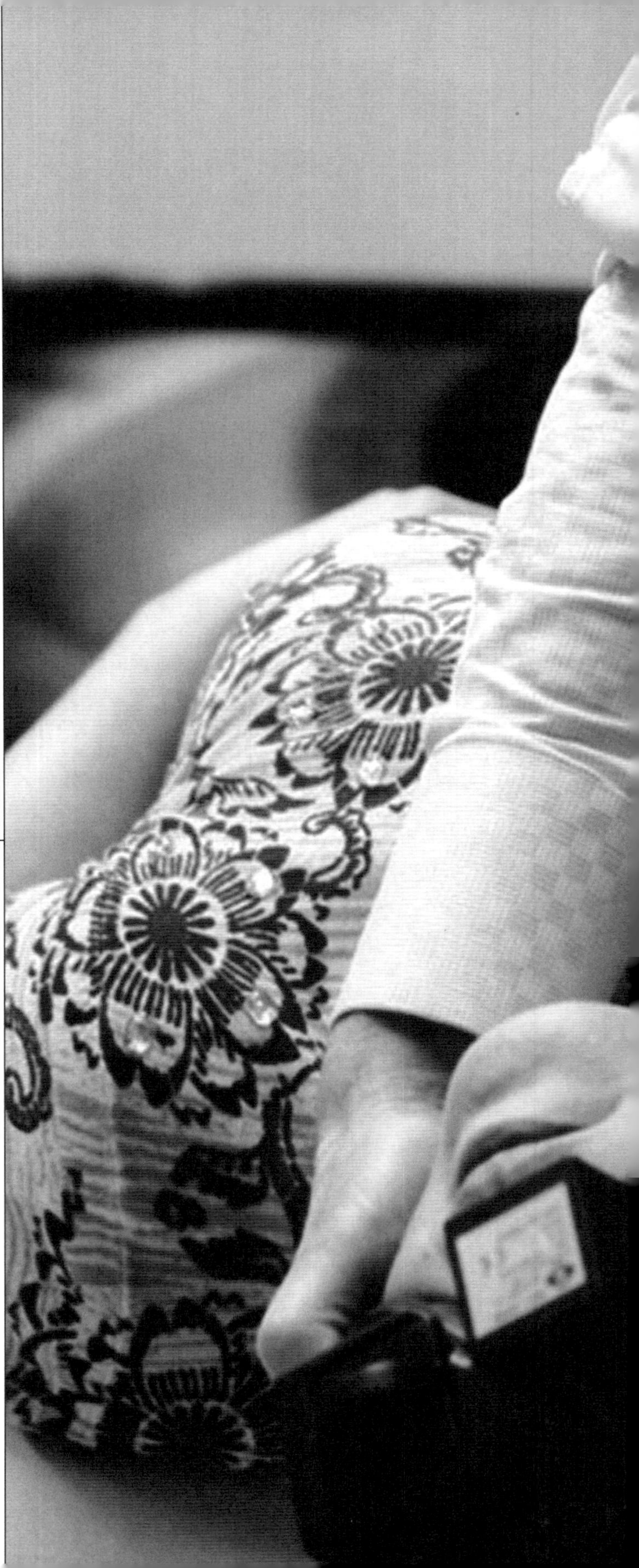

Performing the Dix-Hallpike test with video goggles can be an eye-opener for the clinican to observe more than a BPPV.

Chapter 7

Disease-ABC

A major challenge in medicine is to identify the diagnosis of an ill patient. The difficulty of this challenge is shown especially in patients presenting with vertigo and dizziness. Currently, no biological markers for different vestibular diagnoses exist. In contrast to, for example, a too high cholesterol, which can be measured with a blood test, there are little or no laboratory tests available for detecting specific biological markers for the vertigo-related syndromes. In some cases, imaging can assist the physician in making a clear diagnosis, but this does not apply to the majority of vertigo disorders. So there are only the following options: (1) medical history; (2) clinical investigations; and (3) laboratory tests, such as vestibular and hearing tests, blood tests (in some cases), imaging where appropriate, and other tests to rule out certain diseases (*e.g.*, cardiovascular problems, etc.).

Another complicating factor is the occurrence of several diseases at the same time (*i.e.*, comorbidity), with or without similar symptoms. Ménière disease (MD) can occur in combination with vestibular migraine, both causing vertigo spells. MD causes spells of longer than twenty minutes, while vestibular migraine can cause spells lasting seconds to minutes to hours. Only a profound and systematic anamnesis can protect from jumping to conclusions and missing some diseases. The SO STONED anamnesis tool (table 1), which is discussed earlier in this book, is a possible approach to identify different concomitant diagnoses more easily.

The recent proposed list of clinical vestibular diagnoses offered in the beta version of the International Classification of Diseases (ICD-11-Beta) by the World Health Organization mentions three classes of vertigo: acute, episodic and chronic (see website of the WHO and search for ICD 11 Beta draft: Diseases of inner ear). Each of these classes comprises different diseases such as MD, BPPV, etcetera. Such an approach is useful to improve the consistency between different clinical centers to delineate and identify the same illness. Unfortunately, there are still differences between medical practitioners as well as clinical centers in the world regarding the interpretation of the same symptoms. In some cases they lead to diagnosing a patient with 'hyperventilation syndrome' where in other centers the same symptoms may be interpreted as 'vestibular paroxysmia'. These differences are not only bad for the patient but also hamper clinical studies to investigate for example the effect of a specific medication.

In the next paragraphs we will describe the different vestibular syndromes in global terms, followed by a detailed description of the most frequent clinical syndromes with concomitant symptoms, clinical as well as laboratory findings and treatment strategies.

A. Acute vestibular syndromes

An acute vestibular syndrome is described according to the WHO ICD-11 beta draft version, as a clinical syndrome of acute onset, with continuous vertigo, dizziness, or unsteadiness lasting days to weeks. This is accompanied by typical acute vestibular failure symptoms such as vomiting, nystagmus and severe postural instability. There may also be symptoms or signs that suggest an impairment of the cochlea or the central nervous system. Acute vestibular syndrome is often associated with a single cause, but it may punctuate a relapsing-and-remitting or stepwise progressive illness course. Typical acute vestibular syndrome disorders are vestibular neuritis, acute labyrinthitis, traumatic vestibulopathy, demyelinating diseases (multiple sclerosis) with vestibular involvement and strokes affecting central or peripheral vestibular structures.

A1. Vestibular neuritis

Vestibular neuritis is a condition in which a viral infection of the vestibular nerve causes a total or partial loss of the vestibular afferent input from one of the two labyrinths. It occurs suddenly, spontaneously and isolated. In other words, the nerve along which the signals from the vestibular system are constantly transmitted to the brain - the afferent signals - is inflamed and therefore the nerve does not function properly or only partially. It has been found that the inflammation in the majority of cases affects only the superior branch of the vestibular nerve. The nerve bundle consists of two parts, an upper and a lower branch, as seen in Figure 14. The upper branch is responsible for the innervation of the horizontal semicircular canal, the utricle and the anterior semicircular canal. The posterior canal and sacculus are largely innervated by the inferior branch, as guided by the mnemonic HAUSSPI (**H**orizontal, **A**nterior, **U**tricle →

Superior branch; **S**accule, **P**osterior → **I**nferior). A reason why predominantly the superior branch seems susceptible for vestibular neuritis could be the fact that the bony canal through which the superior branch travels, is longer and narrower than that of the inferior division, so that the superior vestibular nerve is more vulnerable to entrapment when it is inflamed.[33]

A vestibular neuritis can be considered pathophysiologically as an acute unilateral vestibular deafferentiation (uVD).

Vestibular neuritis occurs in 7% of the patients visiting a service specialized in vertigo. It is the third leading cause of peripheral vestibular vertigo. Despite the fact that it has a tremendous impact on the patient, there are only a few studies. The most recent one reports 11.7 to 15.5 cases per one hundred thousand inhabitants.[34]

Complaints. Symptoms include dizziness or vertigo, instability, nausea and often vomiting. During the first days the vertigo, *i.e.*, the sensation of spinning, can be very intense and acute, and patients hardly get out of bed. These sensations are aggravated strongly with each head movement. When the patients stands upright or walks, he or she will experience 'lateropulsion', *i.e.*, will deviate towards the affected side, as if the 'healthy' labyrinth pushes without there being a counter pushing of the diseased labyrinth. In the following days, the vertigo gradually decreases in intensity. Particularly in the beginning, there is indisputably a nystagmus present with the fast phase beating to the healthy side. Looking in the direction of the fast phase will intensify the nystagmus. When looking straight ahead, the nystagmus becomes a little less intense. Looking to the side of the 'affected' labyrinth, the nystagmus is the least clear. This is called the second law of Alexander. Under no circumstances may there be a reversal of the direction of nystagmus, *i.e.*, a left beating nystagmus when looking to the left and a right beating nystagmus when looking to the right. Such 'gaze-evoked nystagmus' is a sign of a central neurological problem and in case of a patient who is suspected of vestibular neuritis, this sign of gaze-evoked nystagmus should immediately alarm the clinician to redirect his diagnosis towards a cerebellar hemorrhage or infarction (see part on HINTS on page 189). Note that the gaze should not exceed thirty degrees. Looking further sideways causes an 'end-point nystagmus' which is perfectly normal in all subjects. In this case, the eye is drawn back to the center position by the elastic forces of the eye muscles. Visual fixation should suppress nystagmus in case of a patient with vestibular neuritis since visual information is of a higher order than vestibular information. By looking at an object and focus on this, the nystagmus usually must reduce, as well as the feeling of 'spinning'. If this is not the case, and the nystagmus contrary gets even bigger by looking at an object, then a central neurological disorder is present, involving for example the vestibulo cerebellum.

Vestibular neuritis is a condition that can make a patient suddenly completely immobile but what is the pathophysiology of such a failure of the vestibular nerve and why does it have such an impact on a patient?

First we briefly outline how the vestibular system works. In the left and right vestibular systems, motion detectors are situated, consisting of hair cells that are encased in a gelatinous mass and moving back and forth when the head moves (see 'Hardware and software of the vestibular organ'). Even if we do not move, the hair cells are continuously firing signals (action potentials) to the brain, about a hundred times per second, like two metronomes or pacemakers. That means that at rest the hair cells on the left and right side fire just as hard. Let us, in order to keep it simple, consider the horizontal semicircular canals only. Suppose one moves the head to the left while targeting an object (for example this text), then in the left labyrinth the discharge frequency increases from 100 spikes per second to say 400 spikes per second while on the right side the discharge frequency decreases (Fig. 13) from 100 to 20 or zero spikes per second. The excitation at the left side causes in the vestibular nuclei in the brain stem a number of chain reactions, so that the appropriate eye muscles (medial and lateral recti) will contract while the decreasing action potential firing rate on the other side will ensure the relaxation of the 'antagonistic' eye muscles. Indeed, in order to look right, the lateral rectus eye muscles on the right have to contract (agonists) and simultaneously the medial rectus muscles on the left of the eyeball should relax (antagonists), otherwise the eye would become 'flattened '. The left and right vestibular nuclei in the brainstem communicate further with each other via commissural fibers to confirm those reflexes. The effect of this whole mechanism is the VOR, to ensure gaze stabilization when the head is turned to the left. The eyes make a compensatory eye movement. However, when a vestibular system has been attacked by a virus, such as during a vestibular neuritis, it fails. This results in oscillopsia, *i.e.*, blurred vision due to a failing gaze stabilization system.

In the acute stage, the following occurs. Suppose that the right balance organ is suddenly affected by vestibular neuritis. This implies that the spontaneous activity of one hundred spikes per second in the right system acutely has fallen back to zero, while the activity on the left side still is one hundred spikes per second. This causes a tonic imbalance between the left and right side. The fact that there are a hundred action potentials more on the left than on the right side, is interpreted by the brain as if there is a movement of the head to the left. Therefore, there will be a nystagmus to the left. If the brain namely 'thinks' there is a movement to the left, eyes will drift to the right, as it were, to look at the objects passing to the right, while turning to the left with your head. At the edge of the eye sockets, the eyes make a quick maneuver to the left, and then drift again to the right, followed by another quick reset movement and so on. As such a spontaneous nystagmus is generated, because it appears without any motion, neither of the environment nor the person. Thus the patient with vestibular neuritis in the acute phase will experience spinning because his or her eyes constantly behave as if he or she is moving, causing the illusion of movement called vertigo. These sensations will be in conflict with all other senses and also with the awareness of the position in the surroundings, which means that the patient in the acute phase suffers from vertigo as well as nausea and in frequent cases also vomiting.

Compensation. After several hours to days, a compensation process emerges in the vestibular nuclei in the brainstem where an imbalance is caused by unequal peripheral input. This will reduce and eventually make the spontaneous nystagmus disappear in the days to weeks after the occurrence of the neuritis. Basically, a fake signal of one hundred spikes per second is simulated in the vestibular nuclei on the affected side. Consequently, at rest the difference between the healthy and affected side no longer exists regarding rest activity, and no spontaneous nystagmus is elicited. This process is preceded by a period in which the entire vestibular system is relatively silenced, so that the contrast between the working and non-working side is less extreme. That inhibition is centrally imposed through the commissural fibers between left and right vestibular nuclei. The word 'compensation' refers to the coping process whereby the (partially) missing function of a vestibular system is compensated, so that overall functioning can still be quite normal, without too much hindrance from vertigo or instability. In order to stimulate and enhance the process of compensation it is essential that the patient is moving a lot so that the central nervous system is forced to integrate information from the different peripheral sensory systems that feed seemingly contradictory inputs. This is similar to general processes of learning that are caused by conflicts. In fact, visual, proprioceptive and vestibular stimuli need to be reconciled by central adjustments. Hence, the importance of habituation exercises. In patients who generally do not move much or have a sedentary profession, it will generally take longer for their balance system to properly compensate, that is to say, the brain will adapt slower to the partial or total failure of one side. However, people with a very active profession, who move around a lot, will generally recover sooner and smoother. Scientific evidence exists that customized exercise programs have a significant beneficial effect on the time of recovery after acute failure of the equilibrium system, such as after surgical removal of the vestibular or auditory nerve caused by a vestibular schwannoma (also known as acoustic neuroma).[35] Next to following a personalized exercise program, supervised by a physiotherapist, it is highly recommended to perform sports to facilitate the compensation process. Ball games in particular are beneficial because of their complex eye-hand coordination. The brain must calculate the trajectory of the ball and integrate this with the proper body movements, with a coordinated move as a result. That takes time, but is very effective in boosting the overall functioning of the balance system. Especially if the patient has previously practiced a sport, taking up that sport again is very beneficial for the healing process. The recent work of Professor Kathleen Cullen and co-workers have now proven scientifically that movement and exercise contribute to a better balance. Their research has in fact shown that there are signals from other parts of the body, and in particular the neck, that are sent to the vestibular nuclei as a substitute for missing signals from a failed balance organ.[36]

With detailed vestibular tests one can measure the amount of compensation of an individual patient and follow the progress over time. This is done by quantifying gain and phase during rotation tests. This is one of the added values of detailed balance tests (Fig. 18).

Viral infection. Vestibular neuritis is probably mainly due to a resurgence of latent herpes simplex virus type 1 (HSV-1). However, other viruses can also be responsible for a neuritis. The condition can occur simultaneously with or just after any other viral disease, such as causing a sore throat, mononucleosis, influenza or a cold. Sometimes one is not aware of another viral infection and only experiences the symptoms of vestibular neuritis.[37]

Treatment. Vestibular neuritis is often treated with the corticosteroid methylprednisolone, based on a pivotal study published in 2004.[38] However, in the mean time, the emerging truth seems to show that on the long time, *i.e.* after 12 months, there is no added benefit of corticosteroids compared to placebo or vestibular exercises.[39,40] The efficacy of medication in this pathology requires further studies.

In the acute stage, patients are sometimes given vestibular sedative drugs, to ease the symptoms. But these drugs hamper the central compensation, so the sooner patients are without vestibular suppressants, the better.

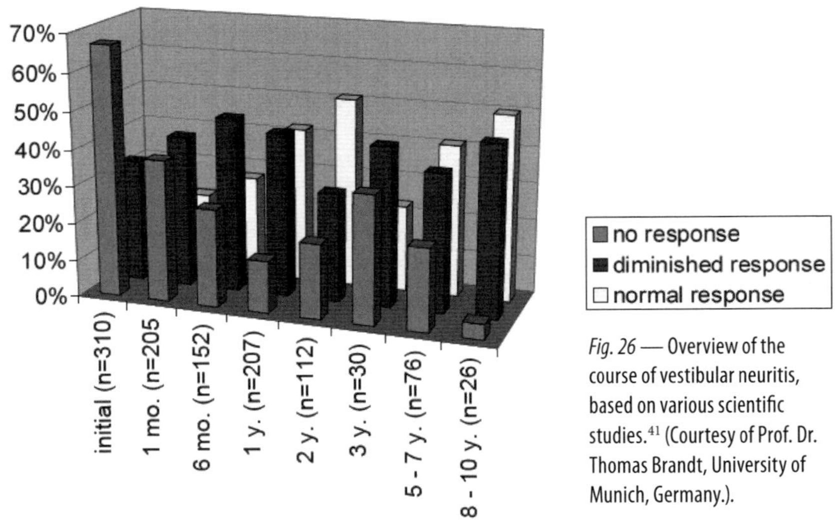

Fig. 26 — Overview of the course of vestibular neuritis, based on various scientific studies.[41] (Courtesy of Prof. Dr. Thomas Brandt, University of Munich, Germany.).

Course. Healing or repair of a vestibular neuritis consists of a combination of (1) a restoration of the function of the peripheral vestibular system; (2) proprioceptive (somatosensory) and visual substitution; and (3) central compensation, promoted by vestibular exercises and or sport. Overall, it can be said that one third of the patients cures partially or entirely within a month, one third within a year and the remaining third is taking much longer or ultimately do not heal. Figure 26 represents a review of several studies, showing that after five to ten years only a small group of 20% still have no response during the caloric test. The remaining 80% is recovered fully or partially. The chances of relapse are very slim with regard to vestibular neuritis, approximately 2%. Vestibular neuritis is an exclusion diagnosis. That means that one should carefully verify if there is no brainstem infarction caused by occlusions in the PICA or AICA regions, as explained before. Also vestibular migraine or the beginning of MD should be considered when a patient is seen with neuritis-type complaints.

A2. Labyrinthitis

Labyrinthitis is an insult of the entire inner ear, comprising the vestibular system and the cochlea. This means that the symptoms are similar to those of a vestibular neuritis, supplemented with hearing-related symptoms, in some cases including total deafness. Labyrinthitis is less frequent than vestibular neuritis. Causes may be both bacterial and viral infections of the entire inner ear. Treatment focuses on possible restoring of the hearing as well as easing the dizziness, depending on the cause. If it is a bacterial infection, targeted antibiotics are needed. Typically, the complaints and symptoms diminish in a relatively short period of a few weeks. Here, too, the possibility of a stroke at the level of the posterior cerebral circulation should be excluded by means of clinical examination and additional imaging.

B. Episodic vertigo

An episodic vestibular syndrome is a clinical syndrome of transient vertigo, dizziness or unsteadiness lasting seconds to hours or occasionally days. The associated symptoms are mostly temporary and are typical for short-term vestibular disorders: nausea, nystagmus or sudden falls. There may also be symptoms that suggest a dysfunction of the cochlea or the central nervous system. An episodic vestibular syndrome usually implies multiple, recurring complaints caused by an episodic disorder with repeated spells (triggered or spontaneous), but the syndrome may already be present after the first event. Disorders typical of this syndrome are benign paroxysmal positional vertigo (BPPV), Ménière's desease (MD), vestibular migraine (VM), vestibular paroxysmia (VP), panic attacks, hypoglycemia and transient ischemic attacks (TIAs) affecting central or peripheral vestibular structures (WHO ICD-11 Beta definition).

B1. Benign Paroxysmal Positional Vertigo (BPPV)

The second most common cause of vertigo is benign paroxysmal positional vertigo (BPPV), a benign, suddenly emerging vertigo that occurs when moving into a certain position. The movement itself from one position to the other is essential, as well as the final position. Hence the word 'positional' that is used in the definition of BPPV rather than 'position'. The symptoms associated with BPPV can be explained based on a purely mechanical model. BPPV is in fact caused by loosened otoconia (1 to 30 micrometer large calcite crystals composed of calcium carbonate) of the utricular macula (Fig. 8) in the vestibule, which accidently ended up in one of the semicircular canals. Otoconia have a higher density (otoconial density $\approx$ 2710 kg/m^3) than that of the endolymph ($\approx$ 1000 kg/m^3) or the gelatinous mass they normally lie on.

There are two places where the otoconia may end up, namely, free floating in the endolymph in the semicircular canals or embedded on the cupula of one of the canals. One speaks respectively about canalolithiasis or cupulolithiasis. When the otoconia swirl around freely in the viscous endolymph of the semicircular canals, and a position change occurs, they seek the lowest point. During that migration of the otoconia, they create a convective flow in the endolymph, resulting in a movement of the cupula, which is the motion sensor of the semicircular canal. This cupular deflection will evoke not only a sensation of self-movement, but also an eye movement typical for stimulation of that particular canal during head motion. In case of debris in the right posterior semicircular canal for example, the concomitant eye movement upon lying down will be counter-clockwise (from the examiner's viewpoint) and upbeat. Because the sensation of movement lasts a little longer than the actual head movement, the illusion of motion is generated, *i.e.*, vertigo. This vertigo typically last a few seconds, until the otoconia floated down to the lowest point of the semicircular canal. This phenomenon is similar to a liquid-filled snow globe, in which snowflakes whirl up when shaken. Within a few seconds the flakes settle back down at the bottom of the globe, until it is shaken again.

To resolve this disorder, the loosened otoconia have to be moved back to the vestibulum where they can be re-attached to the otoconial layer of the utricle as well as absorbed or broken down in the dark cells - the recycling plant in the inner ear. Typical daily movements, however, will not suffice to move the debris back to the vestibulum because it requires bending the head in such a sequence of positions that the otoconia can find their way out through the semicircular canals, for example by performing a somersault. The patient suffering from BPPV will, however, refrain from making somersaults spontaneously because it causes dizzyness instantly. Therefore, the complaint can persist usually for days, weeks or sometimes even months.

Dispite the fact that BPPV is one of the most common vestibular disorders, there are ample studies that actually prove that the free floating otoconial particles are the geniune cause of this disorder. Recently a group of researchers used electron microscopy methods to study the material that was found in the semicircular canals of 2 patients with intractable BPPV.[42] These authors state that "in BPPV, fragments of the otolithic membrane become displaced from the utricle en bloc. That is, otoconia embedded within the gel matrix and interconnected with linking fibrils dislodge together as a unit from the utricular otolith organ." These observations may be generalized, but on the other hand, one should be carefull with such a generalisation since the fact that the studied patients had intractable BPPV, may be caused by the large size of the dislodged material. In the majority of cases where BPPV is resolved within weeks to months, the particles may be individual otoconia in stead of lumps of the otolith membrane.

The debris can fall into the three arched hallways, but there is a clear preference for the posterior *i.e.* rear canal (*posterior canal* = PC), followed by the horizontal canal (*lateral or horizontal canal* = HC) and then the anterior canal (*anterior canal* = AC). The posterior canal is by far the most frequently affected canal (80–90%); next is the horizontal canal (5–30%). Involvement of the anterior canal is rare, accounting for only 1% to 2% of patients in large case series.[43]

The fact that the most common form is BPPV-PC, is probably attributable to the orientation of the entrance to the posterior canal relative to the vestibulum, in a lying condition. As a consequence, loose otoconia preferably just fall in the posterior canal. Additionally, they will remain there longer since the otoconia seem to be trapped in that canal. This is not the case when debris has entered the horizontal canals. Due to the orientation of the horizontal canal, free floating otoconial debris can more easily re-enter the vestibulum with the utricle when the patients shakes his or her head from left to right, resolving as such the BPPV.

In 50 to 70% of the cases, BPPV is idiopathic, *i.e.* without a know cause. In the remaining cases, the most immediate cause of BPPV is a head trauma, thereby detaching some otoconia of the utricular maculae. Sometimes this detachment is delayed, *i.e.*, it may occur a certain time after the initial head trauma event. In extremely rare cases, bilateral BPPV may occur due to a severe head trauma. Inner ear disorders, such as MD or vestibular neuritis, can explain BPPV only in 6% of the cases.

BPPV is one of the most frequent causes of balance problems in the ENT practice, recently pushed away from the first place in prevalence by vestibular migraine.[44] The prevalence for the past year, or in other words the number of patients who had BPPV during the past year in the total population is 2.3% for women and 0.9% for men. At the age of eighty years, the cumulative prevalence is 10%, *i.e.*, 10% of octogenarians have ever had BPPV. It is estimated that a large percentage of BPPV in the elderly is unrecognized and this constutues a significant risk factor for falls. The one-year prevalence is 3.4% among persons over sixty years old.[45] BPPV is nearly twice as common in women as in men. The symptoms often disappear spontaneously after a few weeks or months. Patients may relapse during the following years, but there rarely are persistent symptoms.

As with all vestibular disorders described in this book, we list the diagnostic criteria as they are published in peer reviewed papers. For several disorders these published criteria can be found on the website of the Barany Society through the Journal of Vestibular Research website: *www.jvr-web.org*.

Criteria of BPPV:

1. Canalolithiasis of the posterior canal (pc-BPPV)[43]

- *A. Recurrent attacks of positional vertigo or positional dizziness provoked by lying down or turning over in the supine position.*
- *B. Duration of attacks < 1 min*
- *C. Positional nystagmus elicited after a latency of one or few seconds by the Dix-Hallpike maneuver or side-lying maneuver (Semont diagnostic maneuver). The nystagmus is a combination of torsional nystagmus with the upper pole of the eyes beating toward the lower ear combined with vertical nystagmus beating upward (toward the forehead) typically lasting < 1 minute.*
- *D. Not attributable to another disorder*

2. Canalolithiasis of the horizontal canal (hc-BPPV)

- *A. Recurrent attacks of positional vertigo or positional dizziness provoked by lying down or turning over in the supine position.*
- *B. Duration of attacks < 1 min.*
- *C. Positional nystagmus elicited after a brief latency or no latency by the supine roll test, beating horizontally toward the undermost ear with the head turned to either side (geotropic direction changing nystagmus) and lasting < 1 min.*
- *D. Not attributable to another disorder.*

3. Cupulolithiasis of the horizontal canal (hc-BPPV-cu)

- *A. Recurrent attacks of positional vertigo or positional dizziness provoked by lying down or turning over in the supine position.*
- *B. Positional nystagmus elicited after a brief latency or no latency by the supine roll test, beating horizontally toward the uppermost ear with the head turned to either side (apogeotropic direction changing nystagmus), and lasting > 1 minute.*
- *C. Not attributable to another disorder.*

4. Probable benign paroxysmal positional vertigo, spontaneously resolved

- *A. Recurrent attacks of positional vertigo or positional dizziness provoked by lying down or turning over in the supine position.*
- *B. Duration of attacks < 1 min.*
- *C. No observable nystagmus and no vertigo with any positional maneuver.*
- *D. Not attributable to another disorder.*

5. Canalolithiasis of the anterior canal (ac-BPPV) (being a rare variant of BPPV)

- *A. Recurrent attacks of positional vertigo or positional dizziness provoked by lying down or turning over in the supine position.*
- *B. Duration of attacks < 1 min.*
- *C. Positional nystagmus elicited immediately or after a latency of one or few seconds by the Dix-Hallpike maneuver (on one or both sides) or in the supine straight head-hanging position, beating predominantly vertically downward and lasting < 1 min.*
- *D. Not attributable to another disorder.*

What type of examinations are needed to identify BPPV? In depth anamnesis (SO STONED) allows to identify whether the vertigo has a positional cause or whether it has other causes. Particularly the duration and triggers are of great importance to discriminate between, for example, vestibular migraine and BPPV, both causing vertigo spells.

Also, it is very useful to determine the side of the involved canal, based on the experience of the patient. Usually, patients can tell if either the left or the right side is affected. But the key approach to establish if BPPV is the cause of the vestibular problems is the Dix-Hallpike maneuver.

Dix-Hallpike maneuver. The diagnosis of posterior SCC BPPV is realized by means of the clinical test called Dix-Hallpike maneuver for which the patient is positioned lying down on a diagnostic table with his or her head hanging over the upper edge. Typical of BPPV is that it is 'exhaustible', so for obvious reasons it is not advised to try out if the seating position of the patient is appropriate. By verifying that upon lying down, the head hanging over the edge causes the

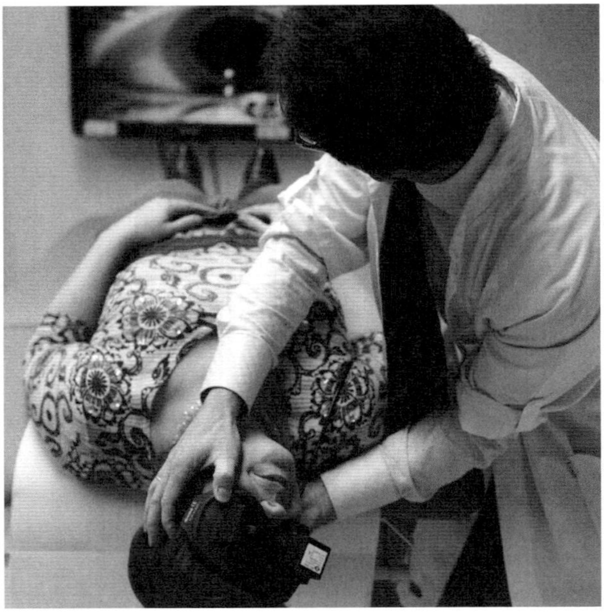

Fig. 27 — The Dix-Hallpike-maneuver, with the patient's head hanging over the upper edge of the table. Based on this maneuver, BPPV of the posterior semicircular can be diagnosed.

otoconia to swivel around and be dispersed in the canal. The next time this head-hanging position is evoked, much less otoconia will disturb the endolymph flow. Indeed, the visible effect of the migrating crystals may be most obvious when they move as a clot or 'en bloc' in the canal. Are they disintegrated into individual crystals, and distributed in the canal, then the effect of whirling up is much less disruptive. Hence BPPV is always most apparent for patients after they adopted the same posture for a while, like an evening watching TV, or a night in bed. When getting up, the clot of crystals will obviously cause more disruption in the semicircular canal. During a busy day, the crystals are constantly dispersed with much less disturbance and vertigo as a consequence.

This 'exhaustible' aspect of BPPV is why it is important to start the clinical investigation with the (suspected) affected side.

A Dix-Hallpike maneuver is considered positive for the posterior semicircular canal when a torsional and upward nystagmus occurs with a crescendo diminuendo profile within a time span of about one minute. Important is the concomitant vertigo that the patient should experience that is typical of his or her complaints. The torsional nystagmus is characterized by a torsional beating of the top of the eyes towards the ground (geotropic). A BPPV of the right posterior semicircular canal has a typical upbeat nystagmus as well as counter-clockwise nystagmus as seen from the perspective of the clinician. A BPPV of the left posterior semicircular canal results in a torsional clockwise and upbeat nystagmus. When the patient is put back upright in the initial position, the nystagmus is reversed, but it is often less intense (inversion phenomenon).

The much less common anterior canal BPPV is characterized by a similar torsional nystagmus, but with a downbeat nystagmus, which is more dominant than the torsional nystagmus, because the anterior canal is much more in the sagittal plane.

Since the endolymph flows through very thin channels, this fluid can be considered as viscous, causing the otoconia to start moving with a delay. Hence, vertigo and nystagmus sometimes only emerge after about ten seconds.

Roll-test. The Dix-Hallpike maneuver test only determines whether debris is located in the posterior or anterior semicircular canals. The horizontal canal, however, can also contain loosened particles. Hence, each negative Dix-Hallpike maneuver should be followed by the roll test.

The patient is in a supine position, *i.e.*, lying down on his or her back, but the head is flexed at 30 degrees. This way, the horizontal canals are positioned in the vertical plane. Then the clinician turns the head about ninety degrees to one side while observing the eye movements for at least ten seconds with the head maintained in that position. Then the head is turned to the other side and again possible nystagmus is noted. A horizontal nystagmus should be observed during the head turns, since this is the VOR, but when the nystagmus persists longer than the head movement, and the patient recognizes the symptoms of vertigo, then a horizontal canal BPPV is likely. The clinical criteria for both the variants, canalolithiasis and cupulolithiasis are described earlier in this section. However, it is not always obvious to identify the side of the lithiasis, *i.e.* right or left. This jeopardizes the right treatment. It depends also on whether the patient suffers from canalolithiasis or cupulolithiasis. In case of cupulolthiasis, clinicians usually choose the most symptomatic side for treatment, but one can also be guided by the search for the zero position. Starting in a position – either head left turned or right turned, one seeks the position where the nystagmus disappears. When turning the head further causes a reverse of the nystagmus one can identify the null position. This requires however knowledge of the position of the horizontal canal in the skull of the patient and more specifically the position of the cupula of that canal.

In this way one can determine on which side the problem is located. In my experience, patients with horizontal canal BPPV usually have the variant of cupulolithiasis rather than canalolithiasis, since the latter variant often is resolved by itself. Just shaking the head will move the dislodged otoconia back to the vestibule where they are captured by the dark cells or get stuck back on the macula.

Treatment of BPPV. Treatment of BPPV with drugs is of no use, it has no effect. BPPV has a purely mechanical cause: loosened otoconia that are residing in the wrong place in the vestibular system and have to be relocated in the vestibule through a specific sequence of movements. It is important to first find out in which part of the vestibular system the otoconia are located in. This is done by the aforementioned Dix-Hallpike maneuver and the roll test. Depending on these findings, the clinician determines the appropriate maneuver to relocate the otoconia. As BPPV of the posterior canal is most common, the most frequently used maneuvers to relocate otoconia are the Epley and the Semont maneuvers. The main difference between the Epley and the Semont-maneuver is the speed of implementation. The Epley-maneuver is a slow maneuver, based on the migration of the debris to the lowest point of the semicircular canal, purely by the action of gravity on the debris. This is a very suitable maneuver for elderly or obese patients. In addition, it allows the researcher to observe the eye movements well during the maneuver, for example, with video-oculoscopy. The Semont-maneuver should be performed fast, as it uses inertia and gravity to evacuate the crystals from the canal.

BPPV of the horizontal canal is treated by for example the Lempert maneuver (or BBQ roll) and the maneuver of De La Meilleure. For BPPV of the anterior canal, one has to apply a modified maneuver.

However, if the wrong maneuver is applied, it can provoke migration of dislodged otoconia in different semicircular canals causing even more complaints. Therefore, it is rather obvious to apply the appropriate maneuver being an Epley or Semont maneuver for posterior SCC BPPV and the BBQ roll for horizontal canal BPPV. Randomized clinical trials show that the repositioning of the crystals with an Epley maneuver or a Semont maneuver have significantly more success than a sham treatment (see box). According to a systematic overview study, there is no significant difference in efficiency between an Epley and a Semont maneuver,[46] but most of the studies just look for short-term evaluations. In a long-term study, it was shown that the Epley maneuver had a lasting beneficial effect after one year in 91% of treated patients, while a sham maneuver only had a success rate of 46% after one year.[47] The success rate of vertigo control after the initial canal repositioning procedure is high. Typical numbers are more than 80%, like reported *e.g.* by Su and co-workers who obtained a value of 83% success rate after the first treatment in their study including 243 patients.[48]

Epley maneuver for the right posterior semicircular canal: detailed procedure. The patient is sitting upright on a table, straightened legs in front of him or her, and with the head turned 45^{0} to the affected side – in our example the right side. This is called the zero position (Fig. 28a). The first position of the Epley maneuver consists of the Dix-Hallpike position with the patient's head hanging over the edge of the table (Fig. 28b). A counter-clockwise (CCW) nystagmus (from the clinician's viewpoint) and an upbeat nystagmus should be seen, in combination with the patient reporting vertigo. The time course should be crescendo-diminuendo within approximately 30 seconds. This position has to be maintained at least for 30 seconds longer or as long nystagmus is visible. This applies to all subsequent positions. Position two of the Epley maneuver is obtained by slowly rotating the head 90 degrees towards the opposite side - in this case the left side - while still in the head-hanging position (Fig. 28c). Again nystagmus is to be observed, although - in my experience - in several occasions no nystagmus is seen, nor does the patient experience a distinct vertigo. For the next position, the patient is rolled over on his/her left side. The head is also turned left, in exactly the same angle as in the previous position. The nose is now pointing down (Fig. 28d). Often this generates a distinct nystagmus as well as vertigo. After waiting another 30 seconds, the patient is asked to sit upright, with both legs hanging over the side of the table (Fig. 28e). Important is not only to observe nystagmus, but also to firmly hold the patient. This safety precaution is needed since otoconia falling onto the macula of the utricle in this fourth position, may generate a severe feeling of linear sensations, (utricle is mainly about linear sensations), and the patient may feel pushed forward or backward. This sensation is comparable to a Tumarkin crisis (see B.2 Ménière's disease , p. 259).

The Epley maneuver is ended by turning the head in the neutral position in the upright position. Each of the previous positions has to be maintained for about thirty seconds to allow the debris to migrate to the lowest point. As such, the debris is guided toward the vestibulum through the subsequent positions. At the second, third or fourth position, one can sometimes observe a reversal of the nystagmus. This may suggest that the debris floats back to the original position, creating a reverse endolymph flow, with a reverse eye movement as a result. Still, it is best to continue the original sequence of movements and complete the procedure as intended. But it is of utmost importance to observe any aberrant eye movements, since they may suggest that other canals are involved, or even that BPPV may not be the underlying cause of the problems (See the special paragraph: 'Inconsistencies do not match').

Inconsistencies do not match

It cannot be stressed enough that the presence of a given nystagmus during a lying-down position does absolutely not imply that the patient suffers from BPPV. When an liberatory Epley maneuver is performed, it is imperative that the observed nystagmus in the different positions corresponds with the migrating otoconia in the respective semicircular that is treated. A horizontal nystagmus does not fit the picture of BPPV of the posterior canals. Neither does a persistent torsional nystagmus, either clockwise or counter-clockwise, and neither does a persistent pure vertical nystagmus. In short, an atypical nystagmus should alert the clinician that other etiologies are much more likely than BPPV. The same goes for a repeated treatment of BPPV. When repeated treatment is needed to try to resolve the BPPV, it is presumably not BPPV. The new diagnostic entity 'vestibular paroxysmia' (see later in this chapter), provokes very similar complaints of short-lasting dizziness spells, often occurring during certain positions like lying in bed on one side. It resembles BPPV very much since the symptoms usually last seconds and they are very often position-dependent. Yet, when the disorder is vestibular paroxysmia instead of BPPV, in positions like Dix-Hallpike or during the roll test the patient will have a non-BPPV type nystagmus, *i.e.*, either persistent or not in the plane of the stimulated canal. A typical example is the occurence of a persistent horizontal nystagmus in the Dix-Hallpike position. During the Dix-Hallpike maneuver, the horizontal canal of the investigated side is virtually in the horizontal plane, so it is very unlikely that it would generate a horizontal nystagmus due to floating otoconia. In a pilot study [presented at the IFOS meeting in Paris, 2017] which we performed in around forty vestibular paroxysmia patients visiting our ENT clinic, 80% had a non-BPPV type nystagmus.

Immediately after the treatment. Since it takes about two days before the otoconia are resorbed or recaptured by the maculae of the otolith organs, it may occur that the patient experiences a floating sensation (walking on clouds) during the first few days after treatment, clearly distinct from the initial rotary vertigo that the debris caused when moving in the semicircular canals. Some clinicians and physiotherapists even ask the patient not to make any sudden head movements, keep the head up, even at night, wearing a neck collar, not to sleep on the side of the affected ear or other limitations and postural restrictions. Yet, there is no scientific proof of the usefulness of these restrictions, so it makes no sense to impose them.[49-51] On the day of the treatment itself, the patient should be careful, since the treatment can cause some feeling of instability.

a

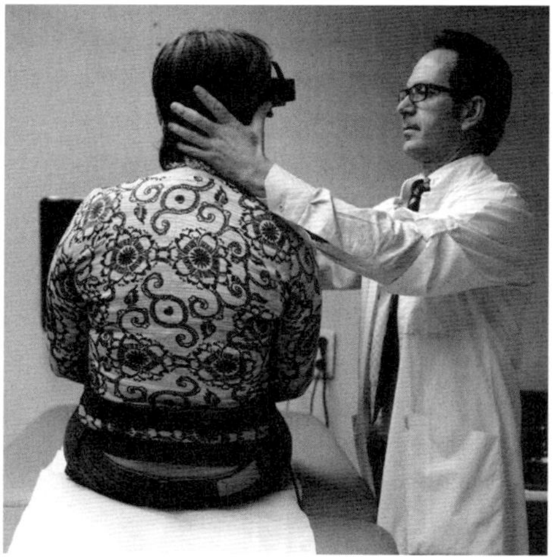

b

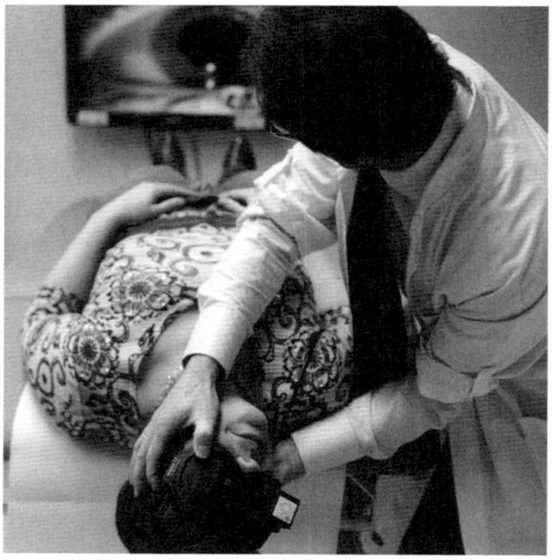

c

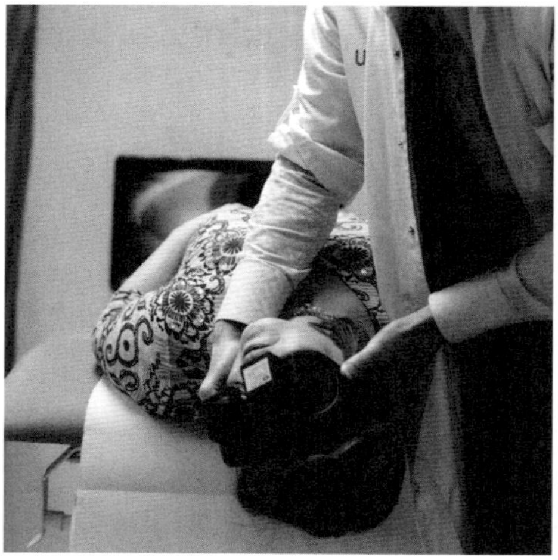

d

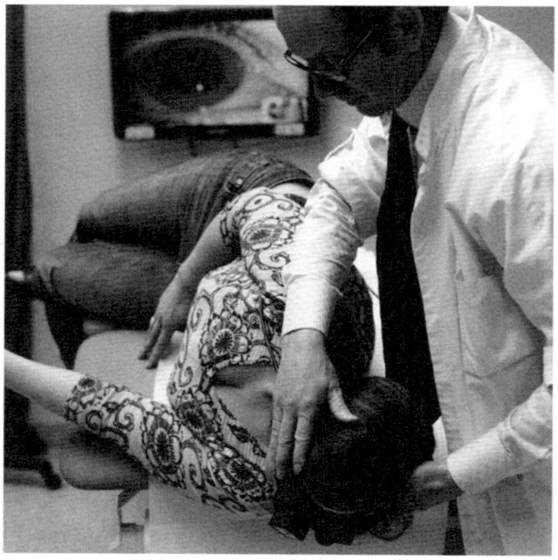

e

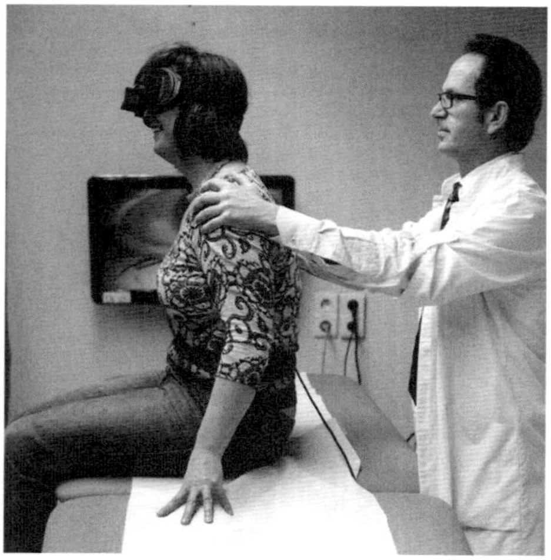

Fig. 28a-b-c-d-e — Subsequent positions during the Epley maneuvre. Each position is maintained about 30 seconds, unless the patients experience longer vertigo, or a nystagmus is observed

We typically perform the Epley maneuver only once per session, to avoid the risk of entering the free swirling otoconia in other parts of the labyrinth. One week after the first treatment, the patient is examined again by a control Dix-Hallpike maneuver, possibly followed by an Epley maneuver. As the first position of the Epley-maneuver essentially is identical to the Dix-Hallpike position, it is evident to immediately continue with positions two, three and four of the Epley-maneuver instead of having the patient sit upright again.

Obviously, the Epley-maneuver for a BPPV of the left posterior canal mirrors the positions described above. After successful treatment, *i.e.*, no further nystagmus is observed during the Dix-Hallpike maneuver and the patient does not experience vertigo upon lying down or similar provoking positions, one may start with Brandt Daroff exercises (see below). This is a profylaxis to prevent one would relapse in the next few months, but it does not cure the BPPV.

Semont maneuver for the right posterior semicircular canal

The patient sits upright with his/her legs over the long side of the examination table. Rotate the head 45 degrees to the patient's left, so that the right posterior canal is situated in the plane of the subsequent movement (Fig. 29a). Then, have the patient lean aside to the patient's right , so that the patient's back of the head rests on the examination table (Fig. 29b), and the patient looks up. This movement is provocative and sweeps the otoconia around causing vertigo and nystagmus. Wait until the patient has no nystagmus or vertigo any more. Typically, that lasts from one to three minutes. Subsequently, swing the patient with a very quick jerk in the other direction (Fig. 29c, d), keeping the head in exactly the same position. (That means that the patient's nose points in the direction of the examination table (Fig. 29e.)

Wait again until nystagmus and possible vertigo disappear. Then bring back the patient into upright sitting position (Fig. 29f). Hold the patient for a little while, because some debris may drop on the utricle and provoke linear sensations. Repeat this two more times.

It is important that the movement from one side to the other is done quickly, because otherwise the particles reverse back in the canal and the maneuver fails. Because of the rapid movement, the crystals are moved together with the endolymphe in the canal. Hereto, one uses the centrifugal force, the principle

a

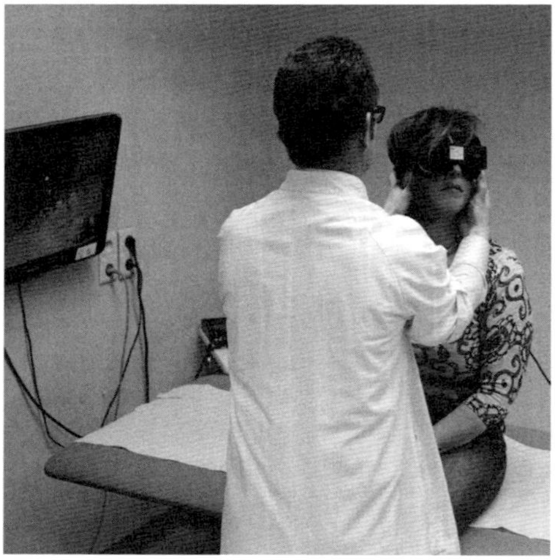

b

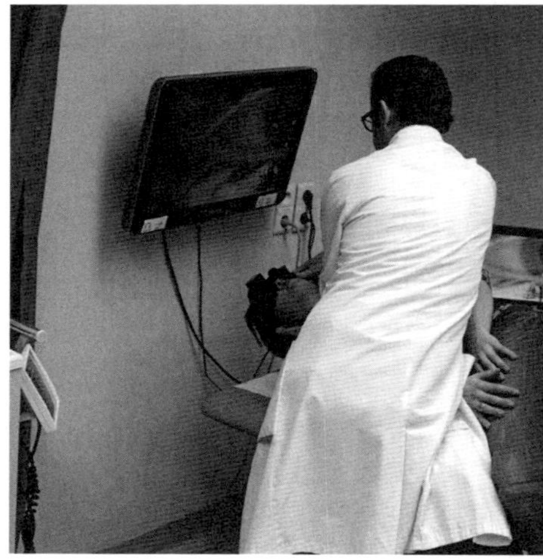

c

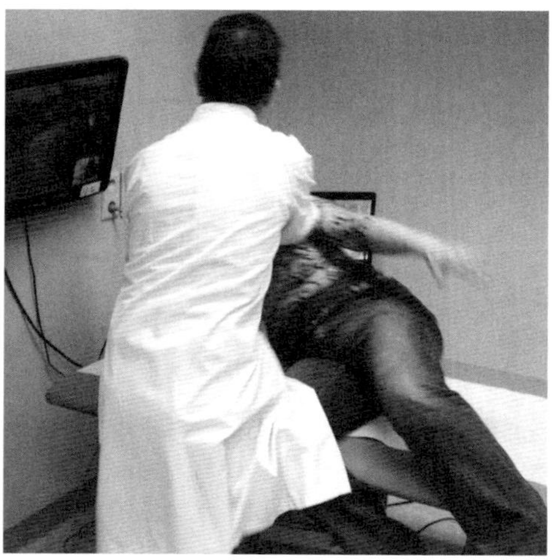

d

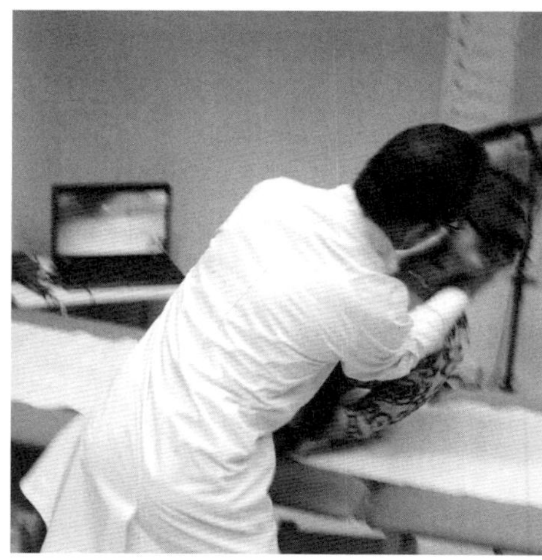

e

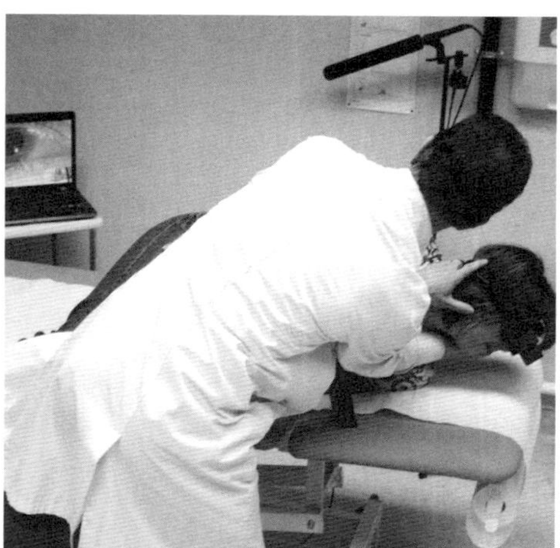

f

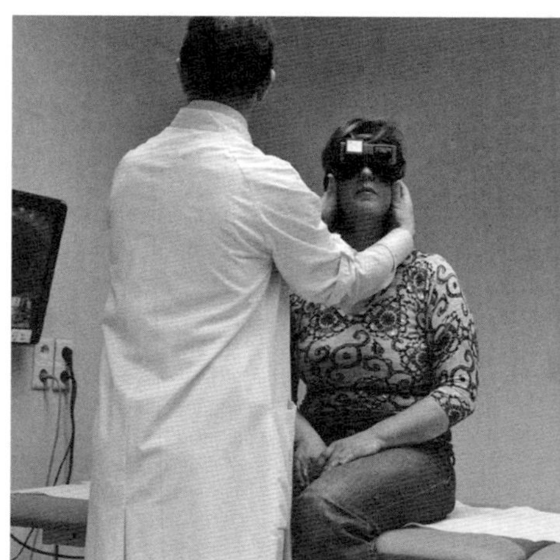

of physics that manifests itself when swinging around a bucket of water. If that happens fast enough, the water will not be spilled, not even when the bucket is upside-down. The same applies for the crystals in the semicircular canal. Typical of the Semont manouver is 'nose up, nose down'.

Both the Semont and the Epley maneuver have the same success for solving BPPV. The Epley maneuver is a bit easier to perform on elderly or obese people.

What about bilateral BPPV? Bilateral BPPV means that both ears are affected simultaneously. It occurs in less than ten percent of patients with BPPV and is therefore quiet rare . It is mostly found after a considerable head trauma. In this case, it is recommended to first apply the maneuver to the most affected side. Then wait a week. When the symptoms have disappeared in the treated side, one can treat the other side.

Brandt-Daroff exercises. A few decades ago, Brandt-Daroff exercises were often applied to cure BPPV, but this treatment is clearly less effective than the Epley or Semont maneuvers, as evidenced by the review of Helminski.[29] However, when the BPPV problem is solved, *i.e.*, the patient is free of symptoms, then Brandt-Daroff exercises can be applied as a prophylactic. The treatment mainly aims at preventing possible leftovers from otoconia to form a clot during the months after treatment. The Brandt-Daroff movements stimulate the spread of any remaining otoconia in the endolymph, making them easier to resolve.

Position 1. Begin sitting on the edge of your bed, for about thirty seconds.

Position 2. Turn your head 45 degrees to the right (to situate the left posterior canal in the plane of the movement that follows).
Then quickly lie down on your left side - the movement should take no more than two seconds.
Keep your head turned to the right 45 degrees.
Hold that position for thirty seconds.

Position 3. Sit back up. Hold that position for thirty seconds. Then turn your head 45 degrees to the left.

Fig. 29a-b-c-d-e-f — Subsequent positions of the Semont maneuver. Position b (nose up) and e (nose down) should be maintained at least 30 seconds or as long as vertigo or nystagmus is present.

Position 4. Quickly lie down on your right side. The movement should take no more than two seconds.
Keep your head turned to the right 45 degrees.
Hold that position for thirty seconds.

Position 5. Sit straight up again.

Another origin for positional nystagmus can lie in the occurrence of vestibular migraine. This also causes atypical patterns of nystagmi that are elicited or triggered by specific positions. The most prominent signs to discriminate peripheral from central positional nystagmus are based on the following inconsistencies:

- A distinct nystagmus is observed without any subjective signs of vertigo by the patient;
- A nystagmus that is not corresponding with the stimulation of the investigated canal. Example: a torsional nystagmus during the roll test or a pure horizontal nystagmus during the Dix-Hallpike maneuver.

Persistence of a horizontal nystagmus is not necessarily a sign of a central cause, since horizontal canal BPPV of the type of cupulolithiasis generates persistent horizontal nystagmus, but it should be ageotropic. When during the roll test a persistent geotropic nystagmus is observed, *i.e.*, beating to the ground, this cannot be explained by horizontal canal BPPV so it is probably of central origin.

In conclusion: possible diagnoses for positional vertigo are BPPV, but also vestibular paroxysmia, vestibular migraine, MD, medication and alcohol intoxication.

Evolution of BPPV. BPPV is systematically more common in patients who have had a vestibular neuritis (10% of cases). In some cases, in the course of months to years after the first attack of BPPV, a patient may suffer again from the same symptoms, for which he or she should contact the doctor again. It is important to realize that it does not need to be BPPV again on the same side: it can also occur on the other side, or even be some other condition. Therefore, it is necessary to repeat the clinical exam and anamnesis. Epley or Semont maneuvers have proven their effectiveness as treatment, but for persistent cases, surgery like canal plugging of the affected canal offers a permanent solution.

Surgical treatment of BPPV: canal plugging
—Prof. Van de Heyning and Prof. Van Rompaey

Surgical treatment consists of a delicate and technical surgery under general anesthesia in which the posterior semicircular canal of the vestibular system is located and plugged. The surgery is done through an incision behind the ear, followed by the opening of the bone behind the ear (mastoid). After finding the position of the bony rear canal, the membranous labyrinth at the height of the canaliths is closed and the canal is filled with fat and bone glue products. Care should be taken that only the semicircular canal that is responsible for the symptoms is occluded. At the same time, medication is administered to avoid hearing loss.

At the time of surgery, patients may not have an ear infection or upper or lower respiratory tract infection. The patient should not have blood clotting disorders and the use of aspirin should be discontinued ten days before surgery.

After the operation, a pressure cushion is applied to the head, which must be kept in place for 24 hours. A hospital stay of a few days is necessary, depending on the vertigo symptoms, as there is a sudden failure of part of the equilibrium system, which is to be compensated centrally by, for example, equilibrium exercises. Possible instability decreases gradually over four to six weeks. Usually, there is very little pain. Water in and around the ear should be avoided until the scar has healed, approximately ten days later. The first two weeks after surgery, it is advised to avoid lifting weights, practising sports, strain and blowing the nose. Usually, people are incapable to work for about three weeks, but this period may vary depending on the kind of work one does.

B2. Ménière's disease (MD)

A patient with MD will suddenly have a prolonged attack of vertigo in combination with hearing-related complaints. Typically, attacks last for at least twenty minutes and are accompanied by severe vertigo, nausea and frequently vomiting, as well as fluctuating hearing loss, tinnitus and/or a sensation of pressure in the affected ear. MD has become overly diagnosed, which means that patients are being labeled with MD, when in fact they have a different disorder. The disease is much less common than BPPV, for example, or vestibular migraine. The prevalence is 190 per 100,000 patients, with women having 1.9 times more chance to have the disease than men.[53] MD was named after the French discoverer of the disease, Prosper Ménière (1799-1862). In 1861, he was the first physician to describe the combined attacks of vertigo, hearing loss and tinnitus, seen in such patients. Prosper Ménière died of pneumonia a few months later.

Cause. The real cause of MD is still unknown. The disease is always accompanied by an increase of pressure in one of the parts of the cochlea - the scala media - which is filled with endolymph. Therefore, MD is also referred to as endolymphatic hydrops, where 'hydrops' stands for 'fluid accumulation'. When the pressure in the scale media builds up and eventually becomes too high, it causes fissures in the wall of specific compartments. Because of these ruptures, a mixing of endolymph and perilymph is caused and in particular the excess of potassium (K^+) ions in the endolymph provokes a neurotoxic contamination of the peripheral neurons (vestibular and cochlear). This leads to a massive stimulation of the hair cells in the different parts of the system, and thus may cause ringing in the ears, hearing loss, and a feeling of pressure in the ear, as well as sudden vertigo and instability. The attacks last for at least twenty minutes, but often several hours, until the ruptured membrane is healed again. Not all endolymphatic hydrops cause the symptoms of MD. Recent research[54] suggests that it is rather a combination of excess pressure, together with genetic factors, infections, vascular factors, diet, allergy, autonomous, endocrine and auto-immune disorders which ultimately cause MD. It is mainly the suddenly onset of dizzy spells that has an impact on the quality of life of the patient, rather than the tinnitus or fluctuating hearing loss. When the pressure is stabilized, there are hardly any symptoms, although in the course of years, the hearing decreases gradually, as well as the vestibular function. The disease usually begins between the ages of thirty to fifty years. In half of the patients with MD, the number of vertigo attacks is severely reduced over the course of ten years after the onset of the disease. The longer a patient has the disease, the fewer the attacks occur per year, until ultimately, no attacks occur anymore. In 32% of cases, MD will arise in the other ear (median of 24 follow-up studies).[53]

Symptoms. A typical MD attack lasts for several hours and is accompanied by nausea and/or vomiting. Hearing loss and tinnitus, and sometimes a feeling of pressure in the inner ear are also present to a certain extent during a typical attack. A typical attack starts with a unilateral vestibular excitation (intensified activity) causing a horizonal or horizontal-torsional nystagmus towards the affected side. This irritative nystagmus is only seen in the acute phase. Then, in a later stage, the vestibular function is reduced on the affected side and an imbalance at the level of ipsilateral and contralateral vestibular nuclei in the brainstem generates a nystagmus to the healthy side, similar to the one that occurs during a vestibular neuritis. This can last many hours. However, the imbalance at the brainstem will trigger a compensation mechanism to reduce the difference between left and right vestibular nuclei, and this will diminish the nystagmus beating to the healthy side. In the meantime, the healing of the fissures in the hydropic inner ear will cause a restoration of the vestibular and cochlear function. This recovering function is added to the central compensation mechanism, leading to an 'overcompensating' nystagmus to the affected side again. This nystagmus may exist for several days.

It has to be noted that many attacks are not as 'typical' as described in text books. There are numerous variations.

Hearing loss. During the initial phase of the disease, a low-frequency hearing loss is seen on the audiogram. As the disease progresses, the medium - and high frequencies are also affected. In the early phase of the disease, the fluctuating nature of the hearing loss is a key factor of MD. In other words, the hearing loss is most severe during the attack, and then improves again. However, the recovery is usually not complete, so that there is permanent hearing loss after several attacks. In the beginning, there is a clear deterioration of hearing, but after five to ten years, the hearing stabilizes at a level of 50 to 60 dB. A patient may suffer from tinnitus, at first only during an attack, but in a later stage it can become permanent.

Tumarkin crisis. A Tumarkin crisis - also called otolithic crisis - is a special form of a vertigo attack, thought to be related to MD. During such an attack, the patient suddenly gets a strong sensation of linear motion, either sideways or downwards, in which it feels as if he or she is pushed to the side or to the ground. Only 3-7% of Ménière patients experience Tumarkin crises. This phenomenon is very likely caused by a mechanical deformation and even disruption of the otolith (utricular) membrane, as a result of pressure differences in the inner ear.[55] This explains why the sensations are predominantly linear in nature, as opposed to typical Ménière attacks, which are rotatory in nature and in which the hair cells are stimulated in the cupula of the semicircular canals. A Tumarkin crisis is a special case of a drop attack, which is characterized by a sudden onset for no apparent reason and usually without loss of consciousness. Drop attacks can be caused by heart problems, circulatory disorders, neurological disorders such as epilepsy, or some vestibular disorders such as superior semicircular canal dehiscence syndrome.

Diagnosis. Since the main diagnostic criteria are subjective and not based on objective measurements, it is often difficult to diagnose MD with one hundred percent certainty. In 1995, the American Academy of Otolaryngology - Head & Neck Surgery has therefore proposed a 'diagnostic scale ', with four types of MD: certain, definite, probable and possible MD.[56]

In 2014, the earlier criteria and definitions were revised by a group of experts from the Barany Society and in 2015 new criteria were published where only two categories were retained (*http://www.jvr-web.org/ICVD.html* and Lopez-Escamez 2015.[54]

The new criteria of Ménière's Disease (MD) (as of 2015) are:[54]

Definite MD:

- *Two or more spontaneous episodes of vertigo each lasting 20 minutes to 12 hours;*
- *Audiometrically documented low- to medium-frequency sensorineural hearing loss, in one ear, defining the affected ear on at least one occasion before, during or after one of the episodes of vertigo;*
- *Fluctuating aural symptoms (hearing, tinnitus or fullness) in the affected ear;*
- *Not better accounted for by another vestibular diagnosis.*

Probable MD:

- *Two or more episodes of vertigo or dizziness, each lasting 20 minutes to 24 hours;*
- *Fluctuating aural symptoms (hearing, tinnitus or fullness) in the affected ear;*
- *Not better accounted for by another vestibular diagnosis .*

Remarks

The scientific paper[54] *with the diagnostic criteria reports some additional remarks that are important to keep in mind when considering MD. Here are some of these listed.*

- *Episodic dizziness and unsteadiness are not considered as criteria to define MD, although patients with MD can report dizziness and unsteadiness at the long term.*

- *Low-frequency sensorineural hearing loss (SNHL) is defined as increases in pure tone thresholds for bone-conducted sound that are higher (i.e., worse) in the affected ear than the contralateral ear by at least 30 dBHL at each of two contiguous frequencies below 2000 Hz. In cases of bilateral low-frequency SNHL, the absolute thresholds for bone-conducted sound must be 35 dBHL or higher at each of two contiguous frequencies below 2000 Hz. If multiple audiograms are available, demonstration of recovery of low-frequency SNHL at some point in time further supports the diagnosis of MD. Bilateral synchronous SNHL (symmetric or asymmetric) can occur in some patients, although such a pattern should raise concern for the possibility of auto-immune inner-ear disease and when progressing slowly over years, may favor migraine as an alternate explanation for the vertigo episodes or a comorbid condition. Bilateral low-frequency SNHL may also be observed in early stages of non-syndromic progressive deafness (DFNA6/14) due to mutations in the WFS1 gene, but vertigo attacks have not been associated with this group of mutations. SNHL in MD can also involve mid and high frequencies after several episodes of vertigo, leading to pantonal hearing loss.*
- *Regarding the non-simultaneous onset of vertigo and hearing loss the following should be noted. "Sensorineural hearing loss may precede the onset of vertigo episodes by several months or years. This clinical variant has been called 'delayed hydrops', but the preferred term should be delayed MD, since endolymphatic hydrops (EH) is a pathological finding. Episodic vertigo may precede the onset of hearing loss by several weeks or months, but tinnitus or aural fullness is usually associated with the first episode of vertigo."*
- *A temporal association between hearing loss and the vertigo episode is sometimes observed by the patient, generally as a change in hearing within 24 hours of the vertigo episode. Hearing loss typically fluctuates spontaneously in the first few years of the disease. After repeated attacks, the hearing loss may progress and become permanent, and the episodes of vertigo may no longer be related with the aural symptoms.*
- *An increase in tinnitus intensity or aural fullness in the affected ear is often associated with the episode of vertigo in the first years. Tinnitus may be persistent once the hearing loss has become permanent.*

An increase of pressure or hydrops can be documented using electrocochleography, a special hearing test to measure the reaction of the inner ear and the auditory nerve to different sounds. As with many tests related to vestibular disorders however, is the specificity or sensitivity relatively low. This is part of the reason why among the criteria of MD, no reference has been made to balance tests. This means that the diagnosis of MD cannot be based on ENG/VNG or other balance tests, as described in the Chapter Balance Tests . The reason for this is that during the initial stages of the disease, one can obtain hypersensitive reactions during balance tests on the affected side. In later stages, however, it is just the opposite, since a decreased vestibular function on the affected side will be shown in the tests. The basic ENG/VNG tests assess the horizontal canal function. More advanced techniques such as VHIT, cVEMP, oVEMP or unilateral centrifugation may assess if other parts of the vestibular system are impaired (see chapter Balance Tests).

However, regardless of the results of the standard balance tests, the diagnosis will have to be determined by means of thorough anamnesis and hearing tests, and based on the criteria as published by the Barany Society Committee[54] in order to obtain the correct diagnosis as soon as possible.

It is important to discriminate MD from other diseases such as vestibular migraine, vestibular paroxysmia, DFNA9 and other disorders. Hence, it is necessary to carry out further investigations, (MRI, blood or urine tests,...) to rule out other possible diagnoses, such as:

- Autosomal dominant sensorineural hearing loss type 9 (DFNA9) caused by COCH gene;
- Autosomal dominant sensorineural hearing loss type 6/14 (DFNA6/14) caused by WSF1 gene;
- Autoimmune inner ear disease;
- Cerebrovascular disease (stroke/TIA in the vertebrobasiliar system/bleeding);
- Cogan's syndrome. Some cases may have recurrences.
- Endolymphatic sac tumor;
- Meningiomas and other masses of the cerebellopontine angle;
- Neuroborreliosis;
- Otosyphilis Susac syndrome;

- Third window syndromes (perilymph fistula, superior semicircular canal dehiscence, enlarged vestibular aqueduct);
- Vestibular migraine;
- Vestibular paroxysmia (neurovascular compression syndrome);
- Vestibular schwannoma;
- Vogt-Koyanagi-Harada syndrome.

Therapy. In scientific literature, there is no consensus on the best drug therapy for MD. This is due to the fact that very few randomized clinical trials (RCT) have been published that conclusively demonstrate the effect of specific medication on MD. In addition, the identification of patients with MD is mainly based on subjective criteria and not on objective measurements, which makes it even more difficult to come to definite proof. In 2013, a study was published indicating that salt restriction has a beneficial effect on the prevention of the attacks.[57]
A recent review paper[58] states that multiple low evidence-level studies report that oral diuretic therapy may be beneficial in the medical management of MD. Improvement in vertigo episode frequency was consistently reported, with less convincing evidence for improvement in hearing outcomes.The very popular and often prescribed drug Betahistine (in Europe) does not seem to be as effective as previously thought, as recently shown by the group of researchers around Prof. Michael Strupp.[59] In this trial, performed according to the current-day scientific standards for randomized controlled trials (RCT's), (double blind, multicentre, placebo-controlled, randomized) three groups of MD patients were treated with (a) placebo; (b) low-dose betahistine (2 x 24 mg daily); and (c) high-dose betahistine (3 x 48 mg daily) for nine months. The numbers of patients in the three groups were 74, 73 and 74 respectively. The authors concluded that the effects of the two different doses of betahistine could not be distinguished from a patient-reported effect caused by placebo intervention in terms of the incidence of attacks as well as vestibular and audiological function and quality of life. However, it is important that in all groups, including the placebo group, a significant reduction in vertigo attacks was observed by a factor 0.76.

Gonzalez and colleagues,[60] Coehlo and Lalwani[61] and Claes and Van de Heyning[62] published summaries on administered medications and treatments, which are listed below . It should be noted that drug therapy remains the responsibility of the treating physician, who must estimate how much impact possible side effects may have on the entire treatment of the patient.

Treatment in the acute phase, *i.e.*, during the attacks:

- Rest and rehydration;
- Antidepressants or vestibular suppressants such as benzodiazepines (diazepam) and antihistamines (dimenhydrinate), calcium antagonists (cinnarizine) and phenothiazines (chlorpromazine, promethazine).

In the period between the attacks:

- Adjustment of lifestyle, avoiding coffee, stress and alcohol;
- Systemic treatments:
  - Diuretics
  - (Betahistine dihydrochloride, is not better than placebo!).

In case further treatment is needed, topical treatments such as intratympanic administration of medications have become very popular and effective. During this treatment, medication is injected into the space behind the tympanic membrane by means of a syringe while the patient lies on his or her side, so that the medication can slowly permeate the inner ear. The medication then acts selectively on the vestibular hair cells or other cells that control the water balance in the inner ear. The treatment can take place under general anesthesia or local anesthesia. The effect of the medication, which aims to reduce the balance function, takes 24 to 72 hours. The medications with proven effect are corticosteroids[63,64] and aminoglycosides.[65,66] A British group led by Prof. Adolfo Bronstein published recently a study where the two intratympanic drugs are compared with each other.[67] In their double-blind comparative effectiveness trial, 60 patients aged 18-70 years with refractory unilateral MD were enrolled at two different hospitals in the UK. Patients were randomly assigned to two intratympanic methylprednisolone (62·5 mg/mL) or gentamicin (40 mg/mL) injections given two weeks apart, and were followed-up for two years. All investigators and patients were masked to treatment allocation. The primary outcome was vertigo frequency over the final six months (18-24 months after injection) compared with the six months before the first injection. In the six-month period before the treatment the gentamicin group had on average 3.3 ± 0.5 (se) vertigo attacks per month and after treatment 0.42 ± 0.18 (se) attacks per month which is a 87% reduction. The methylprednisolone group had in the same period on average 2.7 ± 0.4 attacks per month and after the treatment 0.27 ± 0.10 attacks per month, representing a 90% reduction. Both gentamicin and methylprednisolone injections controlled vertigo attacks and vestibular-mediated disability in refractory unilateral MD. But the number of patients experiencing a clinically meaningful deterioration in speech perception was higher in those receiving gentamicin than in those receiving methylprednisolone. Thus, corticosteroids would be preferred by many patients because they have no side-effects and, unlike gentamicin, are suitable in bilateral disease .

Lifestyle modifications are important because stress can trigger an MD attack. As with all diseases, it is crucial to give the patient an explanation of the disease as well as the mechanisms that cause it. In the English-language literature it is commonly said to 'avoid CATS', or Avoid Caffeine, Alcohol, Tobacco and Stress. Stress is not always easy to deal with, but basically it should be possible to switch to decaf, to smoke less or to quit smoking altogether and to consume less alcohol.

Surgical treatment

If no drug treatment works and the attacks are too frequent and too incapacitating, a patient may decide to undergo a selective vestibular neurectomy, which means that the vestibular nerve going from the inner ear to the brainstem is surgically cut. Inevitably, this surgical intervention provokes a lot of vertigo and instability because of the abruptly induced unilateral failure of the balance system. This unilateral failure must be centrally compensated which can be enhanced by balance exercises. Still, a certain degree of instability may continue to manifest in case of insufficient central compensation. Also, permanent hearing loss may occur in 10% of the patients. Given the effective options and emerging evidence for intratympanic treatment, the surgical approach has become a last resort.

Alternatively, endolymphatic sac surgery (ESS) has been done in the past decades. A recent review study however states that there is currently a low level of evidence for the use of ESS in the treatment of Ménière's disease.[68] This was earlier also already indicated by Pullens and coworkers,[69] who state that only 2 studies were performed according to the standards for RCT's and that neither study reported any beneficial effect of surgery either in comparison to placebo surgery or grommet insertion. So there is a clear need for future RCTs and/or controlled studies to fully evaluate endolympahic sac surgery. However, there are difficulties in designing a valid placebo and achieving adequate blinding of observers and investigators.

Course. The way MD presents itself varies greatly from patient to patient. In one patient, it can emerge with a slow start followed by a gradual increase of symptoms; in another patient, MD can start suddenly and in full force: heavy attacks, severe tinnitus and from the start a certain degree of hearing loss. The later phase also has differences in appearance, not only between individuals but also within the same person. Periods of frequent and violent attacks are interspersed with periods of relative calmness. Hearing loss fluctuates greatly, especially in the beginning. Additional complaints are also not the same between patients. Some may experience loud sounds as painful, while others report a fullness in the ear, a constant light-headedness (also between attacks), fatigue or head and neck pain and eye problems. In several cases, the attacks occur frequently during a period of approximately five years and then they occur less and less frequent until they disappear almost completely. Yet, tinnitus and hearing loss will remain, as well as, in some cases, a decreased vestibular function on the lesioned side. Because of the various forms and experiences and the relative rarity of the disease, the diagnosis is not always easy. Therefore, a good patient history and additional testing is important, particularly with regard to the exclusion of other causes. Moreover, in some patients, MD is not the only vestibular disease that is present. A combination with vestibular migraine is often present, making it even more complicated to address it accurately.

Coping with MD. For MD, there is currently no effective cure. Treatment can at most combat the symptoms and keep them under control. It is important to accept the disease, however difficult that may be. Understanding the disease and adopting appropriate living conditions can help alleviate the suffering of someone with MD. Additionally, psychosocial support can help to cope with the stress and emotions that can triggers a MD attack.

Contact with peers. Many MD patients search for recognition of their disease as well as the right information. The first contact with peers is often a revelation: finally someone who knows exactly what the other feels, having gone through the same things, and who perhaps has found solutions that the other has not thought of. Also, partners of MD patients need contact with eachother and with other MD patients. There are self-help groups, websites, forums and discussion groups. Fellow sufferers often meet in specially organized weekend meetings.

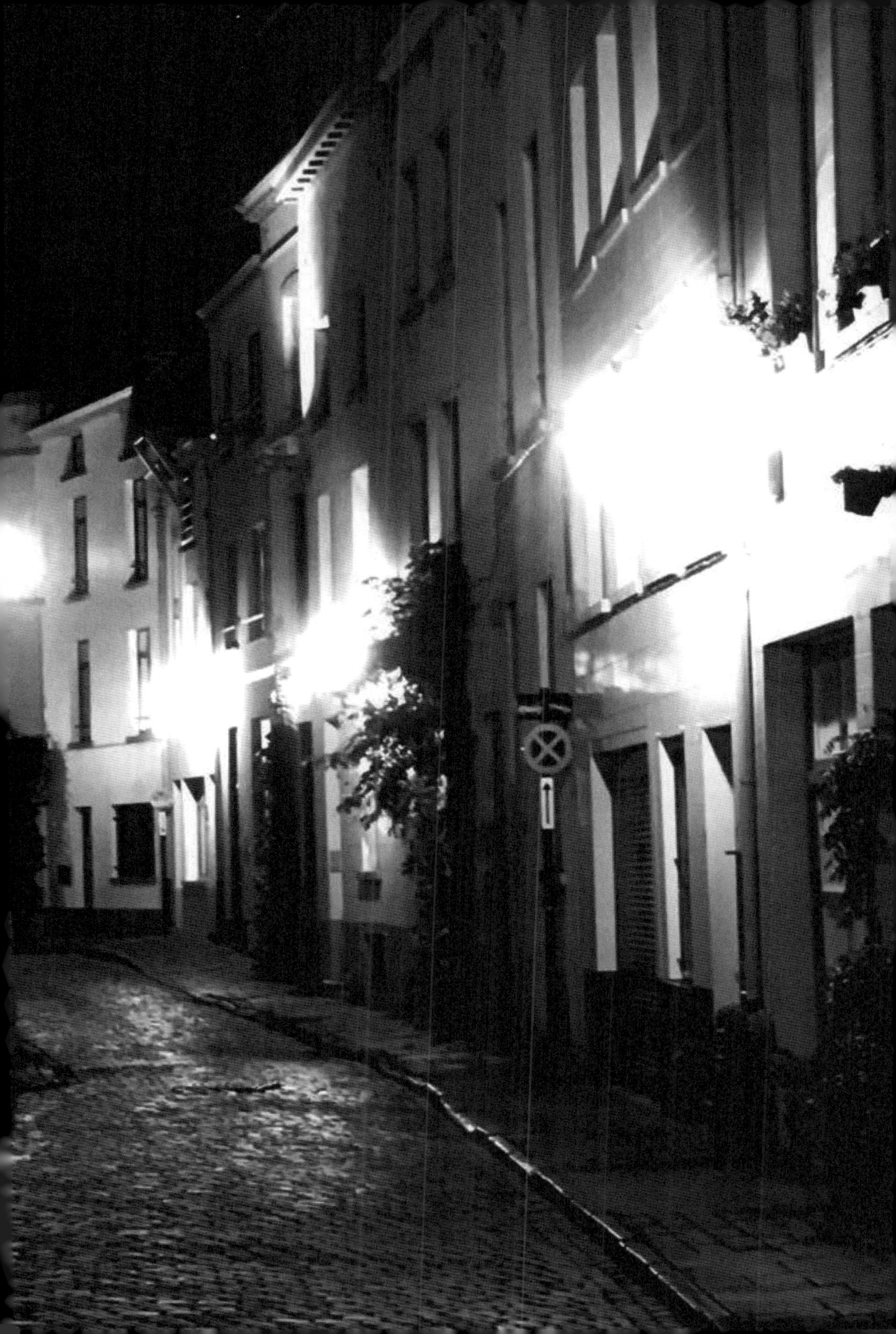

B3. Vestibular Migraine (VM)

Taking into account that the clinical criteria for vestibular migraine were only published in 2012,[15] it is a striking observation that vestibular migraine appears to be the most common cause of dizziness[44] affecting 1% of the population. Vestibular migraine, also known as migrainous vertigo/dizziness, migraine-related vestibulopathy, and migraine-associated dizziness or vertigo was first described by Dieterich and Brandt[70] soon followed by Neuhauser and colleagues[71] and others. Vestibular migraine patients constitute about 10% of patients visiting a ENT clinic, and this number is still an underestimation of the real occurrence.[72]

Clinically, vestibular migraine patients present with attacks of spontaneous or positional vertigo and dizziness lasting seconds to days, accompanied by migraine symptoms such as headache and hypersensitivity to light (photophobia) and sound (phonophobia) or auras. Approximately two thirds of VM patients have spontaneous rotational vertigo whereas one quarter has positional vertigo.[73] It should be noted that the headache does not necessarily have to occur at the same time as the vertigo symptoms. Actually, less than 50% of VM patients have vertigo and headache in every attack.[71] Cochlear symptoms, such as hyperacusis, are not prominent but can also occur and are mostly mild. Furthermore, there is a well-known female preponderance of 5 to 1.[74]

Up to today, there are no biological markers in blood or urine that are indicative for vestibular migraine, although more and more studies show distinct differences at group level between vestibular migraine patients and controls as well as other disorders. Recently, for example, an MRI study showed that differences are noticable regarding grey matter volume in specific brain areas.[75]

Without biological markers, the diagnosis is based on a detailed anamnesis. The diagnostic criteria for vestibular migraine have only recently been published in a consensus document formulated by the Committee for Classification of Vestibular Disorders of the Barany Society and the Migraine Classification Subcommittee of the International Headache Society.[15] This classification suggests two entities: definite vestibular migraine and probable vestibular migraine. These criteria have recently been published as an appendix of the third edition of the International Classification of Headache Disorders. This classification should allow for a broader acceptance of the disorder and lead to more accurate diagnoses and treatment options.

Diagnostic criteria for Vestibular Migraine (VM)[15]

Vestibular migraine

A. At least five episodes with vestibular symptoms (see below for a clarification) of moderate or severe intensity, lasting five minutes to 72 hours.

B. Current or previous history of migraine with or without aura according to the International Classification of Headache Disorders (ICHD).

C. One or more migraine features in at least 50% of vestibular episodes:

- *Headache with at least two of the following characteristics: one-sided location, pulsating quality, moderate or severe pain intensity, aggravation by routine physical activity;*
- *Photophobia and phonophobia;*
- *Visual aura.*

D. Not accounted for by another vestibular or ICHD diagnosis.

Probable vestibular migraine

A. At least five episodes with moderate to severe vestibular symptoms, lasting five minutes to 72 hours.

B. At least one of the following characteristics:

- *Current or previous history of migraine with or without aura according to the International Classification of Headache Disorders (ICHD);*
- *One or more migraine features with at least 50% of the vestibular episodes:*
  - *Headache with at least two of the following characteristics: one sided location, pulsating quality, moderate or severe pain intensity, aggravation by routine physical activity;*
  - *Photophobia and phonophobia;*
  - *Visual aura.*

C. Not accounted for by another vestibular or ICHD diagnosis.

Taking into account that the clinical criteria for vestibular migraine were only published in 2012, it is a striking observation that this disorder appears to be the most common cause of dizziness.

In several cases, migraine headache occurs much earlier in life than the vestibular attacks and therefore, it can be difficult to make a link between both. Vestibular symptoms start typically 8-19 years after migraine with or without aura.[76]
The fact that the symptoms of dizziness not always occur at the same time as the headache makes it difficult to make the diagnosis too. The number of patients who consistently have headache and vertigo at the same time appears to be only 5%. The mean age of onset for women is 38 and 42 in men.[71] VM attacks can actually last from seconds to 72 hours. The 5 minute criterion can be considered also as an accumulated time of several attacks lasting seconds.

The choice of five minutes as a duration criterium is used to make a distinction between the typical complaints of BPPV-nature, which are several seconds and position triggered, and the typical MD symptoms that last for at least 20 minutes.

According to a recent review study by Liu and Xu[77] one of the reasons that physicians were so reluctant to accept vestibular migraine as a distinct disorder was that it produced so many symptoms overlapping with various well-established vestibular disorders such as MD, benign paroxysmal positional vertigo (BPPV), and for example basilar migraine. In some cases, vestibular migraine may be indistinguishable from MD based on history and symptoms. To make it even more complicated, vestibular migraine may be comorbid with MD, *i.e.*, occur at the same time in the same patient.[78] According to these authors, 38% of patients who have VM presented also with subjective hearing loss, aural pressure, and tinnitus during episodes of dizziness and headaches. On the other hand, 59% of the patients with MD, had vestibular migraine, migraine symptoms or migraine risk factors along with their MD.

The prevalence of MD is five to ten times lower than that of vestibular migraine and has a higher female to male preponderance of 1.3 : 1[79] Like VM, the diagnosis of MD is based mainly on history, especially when audiological tests are normal.

The reason behind this overlap is presumably due to the fact that migraine is linked very much both to VM as well as to MD.

Vestibular testing and vestibular migraine. Currently, there are no laboratory tests, such as blood tests, that can indicate whether someone has vestibular migraine. Also vestibular tests are not sensitive for VM.[80] On the other hand, vestibular testing is meant to rule out other disorders. In the symptom-free interval, however, oculomotor abnormalities occur in up to two thirds of patients, including gaze-evoked nystagmus, saccadic pursuit, central positional nystagmus and dysmetric or slow saccades.[81] Our experience in the clinic corroborates in particular the regularly observed central positional nystagmus being nystagmus which is observed during Dix-Hallpike testing, but which is not compatible with BPPV. Most importantly, one should pay attention to whether or not a persistent nystagmus is present in different positions as well as whether this nystagmus is accompanied by vertigo or dizziness. During the attacks, 70% of patients develop spontaneous or positional nystagmus.[82] VEMPs are currently not yet clinically useful as vestibular tests since different studies show inconsistent results.

Pathophysiology of vestibular migraine. Several different hypotheses have emerged in the past decade, but the mechanism underlying vestibular dysfunction that is related to migraine still needs furter research. One theory proposes a parallel activation of nociceptive and vestibular pathways referring to the tight connection between vestibular structures and brainstem areas related to the processing of pain. Also the concept of 'cortical spreading depression' may partly explain the pathophysiology of vertigo in VM. Other explanations focus on trigeminovascular reflex-mediated vasodilatation of cranial blood vessels and subsequently plasma extravasation causing meningeal inflammation which are the key features of pain in migraine.[83] The trigeminovascular system also innervates the inner ear.[84] Dieterich *et al.*[44] conclude that migraine-related vestibular disorders like VM may be caused by enhanced excitability occurring during the processing of sensory information, which is due to a genetic susceptibility. This enhanced excitation induces interactions of vestibular and pain pathways on several levels, from the inner ear to the thalamus and cortical level. A recent review on this topic further elaborates on several aspects of this complex disorder.[85]

Therapy. Avoiding so-called 'migraine triggers' is very important, and changes in lifestyle can make a huge contribution. It is known that fatigue is a migraine trigger, so having a good night's sleep is essential. However, various kinds of food can also cause migraine, as well as specific smells, and so forth. Caffeine sessation for example can relieve symptoms.[86] To date, there is only one RCT study for the prophylaxic treatment of vestibular migraine that matches the current standard criteria and at the updating of our book, it is still ongoing (Strupp M (2008) Prophylactic treatment of vestibular migraine with metoprolol: a double-blind, placebo-controlled trial ISRCTN72824329-2009). Most clinicians treat vestibular migraine successfully with the same medication as for standard migraines. For example, a recent retrospective study showed that 70% of patients are better when treated with either propranolol or flunarizine.[72] But there are other medications that are applied based on expert opinion, but are not yet supported by clinical trials.

Commonly used medications include beta-blockers such as propranolol or metoprolol, calcium channel blockers such as flunarizine, antidepressants such as amitriptiline, nortriptyline, sertraline, fluoxetine or paroxetine, anti-epileptics such as topiramate or carbonic anhydrase inhibitors such acetazolamide.[87-89]

B4. Vestibular Paroxysmia (VP)

Vestibular paroxysmia (VP) is the more recent name of what for years was called a neurovascular conflict of the vestibulocochlear nerve. Vestibular paroxysmia presents with repeated brief attacks of vertigo or dizziness, typically lasting a few seconds to several minutes, and occuring several times a day. The attacks may occur spontaneously, but can also be triggered by certain head movements. The latter makes the entity difficult to distinguish from BPPV. Possible additional symptoms include short-lasting tinnitus and hearing loss. During the periods between attacks, mild to moderate hearing loss and balance may occur, which might make it difficult to distinguish from MD. Alternatively, spontaneously occurring short spells of dizziness also occur with vestibular migraine, making it even more challenging to diagnose VP correctly.

The underlying cause of vestibular paroxysmia is a neurovascular conflict, in which a blood vessel touches or compresses the vestibulocochlear nerve (N VIII) (Fig. 30). Along this nerve, which runs from the cochlea and the vestibular organ in the inner ear to the brainstem, all the signals of hearing and balance are transmitted. The compressive blood vessel usually involves the anterior inferior cerebellar artery (AICA), but sometimes the posterior inferior cerebellar artery (PICA) or other nearby blood vessels are involved. At a certain moment, the contact between the blood vessel and the nerve leads to irritation with symptoms of dizziness and hearing-related complaints as a result. The chronic external pressure from the blood vessel presumably leads to demyelination, decreasing its firing threshold and making the nerve susceptible to unwanted stimulation by a mechanism called ephaptic transmission. Ephaptic (from the Greek) means 'touching onto'.

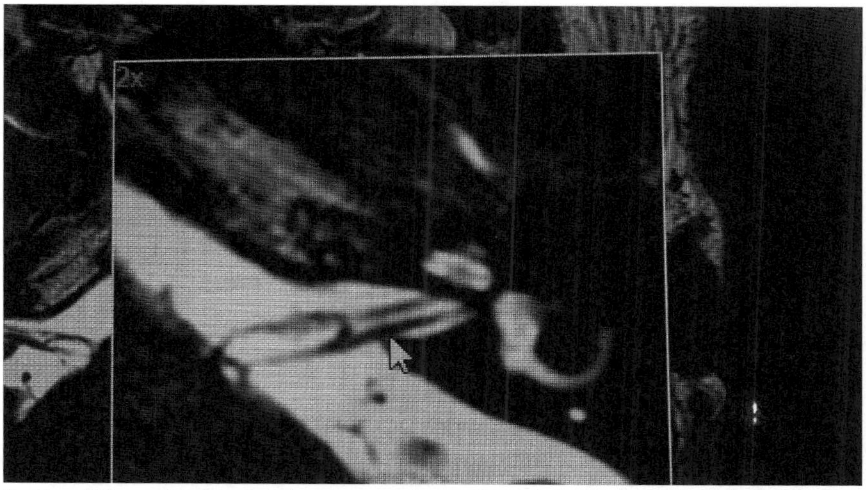

Fig. 30 — MRI scan of the fossa posterior (inner ear and connection to the brain stem). Notice the loop of a blood vessel making contact with the vestibulo cochlear nerve in the internal ear canal causing vestibular paroxysmia. Normally two parallel black lines should run from the cochlea and vestibular organ (on the right side of the picture) to the brain stem (left side of the picture).

Almost 40% of the patients will present with nausea, with or without vomiting. Movements in which the force of gravity (lying down) or inertia (rapid head movements), causes more pressure of the blood vessel on the nerve, which typically causes a symptom increase in 50% of cases. Many patients develop nystagmus with hyperventilation,[90] which is hypothetically due to transient changes in conductivity across the demyelinated portion of the nerve during hyperventilation, causing excitatory or inhibitory patterns of nystagmus. Age induced vascular elongation due to increasing atherosclerosis and arterial hypertension that generate stronger pulsations are thought to be possible explanations why VP complaints start between the ages of 40-70.[91] According to Brandt and coworkers, VP accounts for approximately 4% of outpatients in a dedicated vertigo clinic.[91] In 2008, Brandt and his coworkers published clinical criteria for VP,[90] in attendance of the criteria recently proposed by the Barany Society.[92]

There are two types of vestibular paroxysmia: definite and probable vestibular paroxysmia.

The original criteria are still listed here as an example, since to my opinion, they describe nicely the typical signs of VP. Obviously, the new criteria listed below this table are the ones to be used.

Former criteria of definite vestibular paroxysmia[90]

At least five attacks and the patient should fulfil the following criteria:

A. Vertigo spells lasting seconds to minutes. The individual attack subsides without specific therapeutic intervention.

B. One or several of the following provoking factors of the attacks:

1. *Rest;*
2. *Certain head/body positions (not BPPV-specific positioning maneuvers);*
3. *Changes in head/body position (not BPPV-specific positioning maneuvers).*

C. One or several of the following characteristics during the attacks:

1. *No accompanying symptoms;*
2. *Disturbance of stance;*
3. *Disturbance of gait;*
4. *Unilateral tinnitus;*
5. *Unilateral pressure/numbness in or around the ear;*
6. *Unilaterally reduced hearing.*

D. One or several of the following additional diagnostic criteria:

1. *Neurovascular conflict demonstrated on MRI (CISS sequence);*
2. *Hyperventilation-induced nystagmus as measured by ENG;*
3. *Increase of vestibular deficit at follow-up investigations as measured by ENG;*
4. *Treatment response to antiepileptics (not applicable at first consultation).*

E. The symptoms cannot be explained by another disease

New criteria of Vestibular Paroxysmia (VP):[92]

(Definite) Vestibular paroxysmia - (each point needs to be fulfilled)

A. At least ten attacks of spontaneous spinning or non-spinning vertigo

B. Duration less than 1 minute

C. Stereotyped phenomenology in a particular patient

D. Response to a treatment with carbamazepine/oxcarbazepine

E. Not better accounted for by another diagnosis.

Probable vestibular paroxysmia (each point needs to be fulfilled)

A. *At least five attacks of spinning or non-spinning vertigo*

B. *Duration less than 5 minutes*

C. *Spontaneous occurrence or provoked by certain head-movements2*

D. *Stereotyped phenomenology in a particular patient*

E. *Not better accounted for by another diagnosis.*

Audiovestibular tests have their specific use, because they show a one-sided disorder (for example by caloric examination), as well as a spontaneous nystagmus in the majority of patients. In addition, patients often have a unilateral hearing loss. In our pilot study on this topic, we observed in 84% of the patients with VP (n = 36) a positional non-BPPV type nystagmus during the Dix-Hallpike position, whereas this was only 40% in the group of VM patients (n = 36). Very helpfull, however, is to perform an MRI on which the neurovascular conflict can be determined. On the other hand, in many persons the MRI seems suggestive for neurovascular conflict, without causing complaints. Hence the importance to check the published criteria corroborated with audiovestibular features.

There is a considerable overlap in the complaints between the other episodic vertigo disorders, being BPPV, vestibular migraine and MD. Proper anamnesis and clinical investigations should help to identify the correct diagnose. The SO STONED table (table 2) with the different vestibular disorders shows that in several of the dimensions clear differences exist.

Therapy. Carbamazepine or oxcarbazepine have proven to be very effective to reduce symptoms or even eliminate them.[90, 91] The reduction or disappearance of the symptoms by taking carbamazepine in itself is a clear support of definite VP diagnosis. This is similar to vestibular migraine, which is corroborated as diagnosis when specific anti-VM medication alleviates the symptoms.

B5. Superior Semicircular Canal Dehiscence Syndrome (SSCD)

—Prof. V. Van Rompaey

The superior semicircular canal dehiscence syndrome (SSCD) is a relatively new otovestibular disease, first described in 1998 by the group of Prof. Dr. Lloyd Minor.[93,94] A dehiscence (cut) in the bony capsule around the superior semicircular canal (SSC) creates a mobile third window into the inner ear, next to the oval and round window. The brain membrane of the middle cranial fossa comes into direct contact with the contents of the vestibular organ, with the result that it is sensitive to pressure fluctuations and sound stimuli. The prevalence of SSC dehiscence varies between 0.4 and 0.7%, with a large group of asymptomatic patients.[95] The exact cause is still unclear, but genetics, developmental defects, pressure of the cerebrospinal fluid and head trauma are suggested as the best hypothesis. Extremely seldom the dehiscence is caused by a tumor or a blood vessel.[96,97]

Typical symptoms include hearing loss, autophonia (when one hears his or her own voice in an annoying way), pressure sensation, pulsatile tinnitus, dizziness caused by pressure fluctuations or noise stimuli (respectively Hennebert and Tullio phenomenon) and hyperacousis to bone-conducted sounds. This can lead to, for example, patients hearing their eyeballs move, or when they turn the head it sounds like a thunderstorm. Frequently, there are only auditory complaints, without vertigo. The reason why a mobile third window causes these complaints, is probably by diverting acoustical energy from air-guided sounds from the cochlea to the dehiscence - this leads to a conductive hearing loss at low frequencies and clinical hearing loss. Bone-conducted sounds cause movement of the basilar membrane in the cochlea, which is enlarged at a third window injury due to an impedance difference between the scala tympani and the scala vestibuli. This leads to the fact that bone conduction audiometry is better than expected for the age and additionally to clinical hyperacousis of the bodily sounds.[98]

The diagnosis is suggested by a detailed history. Indeed, patients rarely associate these symptoms with an otovestibular condition. Otoscopy may reveal no abnormalities. Vestibular clinical research (with video oculoscopy) sometimes makes it possible to generate nystagmi by sound or pressure variation in the affected ear. Audiometry can show low-frequency conductive hearing loss, often with a supra-normal bone conduction. Stapedius reflexes are normal. An abnormally low threshold value and high amplitude are recorded during cVEMP tests, which are a reflection of the increased sensitivity of the sacculus or a reduced attenuation of the pressure waves in the inner ear. It is a very important component to confirm SSCD.

The diagnosis of SSCD at electrophysiological level. The diagnosis can only be made by performing a high-resolution CT scan of the temporal bones, with specific reconstructions in the plane of the SSC. With the correct level of detail and correct interpretation, there is a sensitivity of 100% and a specificity of 96%.[99] Additional MRI scans may be useful to exclude rare underlying tumorlike processes in case of simultaneous vertigo or sensorineural hearing loss.[96,100] Several conditions can mimic some of the symptoms, but rarely the entire syndrome. Otosclerosis can present with a similar hearing loss, but the stapedius reflexes can not be provoked. The main reason to perform a CT scan for suspected otosclerosis is the exclusion of a third window injury. Chronic otitis media would reveal otoscopic abnormalities such as tympanic membrane perforation or a cholesteatoma. Complaints that reveal a Tullio or Hennebert phenomenon in a patient with chronic otitis media should alert the clinician to search for a cholesteatoma that enters into the lateral semicircular channel. A tympanic glomus or high jugular bulb in the middle ear can cause pulsatile tinnitus and hearing loss, but are diagnosed based on otoscopy and/or specific abnormalities on CT scans of the temporal bones. Tullio and Hennebert phenomena can also be provoked by syphilis, perilymphatic fistula, trauma, Lyme disease and MD, presumably by a similar pathophysiology, *i.e.*, an impedance difference between the scala tympani and the scala vestibuli.[99]

Therapy. The treatment consists of explaining the pathophysiology of this disorder. Often the complaints, however, are very disturbing, in which case treatment is necessary, consisting exclusively of surgery. Surgery may consist of obliteration (plugging) of the SSC, a procedure in which the region is accessed via the mastoid, similar to the surgical treatment of BPPV.[101] An alternative is 'capping', in which the roof of the SSC is reconstructed. A posterior semicircular channel BPPV is reported in 12% of this type of surgery and is easy to diagnose and treat.[102] Because the labyrinth is opened, there is a risk of sensorineural hearing loss of 1.5.[102] For this reason, methods that preserve the hearing are used which are routinely applied during for example cochlear implant surgery. A recent review study on surgical approaches of SSCD indicates that there is no significant difference between the different approaches, but suggests that plugging via the transmastoid approach is preferred due to lower complication rates and shorter hospital stay.[103]

B6. Mal de débarquement syndrome

Mal de débarquement syndrome (MdDS) is a subjective perception of self-motion after exposure to passive motion, in most cases sea travel, hence the name.[104]

The first real recognition of MdD as a clinical syndrome occurred in 1987 by Brown and Baloh,[105] although the phenomenon is known for centuries.

In most cases, MdD (which freely translates to 'sickness after disembarkment') occurs after sea travel but it can also occur after air or land travel[106] In any case, it is important to make a distinction between transient MdD symptoms (< 48h) and persistent MdDS (> 3 days up to several years), as the latter is pathological, while transient MdD is a common phenomenon (*e.g.*, in naval personnel) and occurs frequently with reported numbers between 72-80%.[107]

Clinically, patients experience a rocking, bobbing or swaying sensation which is often accompanied by unsteadiness and disequilibrium that occurs persistently after cessation of the exposed passive motion stimulus. A high association of MdDS and headache[108] and migraine[109] has been postulated, especially in patients who develop spontaneous MdDS episodes. Previous studies also found associations between MdDS and motion sickness, increased self-motion sensitivity and increased visual sensitivity.[109,110]

In general, no structural abnormalities are found on standard brain magnetic resonance imaging (MRI) scans and inner ear function tests are normal. There is a well-documented female preponderance for MdD, suggesting that the hormonal component is of importance and should be taken into account.[109] To date, treatment options are limited. Counseling and recognition by the clinician of the symptoms and MdDS as a disease is an important start. Unlike most vestibular disorders, MdDS patients suffer mainly from dizziness in a static position (sitting or lying down), whereas moving around and particularly driving a car or using other means of transport, including horseback riding, reduces the symptoms considerably. As soon as the patient comes to a halt, however, all the complaints emerge again. This contra-intuitive complaint, from the vestibular point of view, provokes that MdDS is not yet being taken seriously as a distinct syndrome. Hence the importance of recognition and counseling.

Some pharmaceutical agents (*e.g.*, benzodiazepines, selective serotonin re-uptake inhibitors), stress relief therapy and vestibular rehabilitation have been reported to be beneficial.[109,111] More recently, promising results have been achieved by means of neuromodulation (*i.e.*, repetitive transcranial magnetic stimulation (rTMS)) but this has to be further studied.[112] Less invasive but very promising is the approach by the New York-based group of Professor Bernard Cohen and Dr. Dai. Their approach is based on a modulation of the VOR, which is assumed to be maladapted in MdDS.[113,114] They offer a pattern of moving stripes in front of the patient while the head of the patient is tilted in the frontal plane (from shoulder to shoulder) at the pace of the internal experienced movements or the frequency of swaying as measured with a force platform. This treatment is repeated several times within one week. Centers world wide are currently adopting the same method to study this methodology. Preliminary results of a clinical trial, performed in our lab AUREA in Antwerp, adopting the method of Cohen and Dai, show very promising results.

B7. Perilymph fistula

Symptoms of perilymph fistulas include a varying combination and severity of episodic dizziness, vertigo and instability, often with a gradual deterioration in the (sensory neural) hearing and the occurrence of tinnitus. The episodes are often triggered by changes in head position or pressure-related processes such as coughing, pressing, sneezing, etcetera. The fistula is composed of a leak or tear in the oval or round window in the middle ear, often caused by a barotrauma (for example, as a result of diving or an explosion) or a head trauma.

Therapy. If the perilymph fistula is caused by chronic inflammation (*e.g.*, cholesteatoma), the cause should be treated first (medically or surgically). Surgical obliteration of the oval and round window with plugs is amongst the possibilities, if there is sufficient evidence to confirm the diagnosis.

B8. Auto-immune Inner Ear Disease

Auto-immune inner ear disease (AIED) is a clinical syndrome in which a bilateral sensorineural hearing loss of more than 30 dB occurs at one or more frequencies in a period of three to 90 days. An increase of the hearing loss of more than 15 dB at one frequency or more than 10 dB at two frequencies in at least one ear must be present. Associated vestibular symptoms can occur in half of the patients and systemic autoimmune disease occurs in 30% of the patients. In some patients, AIED begins as a sudden unilateral hearing loss which, however, soon also affects the other ear.

Remark on hyperventilation

In case of an underlying disease like acoustic schwannoma, which is a benign tumor in the peripheral vestibulocochlear system, or vestibular paroxysmia, hyperventilation may generate nystagmus and dizziness. It is, however, never the sole cause of vertigo attacks.

C. Chronic vestibular syndrome

The 3rd type vestibular syndrome, next to acute and episodic, as defined in the ICD-11 Beta classification by the WHO is the chronic vestibular syndrome being a clinical syndrome of chronic dizziness, vertigo or instability that can take months to years and is often characterized by oscillopsia (a 'dancing' image while walking), nystagmus and gait instability. These are typical characters that are suggestive for a permanent loss of the balance system. Also, symptoms consistent with a deterioration of hearing or even the central nervous system can appear in these patients. A chronic vestibular syndrome is one of the few vestibular disorders in which a deterioration of the symptoms occur, or where no evolution of the symptoms is observed. This suggests and incomplete recovery or inadequate compensation after, for example, an acute vestibular disorder. A third form refers to a condition in which a patient experiences vertigo or dizziness even in between the severe vertigo attacks, as a kind of permanent after effects. The conditions that can lead to a chronic vestibular syndrome include an incomplete compensated unilateral vestibular failure, chronic bilateral vestibulopathy, cerebellar degeneration, posterior cranial fossa neoplasms and chronic psychological or behavioral disorders associated with vestibular symptoms.

C1. Persistent Positional Perceptual Dizziness (PPPD)

Persistent positional perceptual dizziness or also PPPD or triple PD is a recent diagnostic entity that brings some earlier diagnoses such as phobic postural vertigo, visual vertigo, chronic subjective dizziness under one heading. This entity is proposed by the Barany Society and further elaborated by Dieterich and Staab leading to the following criteria:[115]

Persistent Positional Perceptual Dizziness (PPPD):[92]

Criteria A - E must be satisfied to make a diagnosis of PPPD.

A. *One or more symptoms of dizziness, unsteadiness, or non-spinning vertigo are present on most days for three months and more.*
   - *Symptoms are persistent, but wax and wane.*
   - *Symptoms tend to increase as the day goes by but may not be active throughout the entire day.*
   - *Momentary flares may occur spontaneously or with sudden movements.*

B. *Symptoms are present without specific provocation but are exacerbated by*
   - *upright posture,*
   - *active or passive motion without regard to direction or position,*
   - *exposure to moving visual stimuli or complex visual patterns,*

   although these three factors may not be equally provocative.

C. *The disorder usually begins shortly after an event that causes acute vestibular symptoms or problems with balance, though less commonly, it develops slowly.*
   - *Precipitating events include acute, episodic, or chronic vestibular syndromes, other neurologic or medical illnesses, and psychological distress;*
     a. *When triggered by an acute or episodic precipitant, symptoms typically settle into the pattern of criterion A as the precipitant resolves, but may occur intermittently at first, and then consolidate into a persistent course;*
     a. *When triggered by a chronic precipitant, symptoms may develop slowly and worsen gradually.*

D. *Symptoms cause significant distress or functional impairment.*

E. *Symptoms are not attributed to another disease or disorder.*

Consequently, PPPD is a form of dizziness and/or instability, that lasts at least three months. The symptoms usually occur daily and typically increase during the day. Patients will report ups and downs of the symptoms that can occur spontaneous or are provoked by sudden movements. Usually the complaints increase when the patient is sitting upright. When visual patterns or complex visual stimuli cause an aggravation of the symptoms, one uses the term visual induced dizziness (VID), formerly known as visual vertigo or visual vestibular mismatch. Examples of typical triggering visual stimuli are crowded areas such as busy crossroads, shopping malls, supermarkets, escalators, etcetera. PPPD patients are often stimulated by both passive and active head movements. PPPD can occur after an acute or periodic vestibular problems caused by migraine, orthostatic intolerance, panic attacks with dizziness, peripheral or central vestibular disorders, head concussion, etcetera. At first, the symptoms occur occasionally, but in the long run they appear more and more.

For the treatment of VID one can desensitize the patient by means of a rotating disc that is placed in front of the subject.[116] On this disc, fluorescent dots are placed in a random pattern. When this disc rotates in total darkness in front of the subject, vection is generated and when offered in gradual doses, this desensitizes the patient ultimately. Additionally, providing information on how balance functions and what a mismatch in essence is, is an important step to cope with this condition. Recent studies show that in VID patients the brain areas that are involved in vestibular integration (the vestibular cortex) and visual interpretation (the visual cortex) are respectively less and more excited than in healthy control sucjects.[2] These findings are important to show that biomarkers exists of VID, and hence therapy effect can be more objectively evaluated.

Patient education, physiotherapy, cognitive behavior therapy, and medications such as selective serotonin reuptake inhibitors (SSRI's) are succesful treatment options for PPPD.

In the following years, the definition of PPPD is likely to be further refined. Identifying a pattern of symptoms is a step in the right direction, so that scientific studies can be designed to evaluate the effect of possible treatments.

As part of PPPD, chronic subjective dizziness pops up as an entity that causes persistent dizziness or instability that do not resemble vertigo and appears almost daily for at least three months. The symptoms increase when standing upright, when the patient moves, or if he or she is exposed to visual stimuli such as shopping centers or precision tasks with the eyes, such as reading. The disorder that lies at the origin of CSD has a neuro-otological cause such as vestibular neuritis, panic attacks, long-lasting BPPV, etcetera. Even when episodic syndromes occur such as MD, one can eventually develop CSD. The real cause of CSD is not yet known, but it appears that it has to do with the fact that a patient after an acute vestibular attack is not able to respond to it in an adequate way, and continues to have problems with the compensation process. It is clear from the previous description that the various syndromes in the chronic vestibular syndrome group show a large overlap. SSRI's often bring symptom relief in case of CSD pathology.

C2. Bilateral Vestibulopathy (BV)

There are a number of terms to describe the condition in which the function of the balance organ is entirely or to a great extent lost on both sides: bilateral vestibulopathy, bilateral areflexia or bilateral vestibular function loss. Areflexia stands for total absence of reflexes. Bilateral vestibulopathy is present in 7% of vestibular patients, according to a German study.[117] It manifests itself in an unstable walk at twilight or darkness or on an unstable surface. Since most or nearly all of vestibular information from the labyrinth is absent, only visual and proprioceptive information is present. When this information is jeopardized as well, like in the dark or on an unstable underground (*e.g.*, on a dry, sandy beach) there is too little information to rely on, and instability is a logical consequence. Such patients do not complain of vertigo or dizziness since this occurs mainly by an imbalance between the left and right balance system. If, however, neither of the two systems is functioning, there is also no asymmetry, and no vertigo or an illusion of movement. In addition to instability in the dark, around 40% of these patients also experience a disturbed gaze stabilization during rapid head movements. For example, they are not able to read street names while they are walking. They will need to stand still, keep their head stable, read and then proceed again.

Bilateral vestibulopathy is determined by a bilateral abnormal (video) head impulse test (HIT or vHIT) or an abnormal caloric test, which is commonly a standard part of the vestibular test battery. The caloric test evaluates the vestibular system at low frequencies, while the vHIT measurement accounts for higher frequencies. Testing the sacculus by the VEMP appears to show fewer defects than testing the horizontal canals.[118] There are several causes of bilateral areflexia or vestibulopathy: aminoglycoside (gentamicin)-ototoxicity, meningitis and an advanced Ménière's disease are the most important causes, but in some cases it is caused by a slow evolving disease with an unknown origin. Gentamycin is an antibiotic that is sometimes given to patients who have a very serious bacterial infection of vital organs such as the heart. If the patient has survived the bacterial infection and returns home after a hospitalization period, he or she notices the signs of bilateral vestibular areflexia. When gentamicin is administered to patients in high doses, it acts as an ototoxic drug, *i.e.*, it is harmful to the inner ear. First, the hair cells of the vestibular organ are impaired, then the hearing is affected and eventually, the patient may become deaf.

There are also a number of genetic disorders, such as DFNA9, which cause bilateral vestibular failure and deafness around the age of 40. These non-syndromic autosomal dominant genetic disorders are rare, but there are certain regions where the gene occurs more than in other regions. MD also causes a bilateral vestibulopathy when the unilateral MD has evolved into a bilateral MD. In addition, degenerative neurological factors in some cases originate bilateral vestibulopathy. Recently it was discovered that in some cases, cobalt ions, coming from *e.g.* metal on metal hip replacement joints, can lead to bilateral vestibular failure.[119]

Course and treatment. The course of bilateral vestibulopathy is generally not favorable: as soon as the function of the two vestibular organs is gone, it rarely comes back (in contrast to unilateral vestibular neuritis) and in most patients, the condition remains stable but bad. Drug therapy makes little sense, because so far there are no drugs that can re-establish that kind of lack of function (although there are drugs under development).

Sports

The role of sports is substantial in vestibular recovery. Ball sports in particular are very beneficial since not only the muscles are trained, but also the integration of proprioceptive, visual and vestibular signals. Without eye-hand coordination and efficient integration, no estimate can be made the brain to calculate where the ball w be in the next moment when the patie needs to return it with for example his or her racket. This paradigm (ball sport) is much more efficient to train the central compensation than anythir else. The rhytm is determined by the game, not by the player. Despite a lesioned peripheral system, some people perform better and better whe they exercise more sports. As a socia activity, it may also help the patient w is socially excluded. Practising sports is a necessity for the dizzy patient. In the beginning it will be tough, but afte a while it will bring joy and more self confidence to the patient.

Actually, treatment relies on two other aspects: information and training. In other words, to give the patient clear information on the issue of the condition and how the lack of balance function can be coped with through proprioception and vision (eye). That is substitution rather than compensation, for compensation usually refers to compensating for the loss of one of the two equilibrium systems in which the healthy side takes over the balance function partly in combination with proprioception and vision. In the event that there is no function in both sides, then substitution is the appropriate word. The use of a walking stick is very appropriate, especially in elderly patients with vestibular problems. That should not be a cane to lean on, but rather an 'antenna'. That, combined with special rehabilitation exercices at the physiotherapist that help feed the substitution process and keep the muscles in shape, is an effective approach, and it can help to gain confidence. A recent study by Prof. Kathleen Cullen has proven the physiological basis of substitution because she showed that signals from, *e.g.*, the neck are sent to the vestibular centers in the brain, replacing the failed balance organs. It appears that these replacement signals only come about after vestibular organ failure.[5]

Vestibular implants

Currently, a lot of research is done in laboratories around the world in the field of vestibular implants, similar to cochlear implants. Over the next few years, this will be implemented in daily routine, when appropriate. Another tool is called a vibrotactile feedback system with vibrating elements (such as those found in mobile phones). When a patient experiences loss of balance while standing or walking, some of these elements vibrate. In this way they generate a sensation that may assist the patient in recovering his/her equilibrium.

The term chronic vestibular syndrome comprises a number of other diagnoses - according to the ICD-11 beta version of the World Health Organization (WHO). We distinguish:

- Persistent unilateral vestibulopathy after vestibular neuritis;
- Persistent unilateral vestibulopathy following a schwannoma (acousticus neuroma or schwannoma);
- Persistent unilateral vestibulopathie after a medical procedure or intervention.

These are different forms of disease which, in essence, generate a very similar pattern of symptoms, as described above.

The treatment is, in general, focused on training of the vestibular system as optimally as possible so that compensation is initiated.

Remaining diagnoses

There are probably a number of other diagnoses that may explain the cause of balance problems, but we will not discuss these here. Examples include multi-deficit syndrome, especially present in elderly patients, or childhood dizziness in children. Some causes are so far unknown, and one should not expect the clinician to know the answer to all problems. Every day, new discoveries may lead to a better understanding of dizziness and what one can do, but it is a slow process, because vertigo is such a complex issue. The syndromes described in this book, however, cover the vast majority of the disorders causing vertigo or dizziness.

Vertigo and serendipity: Diffusion MRI

At a conference on the brain in Copper Mountain in 2009, I attended a key note lecture by a radiologist about the problem of blast injury . This occurs in people who literally are 'blown' away, during a war conflict, a bomb attack or something similar. The radiologist said that after the recovery process, a number of people were no longer the same as before. They were re-examined using various techniques, but neither blood tests, electroencephalography (EEG), CT scans or MRI scans were able to show clear abnormalities. Everything was 'back in place'. It was only through the use of diffusion MRI techniques and so-called tractography, that certain connections in the brains were shown to be missing.

That made me think of a comparison with patients with vertigo. Some patients do fine after an illness such as a neuritis, while others are not able to perform certain tasks without problems. Possible examples are 'visual induced dizziness' or chronic subjective dizziness. Our recent findings have indeed shown that we should use more of these advanced MRI methods also for vertigo patients.[2]

In the near future, the novel MRI methods will unravel more evidence for lacking connections in the brain that may explain the symptoms in patients with for example PPPD, providing such biomarkers.

Neuroplasticity

However, if we want to check if there is a problem with connectivity, we need to know where exactly in the brain we have to look for missing or less optimal connectivity.

After all, we do not have an (NMR) image of everyone's brain in a healthy state. We only see patients with problems after they have developed those problems. So there is no within-subject comparison.

When cosmonauts or astronauts are in space, they experience a lot of dizziness and disorientation during the first days. Also, after coming back from a six-months' stay in the International Space Station, several space travellers experience a lot of dizziness. But that state, which is very similar to that of dizzy patients in an acute phase, fades away within a few hours or days. Cosmonauts who have previously travelled in space, adapt even faster. All this is due to the process of neuroplasticity. Neuroplasticity describes the adaptation to new situations by making new connections or optimizing existing connections. These can be of a structural or functional kind. Riding a bicycle is a good example of this learning process. Children usually need a while before they can ride the bicycle. Sometimes they need training wheels. And then suddenly it works out: they can keep their balance on the bicycle without falling. This is because somewhere in the brain connections are established between various centers, so that one can control what could not be controlled before – in this case the balance on a bicycle.

Because cosmonauts show such obvious signs of dizziness which disappear within a few days, due to neuroplasticity, I just assumed that they were the ideal group to study, especially because of the comparison between their state before they go into space and when coming back on earth. By taking images with advanced MRI diffusion techniques that show the connectivity immediately after they come back, and comparing these images with those that were taken before their flight into space, we hypothesised that we can identify the regions of interest where differences occur. That investigation would then allow to designate areas in the brain where integration occurs between different sensory signals coming from vestibular, proprioceptive and vison inputs. One of the hypotheses is that the 'vestibular cortex' will possibly have undergone changes, but this had to be verified with this type of project. To date, we tested 12 cosmonauts who spent six months to one year in space. Based on the knowledge gained from this, we can look more targeted into patients. The first results from pilot studies already suggest that there are indeed differences in connectivity as seen before and after spaceflight.120-123 Using these techniques, we can investigate some patients with e.g., PPPD-like symptoms to establish whether they show the same differences in connectivity.

In the near future, this research will undoubtedly continue to evolve and become hopefully an important part of the vestibular research.

The inside cover of this book shows images of this highly-advanced MRI diffusion technique.

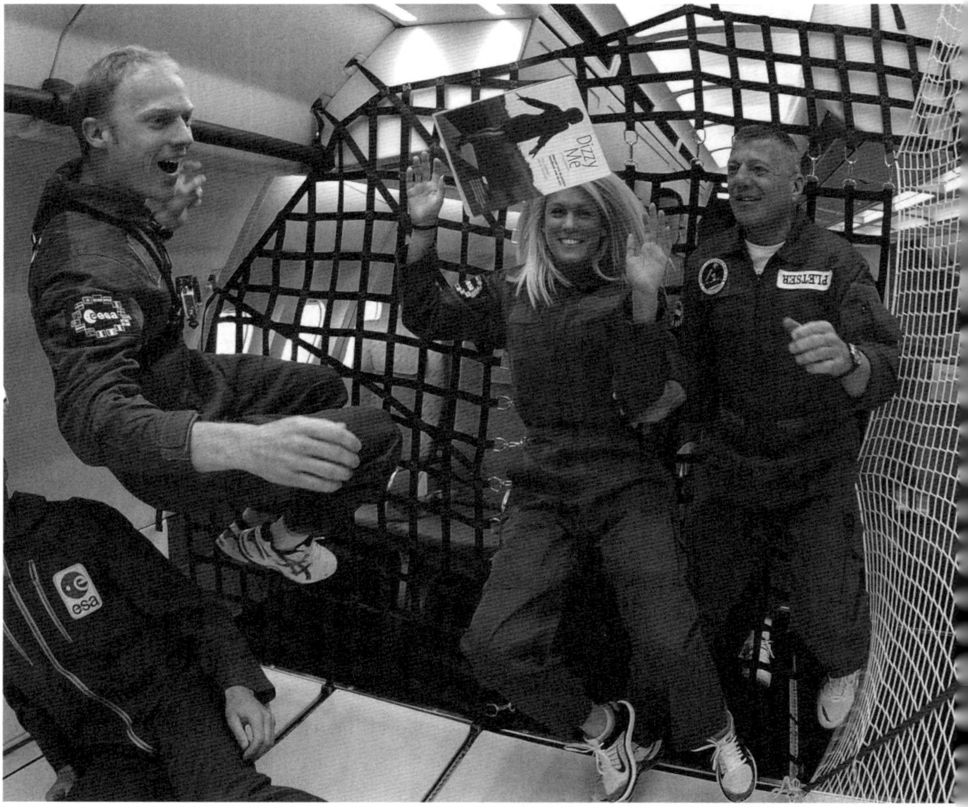

Fig. 31 — Picture made during the 22 seconds of weighlessness on board of the Airbus A310 ZERO-G airplane during the ESA-DLR-CNES parabolic flight campaign in Bordeaux in 2015. The brains of the participants were scanned with MRI method before and after the flight during which 31 parabolas were performed generating subsequent phases of 1g, 2g, 0g, 2g and 1 With these experiments, we have shown that a specific area in the brain - the temporo parietal junction or TPJ - is affected a flight, illustrating evidence of neuroplasticity.[123] In this cortical region, the brain makes sense of verticality, based on visual, vestibular and proprioceptive information. The observed decreased connectivity in this region proves that the brain can reac quickly to disturbing information, and virtually shuts down temporarily the areas that are receiving incongruent informatio The Flemish version of the book Dizzy Me has flown too.

References

1. Hallgren, E., et al., Dysfunctional vestibular system causes a blood pressure drop in astronauts returning from space. Scientific Reports, 2015. 5: p. 8.
2. Van Ombergen, A., et al., Altered functional brain connectivity in patients with visually induced dizziness. Neuroimage Clin, 2017. 14: p. 538-545.
3. van Leeuwen, R.B. and H. van der Zaag-Loonen, Dizziness and neck pain: a correct diagnosis is required before consulting a physiotherapist. Acta Neurologica Belgica, 2017. 117(1): p. 241-244.
4. Brandt, T., Cervical vertigo--reality or fiction? Audiol Neurootol, 1996. 1(4): p. 187-96.
5. Sadeghi, S.G., L.B. Minor, and K.E. Cullen, Neural correlates of sensory substitution in vestibular pathways following complete vestibular loss. J Neurosci, 2012. 32(42): p. 14685-95.
6. Biller, J., et al., Cervical Arterial Dissections and Association With Cervical Manipulative Therapy A Statement for Healthcare Professionals From the American Heart Association/American Stroke Association. Stroke, 2014. 45(10): p. 3155-3174.
7. Bos, J.E. and W. Bles, Theoretical considerations on canal-otolith interaction and an observer model. Biological Cybernetics, 2002. 86(3): p. 191-207.
8. Bos, J.E., et al., Susceptibility to seasickness. Ergonomics, 2007. 50(6): p. 890-901.
9. Hallgren, E., et al., Decreased otolith-mediated vestibular response in 25 astronauts induced by long-duration spaceflight. Journal of Neurophysiology, 2016. 115(6): p. 3045-3051.
10. Bisdorff, A., et al., Classification of vestibular symptoms: Towards an international classification of vestibular disorders. Journal of Vestibular Research-Equilibrium & Orientation, 2009. 19(1-2): p. 1-13.
11. Wuyts, F.L., V. Van Rompaey, and L.K. Maes, "SO STONED": Common Sense Approach of the Dizzy Patient. Front Surg, 2016. 3: p. 32.
12. Kattah, J.C., et al., HINTS to Diagnose Stroke in the Acute Vestibular Syndrome Three-Step Bedside Oculomotor Examination More Sensitive Than Early MRI Diffusion-Weighted Imaging. Stroke, 2009. 40(11): p. 3504-3510.
13. Brandt, T., M. Strupp, and M. Dieterich, Five keys for diagnosing most vertigo, dizziness, and imbalance syndromes: an expert opinion. Journal of Neurology, 2014. 261(1): p. 229-231.
14. Roland, L.T., et al., Utility of an Abbreviated Dizziness Questionnaire to Differentiate Between Causes of Vertigo and Guide Appropriate Referral: A Multicenter Prospective Blinded Study. Otology & Neurotology, 2015. 36(10): p. 1687-1694.
15. Lempert, T., et al., Vestibular migraine: diagnostic criteria. J Vestib Res, 2012. 22(4): p. 167-72.

16. Van der Stappen, A., F. Wuyts, and P. Van de Heyning, Computerized electronystagmography: normative data revisited. Acta Oto-Laryngologica, 2000. 120(6): p. 724-730.
17. Maes, L., et al., Normative data and test-retest reliability of the sinusoidal harmonic acceleration test, pseudorandom rotation test and velocity step test. Journal of Vestibular Research-Equilibrium & Orientation, 2008. 18(4): p. 197-208.
18. Maes, L., et al., The Effect of Age on the Sinusoidal Harmonic Acceleration Test, Pseudorandom Rotation Test, Velocity Step Test, Caloric Test, and Vestibular-evoked Myogenic Potential Test. Ear and Hearing, 2010. 31(1): p. 84-94.
19. Maes, L., et al., Rotatory and Collic Vestibular Evoked Myogenic Potential Testing in Normal- Hearing and Hearing- Impaired Children. Ear and Hearing, 2014. 35(2): p. E21-E32.
20. Maes, L., et al., Clinical usefulness of the rotatory, caloric, and vestibular evoked myogenic potential test in unilateral peripheral vestibular pathologies. International Journal of Audiology, 2011. 50(8): p. 566-576.
21. Van der Stappen, A., F. Wuyts, and P. Van de Heyning, Influence of head position on the vestibule-ocular reflex during rotational testing. Acta Oto-Laryngologica, 1999. 119(8): p. 892-894.
22. Mahringer, A. and H. Rambold, Caloric test and video-head-impulse: a study of vertigo/dizziness patients in a community hospital. European Archives of Oto-Rhino-Laryngology, 2014. 271(3): p. 463-472.
23. Alhabib, S.F. and I. Saliba, Video head impulse test: a review of the literature. European Archives of Oto-Rhino-Laryngology, 2017. 274(3): p. 1215-1222.
24. Colebatch, J., G. Halmagyi, and N. Skuse, Myogenic Potentials Generated by a Click-Evoked Vestibulocollic reflex. Journal of Neurology Neurosurgery and Psychiatry, 1994. 57(2): p. 190-197.
25. Vanspauwen, R., F. Wuyts, and P. Van de Heyning, Improving vestibular evoked myogenic potential reliability by using a blood pressure manometer. Laryngoscope, 2006. 116(1): p. 131-135.
26. Vanspauwen, R., F. Wuyts, and P. Van de Heyning, Vestibular evoked myogenic potentials: Test-retest reliability and normative values obtained with a feedback method for the sternocleidomastoid muscle contraction. Journal of Vestibular Research-Equilibrium & Orientation, 2009. 19(3-4): p. 127-135.
27. Venhovens, J., J. Meulstee, and W.I.M. Verhagen, Vestibular evoked myogenic potentials (VEMPs) in central neurological disorders. Clinical Neurophysiology, 2016. 127(1): p. 40-49.

28. Clarke, A.H. and A. Engelhorn, Unilateral testing of utricular function. Experimental Brain Research, 1998. 121(4): p. 457-464.
29. Buytaert, K., et al., A New Model for Utricular Function Testing Using a Sinusoidal Translation Profile during Unilateral Centrifugation. Audiology and Neuro-Otology, 2010. 15(6): p. 343-352.
30. Hoppenbrouwers, M., F. Wuyts, and P. Van de Heyning, Suppression of the E-effect during the subjective visual vertical test. Neuroreport, 2004. 15(2): p. 325-327.
31. Davalos-Bichara, M. and Y. Agrawal, Normative Results of Healthy Older Adults on Standard Clinical Vestibular Tests. Otology & Neurotology, 2014. 35(2): p. 297-300.
32. Zellhuber, S., A. Mahringer, and H. Rambold, Relation of video-head-impulse test and caloric irrigation: a study on the recovery in unilateral vestibular neuritis. European Archives of Oto-Rhino-Laryngology, 2014. 271(9): p. 2375-2383.
33. Goebel, J.A., et al., Anatomic considerations in vestibular neuritis, otol and nerurotol, 2001, 22(4), p. 512-518
34. Adamec I., et al., Incidence, seasonality and comorbidity in vestibular neuritis. 2015 36(1):91-95.
35. Vereeck, L., et al., The effect of early customized vestibular rehabilitation on balance after acoustic neuroma resection. Clinical Rehabilitation, 2008. 22(8): p. 698-713.
36. Jamali, M., et al., Neuronal detection thresholds during vestibular compensation: contributions of response variability and sensory substitution. J Physiol, 2014. 592(Pt 7): p. 1565-80.
37. Strupp, M. and T. Brandt, Vestibular neuritis. Semin Neurol, 2009. 29(5): p. 509-19.
38. Strupp, M., et al., Methylprednisolone, valacyclovir, or the combination for vestibular neuritis. N Engl J Med, 2004. 351(4): p. 354-61.
39. Goudakos, J.K., et al., Corticosteroids and Vestibular Exercises in Vestibular Neuritis Single-blind Randomized Clinical Trial. Jama Otolaryngology-Head & Neck Surgery, 2014. 140(5): p. 434-440.
40. Fishman, J.M., C. Burgess, and A. Waddell, Corticosteroids for the treatment of idiopathic acute vestibular dysfunction (vestibular neuritis). Cochrane Database of Systematic Reviews, 2011(5): p. 34.
41. Brandt, T., et al., Long-term course and relapses of vestibular and balance disorders. Restor Neurol Neurosci, 2010. 28(1): p. 69-82.
42. Kao, W.T.K., L.S. Parnes, and R.A. Chole, Otoconia and otolithic membrane fragments within the posterior semicircular canal in benign paroxysmal positional vertigo. Laryngoscope, 2017. 127(3): p. 709-714.
43. von Brevern, M., et al., Benign paroxysmal positional vertigo: Diagnostic criteria. Journal of Vestibular Research-Equilibrium & Orientation, 2015. 25(3-4): p. 105-117.

44. Dieterich, M., M. Obermann, and N. Celebisoy, Vestibular migraine: the most frequent entity of episodic vertigo. J Neurol, 2016. 263 Suppl 1: p. S82-9.
45. Neuhauser, H.K., et al., Epidemiology of vestibular vertigo: a neurotologic survey of the general population. Neurology, 2005. 65(6): p. 898-904.
46. Helminski, J.O., et al., Effectiveness of particle repositioning maneuvers in the treatment of benign paroxysmal positional vertigo: a systematic review. Phys Ther, 2010. 90(5): p. 663-78.
47. Bruintjes, T.D., et al., A randomised sham-controlled trial to assess the long-term effect of the Epley manoeuvre for treatment of posterior canal benign paroxysmal positional vertigo. Clin Otolaryngol, 2014. 39(1): p. 39-44.
48. Su, P.J., Y.C. Liu, and H.C. Lin, Risk factors for the recurrence of post-semicircular canal benign paroxysmal positional vertigo after canalith repositioning. Journal of Neurology, 2016. 263(1): p. 45-51.
49. Casqueiro, J.C., A. Ayala, and G. Monedero, No more postural restrictions in posterior canal benign paroxysmal positional vertigo. Otol Neurotol, 2008. 29(5): p. 706-9.
50. Devaiah, A.K. and S. Andreoli, Postmaneuver restrictions in benign paroxysmal positional vertigo: an individual patient data meta-analysis. Otolaryngol Head Neck Surg, 2010. 142(2): p. 155-9.
51. Mostafa, B.E., T.A. Youssef, and A.S. Hamad, The necessity of post-maneuver postural restriction in treating benign paroxysmal positional vertigo: a meta-analytic study. European Archives of Oto-Rhino-Laryngology, 2013. 270(3): p. 849-852.
52. Mandalà, M., et al., Vestibular neuritis: recurrence and incidence of secondary benign paroxysmal positional vertigo. Acta Otolaryngol, 2010. 130(5): p. 565-7.
53. Huppert, D., M. Strupp, and T. Brandt, Long-term course of Menière's disease revisited. Acta Otolaryngol, 2010. 130(6): p. 644-51.
54. Lopez-Escameza, J.A., et al., Diagnostic criteria for Ménière's disease. Journal of Vestibular Research-Equilibrium & Orientation, 2015. 25(1): p. 1-7.
55. Calzada, A.P., et al., Otolithic Membrane Damage in Patients With Endolymphatic Hydrops and Drop Attacks. Otology & Neurotology, 2012. 33(9): p. 1593-1598.
56. Monsell, E.M., et al., Committee on hearing and equilibrium guidelines for the diagnosis and evaluation of therapy in Ménières-disease. Otolaryngology-Head and Neck Surgery, 1995. 113(3): p. 181-185.
57. Luxford, E., et al., Dietary modification as adjunct treatment in Ménière's disease: patient willingness and ability to comply. Otol Neurotol, 2013. 34(8): p. 1438-43.
58. Crowson, M.G., A. Patki, and D.L. Tucci, A Systematic Review of Diuretics in the Medical Management of Ménière's Disease. Otolaryngology-Head and Neck Surgery,

2016. 154(5): p. 824-834.
59. Adrion, C., et al., Efficacy and safety of betahistine treatment in patients with Ménière's disease: primary results of a long term, multicentre, double blind, randomised, placebo controlled, dose defining trial (BEMED trial). Bmj-British Medical Journal, 2016. 352: p. 16.
60. Martín González, C., et al., Medical management of Ménière's disease: a 10-year case series and review of literature. Eur Arch Otorhinolaryngol, 2010. 267(9): p. 1371-6.
61. Coelho, D.H. and A.K. Lalwani, Medical management of Ménière's disease. Laryngoscope, 2008. 118(6): p. 1099-108.
62. Claes, J. and P.H. Van de Heyning, A review of medical treatment for Ménière's disease. Acta Otolaryngol Suppl, 2000. 544: p. 34-9.
63. Phillips, J.S. and B. Westerberg, Intratympanic steroids for Ménière's disease or syndrome. Cochrane Database of Systematic Reviews, 2011(7).
64. Martin Sanz, E., et al., Control of Vertigo After Intratympanic Corticoid Therapy for Unilateral Ménière's Disease: A Comparison of Weekly Versus Daily Fixed Protocols. Otology & Neurotology, 2013. 34(8): p. 1429-1433.
65. Pullens, B. and P.P. van Benthem, Intratympanic gentamicin for Ménière's disease or syndrome. Cochrane Database of Systematic Reviews, 2011(3).
66. Quaglieri, S., et al., Intratympanic gentamicin treatment 'as needed' for Ménière's disease. Long-term analysis using the Kaplan-Meier method. European Archives of Oto-Rhino-Laryngology, 2014. 271(6): p. 1443-1449.
67. Patel, M., et al., Intratympanic methylprednisolone versus gentamicin in patients with unilateral Ménière's disease: a randomised, double-blind, comparative effectiveness trial. Lancet, 2016. 388(10061): p. 2753-2762.
68. Lim, M.Y., et al., Current evidence for endolymphatic sac surgery in the treatment of Ménière's disease: a systematic review. Singapore Medical Journal, 2015. 56(11): p. 593-598.
69. Pullens, B., H.P. Verschuur, and P.P. van Benthem, Surgery for Ménière's disease. Cochrane Database of Systematic Reviews, 2013(2): p. 21.
70. Dieterich, M. and T. Brandt, Episodic vertigo related to migraine (90 cases): vestibular migraine? Journal of Neurology, 1999. 246(10): p. 883-892.
71. Neuhauser, H., et al., The interrelations of migraine, vertigo, and migrainous vertigo. Neurology, 2001. 56(4): p. 436-441.
72. Van Ombergen, A., et al., Vestibular Migraine in an Otolaryngology Clinic: Prevalence, Associated Symptoms, and Prophylactic Medication Effectiveness. Otology & Neurotology, 2015. 36(1): p. 133-138.
73. Neuhauser, H.K., et al., Migrainous vertigo: prevalence and impact on quality of life.

Neurology, 2006. 67(6): p. 1028-33.
74. Lempert, T. and H. Neuhauser, Epidemiology of vertigo, migraine and vestibular migraine. Journal of Neurology, 2009. 256(3): p. 333-338.
75. Messina, R., et al., Structural brain abnormalities in patients with vestibular migraine. J Neurol, 2017. 264(2): p. 295-303.
76. Boldingh, M.I., et al., Comparison of Interictal Vestibular Function in Vestibular Migraine vs Migraine Without Vertigo. Headache, 2013. 53(7): p. 1123-1133.
77. Liu, Y.F. and H. Xu, The Intimate Relationship between Vestibular Migraine and Ménière Disease: A Review of Pathogenesis and Presentation. Behavioural Neurology, 2016: p. 8.
78. Neff, B.A., et al., Auditory and Vestibular Symptoms and Chronic Subjective Dizziness in Patients With Ménière's Disease, Vestibular Migraine, and Ménière's Disease With Concomitant Vestibular Migraine. Otology & Neurotology, 2012. 33(7): p. 1235-1244.
79. Neuhauser, H.K. and T. Lempert, Vertigo: Epidemiologic Aspects. Seminars in Neurology, 2009. 29(5): p. 473-481.
80. Lee, J.W., et al., Clinical manifestation and prognosis of vestibular migraine according to the vestibular function test results. Korean J Audiol, 2013. 17(1): p. 18-22.
81. Radtke, A., et al., Vestibular migraine Long-term follow-up of clinical symptoms and vestibulo-cochlear findings. Neurology, 2012. 79(15): p. 1607-1614.
82. von Brevern, M., et al., Acute migrainous vertigo: clinical and oculographic findings. Brain, 2005. 128: p. 365-374.
83. Moskowitz, M.A., Pathophysiology of headache - Past and present. Headache, 2007. 47: p. S58-S63.
84. Vass, Z., et al., Direct evidence of trigeminal innervation of the cochlear blood vessels. Neuroscience, 1998. 84(2): p. 559-567.
85. Luzeiro, I., et al., Vestibular Migraine: Clinical Challenges and Opportunities for Multidisciplinarity. Behavioural Neurology, 2016: p. 11.
86. Mikulec, A.A., F. Faraji, and L.J. Kinsella, Evaluation of the efficacy of caffeine cessation, nortriptyline, and topiramate therapy in vestibular migraine and complex dizziness of unknown etiology. American Journal of Otolaryngology, 2012. 33(1): p. 121-127.
87. Furman, J.M., D.A. Marcus, and C.D. Balaban, Vestibular migraine: clinical aspects and pathophysiology. Lancet Neurol, 2013. 12(7): p. 706-15.
88. Gode, S., et al., Clinical assessment of topiramate therapy in patients with migrainous vertigo. Headache, 2010. 50(1): p. 77-84.

89. Lepcha, A., et al., Flunarizine in the prophylaxis of migrainous vertigo: a randomized controlled trial. Eur Arch Otorhinolaryngol, 2013.
90. Hüfner, K., et al., Vestibular paroxysmia: diagnostic features and medical treatment. Neurology, 2008. 71(13): p. 1006-14.
91. Brandt, T., M. Strupp, and M. Dieterich, Vestibular paroxysmia: a treatable neurovascular cross-compression syndrome. J Neurol, 2016. 263 Suppl 1: p. S90-6.
92. Strupp, M., et al., Vestibular paroxysmia: Diagnostic criteria. Journal of Vestibular Research-Equilibrium & Orientation, 2016. 26(5-6): p. 409-415.
93. Minor, L.B., et al., Sound- and/or pressure-induced vertigo due to bone dehiscence of the superior semicircular canal. Arch Otolaryngol Head Neck Surg, 1998. 124(3): p. 249-58.
94. Minor, L.B., et al., Dehiscence of bone overlying the superior canal as a cause of apparent conductive hearing loss. Otol Neurotol, 2003. 24(2): p. 270-8.
95. Masaki, Y., The prevalence of superior canal dehiscence syndrome as assessed by temporal bone computed tomography imaging. Acta Otolaryngol, 2011. 131(3): p. 258-62.
96. Crane, B.T., et al., Meningioma causing superior canal dehiscence syndrome. Otol Neurotol, 2010. 31(6): p. 1009-10.
97. Koo, J.W., et al., Superior semicircular canal dehiscence syndrome by the superior petrosal sinus. J Neurol Neurosurg Psychiatry, 2010. 81(4): p. 465-7.
98. Merchant, S.N., J.J. Rosowski, and M.J. McKenna, Superior semicircular canal dehiscence mimicking otosclerotic hearing loss. Adv Otorhinolaryngol, 2007. 65: p. 137-45.
99. Belden, C.J., et al., CT evaluation of bone dehiscence of the superior semicircular canal as a cause of sound- and/or pressure-induced vertigo. Radiology, 2003. 226(2): p. 337-43.
100. Licht, A.K., et al., Vertigo and hearing disturbance as the first sign of a glioblastoma (World Health Organization grade IV). Otol Neurotol, 2004. 25(2): p. 174-7.
101. Agrawal, S.K. and L.S. Parnes, Transmastoid superior semicircular canal occlusion. Otol Neurotol, 2008. 29(3): p. 363-7.
102. Niesten, M.E., et al., Clinical factors associated with prolonged recovery after superior canal dehiscence surgery. Otol Neurotol, 2012. 33(5): p. 824-31.
103. Ziylan, F., et al., A Comparison of Surgical Treatments for Superior Semicircular Canal Dehiscence: A Systematic Review. Otology & Neurotology, 2017. 38(1): p. 1-10.
104. Van Ombergen, A., et al., Mal de debarquement syndrome: a systematic review. Journal of Neurology, 2016. 263(5): p. 843-854.

105. Brown, J.J. and R.W. Baloh, Persistent mal-de-debarquement syndrome - a motion-induced subjective disorder of balance. American Journal of Otolaryngology, 1987. 8(4): p. 219-222.
106. Cha, Y.H., Mal de Debarquement. Seminars in Neurology, 2009. 29(5): p. 520-527.
107. Stoffregen, T.A., et al., Getting Your Sea Legs. Plos One, 2013. 8(6): p. 16.
108. Cha, Y.H. and Y.Y. Cui, Rocking dizziness and headache: A two-way street. Cephalalgia, 2013. 33(14): p. 1160-1169.
109. Cha, Y.H., et al., Clinical features and associated syndromes of mal de debarquement. Journal of Neurology, 2008. 255(7): p. 1038-1044.
110. Tal, D., G. Wiener, and A. Shupak, Mal de debarquement, motion sickness and the effect of an artificial horizon. Journal of Vestibular Research-Equilibrium & Orientation, 2014. 24(1): p. 17-23.
111. Hain, T.C., P.A. Hanna, and M.A. Rheinberger, Mal de Debarquement. Archives of Otolaryngology-Head & Neck Surgery, 1999. 125(6): p. 615-620.
112. Ding, L., et al., Lasting modulation effects of rTMS on neural activity and connectivity as revealed by resting-state EEG. IEEE Trans Biomed Eng, 2014. 61(7): p. 2070-2080
113. Dai, M., et al., Readaptation of the vestibulo-ocular reflex relieves the mal de debarquement syndrome. Front Neurol, 2014. 5: p. 124.
114. Dai, M., et al., Treatment of the Mal de Debarquement Syndrome: A 1-Year Follow-up. Frontiers in Neurology, 2017. 8(175).
115. Dieterich, M. and J.P. Staab, Functional dizziness: from phobic postural vertigo and chronic subjective dizziness to persistent postural-perceptual dizziness. Current Opinion in Neurology, 2017. 30(1): p. 107-113.
116. Pavlou, M., A.M. Bronstein, and R.A. Davies, Randomized trial of supervised versus unsupervised optokinetic exercise in persons with peripheral vestibular disorders. Neurorehabil Neural Repair, 2013. 27(3): p. 208-18.
117. Grill, E., et al., Health services utilization of patients with vertigo in primary care: a retrospective cohort study. J Neurol, 2014. 261(8): p. 1492-8.
118. Zingler, V.C., et al., Saccular function less affected than canal function in bilateral vestibulopathy. J Neurol, 2008. 255(9): p. 1332-6.
119. Leyssens, L., et al., Cobalt toxicity in humans-A review of the potential sources and systemic health effects, Toxicology. 2017. 15;387: p. 43-56
120. Demertzi, A., et al., Cortical reorganization in an astronaut's brain after long-duration spaceflight. Brain Structure & Function, 2016. 221(5): p. 2873-2876.
121. Van Ombergen, A., et al., The effect of spaceflight and microgravity on the human brain. J Neurol, 2017.

122. Van Ombergen, A., et al., Spaceflight-induced neuroplasticity in humans as measured by MRI: what do we know so far? Npj Microgravity, 2017. 3: p. 12.
123. Van Ombergen, A. et al., Intrinsic functional connectivity reduces after first-time exposure to short-term gravitational alterations induced by parabolic flight. Scientific Reports, 2017. 7(1): p. 3061

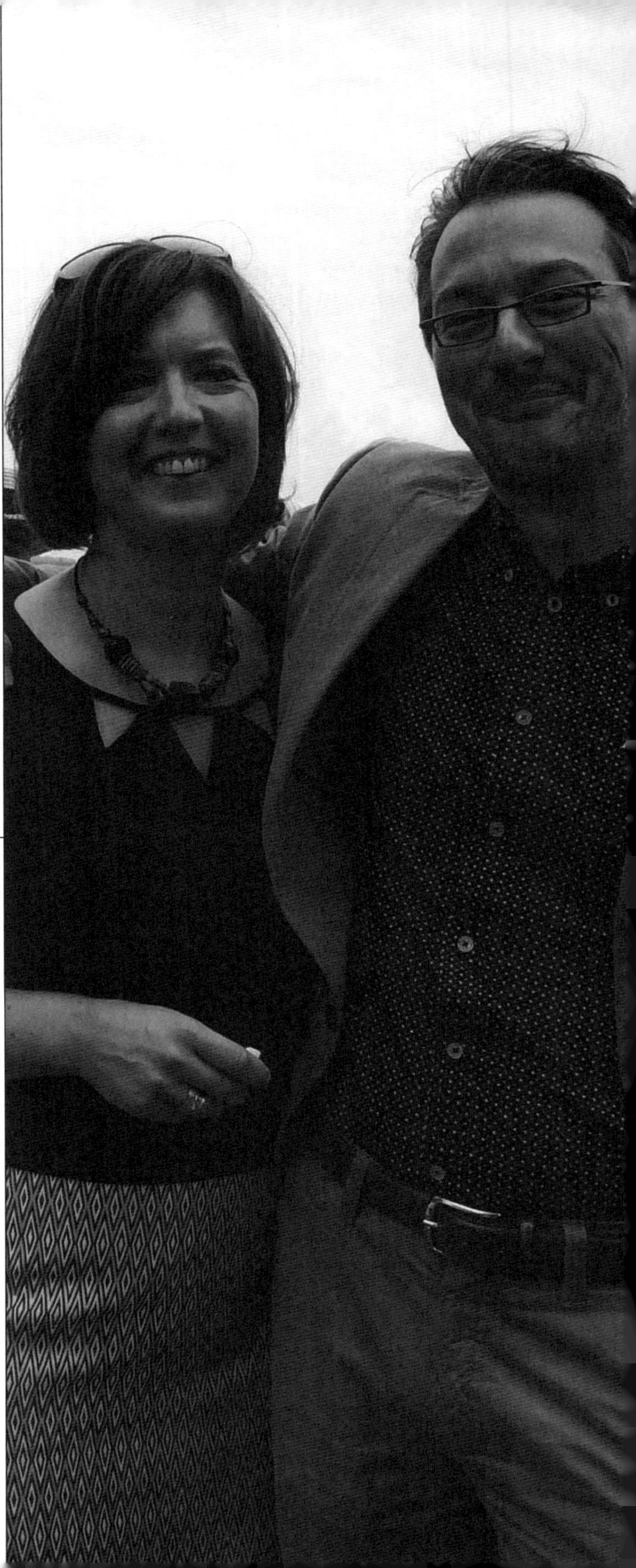

Carry on regardless

David: 'My main purpose in writing this personal history is to show that even a doctor can be confronted with a chronic problem he is unable to resolve on his own.

I encourage physicians, specialists and researchers to continue their efforts to diagnose and treat patients who present with dizziness. Don't just send them home with a bottle of pills. Don't underestimate the seriousness of their condition.

To my fellow sufferers: don't give up, and don't ignore your uncertainty. It took me thirteen years, but I finally got a correct diagnosis - and so, I hope, can you.'

Chapter 8

Patient Voices

DAVID

Being a physician myself, I know how this condition works. I have been living with it for fifteen years.

I am a Belgian physician, forty years old. My story begins about fifteen years ago. At the beginning of my seventh year as a medical student, I was placed in an internal medicine internship at the hospital in Oudenaarde. For several consecutive days, I found myself unable to get out of bed. The world was spinning around me. Finally I was able to stand up again. The experience was a complete shock.
I figured I had developed an infection of my vestibular nerve. And of course I was terrified it might be a tumor, but a CT scan ruled that out. Phew! I decided to see a neurologist and an ENT specialist.

So I made the acquaintance of the incredibly comfortable - please note the sarcasm there - spinning chair and all that caloric hoo-hah. An abnormality on my left side, I was told. That was all. A diagnosis? Well, not really. Possibly Ménière's. But there was no hearing loss. 'Here is a prescription for Betaserc, sir.' And they sent me on my way.

It took me more than a year to get rid of the sensation of having a head full of wadded cotton. I felt insecure. Got tired quickly. I thought I would be stuck with it. But things improved - slooooowly, but still - over a period of months. When my internship put me in the ER, I had a couple of really bad nights, and then it was back again. That sense of spinning. Months passed. I read a lot, did a ton of research, made adjustments in my life. No alcohol - well, almost none. A regular routine, a steady rhythm, not too much stress. Finally decided to specialize in an area that would let me work regular hours, and after my year as an intern I went into occupational health medicine.

Less stress, doctor!

Things got better over the next few years. Occasional attacks. Sometimes I could feel them coming, sometimes not. Sometimes I came home after work and headed straight to bed because of the dizziness. After the umpteenth incident, I finally went to the University Hospital in Ghent for an MRI. My own idea. 'Well, it looks like Ménière's, but we are not sure. You will need to adjust your routine, get plenty of exercise. Less stress. Try Diamox, a diuretic.' And another battery of tests, including the caloric ones.

Years passed, and it was all here again, gone again. And of course the fear. The uncertainty. A touch of dizziness, and the fear would kick in. Was this another attack? No, not this time. Had it been a heavy week? Yeah, lots of emotion, lots of aggravation, that is probably it. And when I felt my neck go stiff, like a block of concrete, I knew an attack was on its way.

You really notice the increased sensitivity to noise during and after an attack – it's like you have got Superman's superhearing! Ordinary sounds were suddenly painful, and I jumped at every noise.

I went to an osteopath. The very next day, I had a major attack. I never went back, even though I knew he was a fine doctor – he is a personal friend of mine. But you don't go asking for trouble.

People just don't understand. You have no idea how many times I have had to explain what I go through. Nobody gets it. No, it's not psychosomatic, and I am not crazy. 'You mean Meunière, like the sauce?' 'No, it's *Ménière*.' 'Ah, well, never heard of it.' 'Is he back in bed again?'

When I have an attack, I think, *This can't last forever, can it? I will survive?* For the next few days, I walk on eggshells. No stress, no coffee – which by the way I am practically addicted to. I roll the wrong way in bed, my eyes go into nystagmus, and there we are again. Shit. A few days' rest, and I can start moving normally.

You want a piece of me?

These days, I sometimes move the wrong way on purpose. Pure orneriness on my part. *You want a piece of me, dizziness?* Well, come and get me! It's like I am daring an attack to begin. And even though the world spins around me for a while, afterwards there's often a kind of relief. I believe you have to test your vestibular system at times like this - within reason, of course. In the middle of an attack, it's basically pointless.

For the last two years, I have been doing a lot of sports. It seems to make my dizziness milder. It's still there, but sport allows me to cope with my daily stress. On top of the reduction in that spinning sensation, I have got more energy. I don't get tired as quickly. It seems clear that stress and exhaustion play a part in my condition.

So I fight against my dizziness. Try to, at least. I look forward to the moment when my head starts to pound. That often means the dizziness is on its way out. But there is so much uncertainty in the wake of an attack. I generally try to give myself two days' rest before I go back to work. And I am often still not fully recovered.

The worst thing is that it's never completely gone. You just have to learn to live with it. If you could, you would cut your own vestibular nerve to make it stop. I understand what Van Gogh must have gone through. Last year I had two really bad attacks, right before summer vacation. I was going through a difficult situation at work, and I was dead tired and extremely stressed out. Right now it's happening again. So I am suffering the dizzy spells more often. I probably ought to lecture about dizziness. I know from the inside how the condition operates. I have been living with it for thirteen years.

Out, out, damned diagnosis!

For years, I was convinced that mine wasn't a typical case of Ménière's. There was no hearing loss. It was a different pattern. More and more, I found myself thinking it had to be something else. To put it crudely, I felt that the diagnoses I was getting were crap. Tania - suggesting the possibility of misdiagnosis - put me in touch with Professor Wuyts two years ago. I decided to screw my courage to the sticking place and, for the first time in years, get another professional opinion. I will not deny that I was nervous, but there I sat in the waiting room. It was strange to be the patient for once, instead of the doctor.

After an intake consultation and some additional tests, the professor told me that what I have is *not* Ménière's, but a type of vestibular migraine. This may seem strange, but my attacks of dizziness are not always paired with headache.
I sometimes experience a serious headache right *after* the attack, but not always. Often, the attacks are brought on by exhaustion and stress. Other triggers include cigarette smoke and strong perfume. What the professor told me matched perfectly my experience of the past – at that moment - thirteen years. Another point is the phonophobia, the fear of noise, which I have during an attack.
So, after all these years, my condition was finally correctly identified. Although it's true that I will have to go on living with my affliction, there is a sort of relief in at least knowing at long last what it *is*. I stopped taking betahistines and eventually went on a beta blocker instead. But I had to give that up because of my asthma.
I took flunirazine, a calcium blocker, as an experimental therapy. Today, I take no mediction anymore.

Carry on regardless

My main purpose in writing this personal history is to show that even a physician can be confronted with a chronic problem he is unable to resolve on his own. For years I searched for a proper diagnosis and a possible solution. I was helped by medication and exercise, and I tried as best I could to reduce the level of stress in my life.

Many specialists are conducting research into the vestibular system. But dizziness remains a symptom with an assortment of possible underlying causes, and this makes diagnosis and treatment challenging. Still, I encourage physicians, specialists and researchers to continue their efforts to diagnose and treat patients who present with dizziness. Don't just send them home with a bottle of pills. Don't underestimate the seriousness of their condition. Take the time to find out what their symptoms are, so you can send the patients along to someone in a position to help them.

I also want to emphasize to my fellow sufferers that, even if you have been wrestling with dizziness for years, it may be advisable to seek out a second opinion if you are not sure you have been properly diagnosed. Don't give up, and don't ignore your uncertainty. It took me thirteen years to feel better, but I finally got a correct diagnosis - and so, I hope, can you.

— David De Keukeleire, occupational health physician and dizziness patient
West Flanders, Belgium

Note from Tania

By the time the English edition of Dizzy Me is being published, David has experienced no more vertigo attacks for more than a year. He found the love of his life and is convinced he has less stress to deal with, now that he is settled and happy again. Sports still play an important role to remain happy and healthy. He takes no more medication.

SHARI

Thirteen and dizzy.

I am Shari, and as I write this I am twenty years old. When I was thirteen, there were days I could not even get out of bed. I had terrible dizzy spells accompanied by vomiting.

My family doctor diagnosed me with Ménière's disease. I had all the symptoms, but I was actually too young to have the condition. They could not come up with any other explanation, though, and they put me on a betahistine. When I had an attack and took the pills, it took three weeks for the symptoms to go away. Even if I took the medicine year round, I still had the symptoms at regular intervals.

In Flanders, schoolkids have to get a medical exam basically every other year in what is called a Pupil Guidance Center. When I went for mine in middle school, they found I had significant hearing loss in my right ear. It did not really bother me, and I did not think anything needed to be done about it. But after a few years, the attacks got worse - and so did my hearing. We made an appointment with an ENT specialist. It turned out there was something wrong with my eardrum. First the doctor thought there was fluid trapped behind it. She tried to drain it, but that did not work, so she decided to do a scan.

The next day, the doctor called to discuss the results. She thought there was more going on than Ménière's disease and referred me to Professor Officiers at the Sint Augustinus Hospital in Wilrijk, and he felt my condition was serious enough to pass me on to Dr. Van Dinter.

It might be a tumor

They rushed me right in for an MRI, and that showed that I had a cholesteatoma. It wasn't cancer, but it was a skin cyst that was attacking my eardrum from the inside. That was affecting my ossicles and had resulted in a hole in my eardrum.

After a long intake interview about my medical history, they concluded that the ear infections I had had as a baby had possibly caused the tumor. I have had bad allergies my whole life, and that is what was making me dizzy. Every time I had an allergic reaction, my sinuses puffed up. They pressed against the tumor, and *it* in turn pressed into my vestibular organ. The result was dizziness - which had been incorrectly diagnosed as Ménière's.

Operation!

So I had to have surgery. It was about an eight-hour operation, and it involved giving me a new eardrum, fixing my ossicles, and getting rid of the tumor. They also had to widen my ear canal, which was too narrow.

The doctor could not promise me my hearing would return to normal but *did* guarantee that the dizziness would go away. Recuperation should normally take a month, but in my case it took three months.

When you have a tumor, you have to go in for a checkup every year at first, and then later every three years and eventually once every five years. It's now almost six years since my surgery. My hearing is better than they thought it would be. The dizziness is gone, and I am completely cured. I do have to go in for the checkups, to make sure the tumor is not growing back, and to clean my ear canal. But otherwise I have been restored to a normal life.

— Shari
Flemish Brabant, Belgium

Note from Tania

After six years, Shari suddenly got a new vertigo attack in September 2015, which kept her sick for a week. She went to the doctor and he said the tumor had not come back. Probably it was BPPV. With good medical care she would get rid of that. In 2016 she went back to the doctor: the tumor had started growing again. It will be followed-up. Thumbs up for her please!

VIV

I have a 'to-do' list and a 'DON'T-do' list for movement.

I was fortunate to get a proper diagnosis quickly, without extensive balance testing. I had BPPV. My first attack was terrifying. I had it in both ears simultaneously. The first two days, I can't even describe how difficult it was. It's like the Earth is a supermagnet pulling you down at warp speed. An uncontrollable feeling of falling. You hardly dare move a muscle. After that first attack, though, I just went on with my life.

The second time, I started asking myself questions. It was not as bad as the first incident: my world spun, but there wasn't that sense of a supermagnet. An examination revealed that, this time, it had only affected one of my ears. I instinctively began to protect myself. I categorized movements as either 'okay to do' or 'not okay'. Over the next few occurrences, I got to know a wide range of types of attack: heavy, medium heavy, light, with or without vomiting, one ear or both, many other manifestations. I gradually came to realize that this wasn't normal, and that I needed help. When you're in the middle of an attack, you just hope it'll be over soon.

After a while, I found that I could not just casually pick up the threads of my life in the wake of an attack. In the beginning, I had maybe one or two incidents a year, each lasting a week or so, but this gradually increased to three to four times a year, and each attack lasted longer. As the occurrences became more frequent and more intense, I began consulting other doctors. What if my original diagnosis and treatment wasn't correct? But I found myself going around in circles. I kept winding up back with my first doctor, who seemed the most competent at running me through the maneuvers that helped me deal with my condition. He taught me the Dix-Hallpike test, the Semont and Epley maneuvers, and the Brandt-Daroff exercises, so that I could perform them myself, without assistance. Sometimes they worked, but other times they made the attacks even worse. If it was a two-ear attack, or an unusually intense one, I could not even work myself into position to *attempt* the maneuvers. I had to wait a few days for the acute phase to pass, and then - with great fear - begin the maneuvers.

The unknown

It's striking that this condition is so little known. The various different ways of executing the maneuvers illustrates the spotty state of the medical profession's knowledge. Some physicians are truly interested in learning more, while others write off the condition as psychosomatic and nothing more than a reaction to stress. Still others see it as a minor inconvenience that will disappear if you swish your head back and forth; they don't even take the *position* of the head into account. You can see in your friends' and acquaintances' eyes that they are convinced you are exaggerating. But they are not there during those first few days of an attack, when you lie there, a pitiful lump of misery. You can tell them your tale of woe maybe once or twice. After that, you are on your own - no one wants to listen to the same sad story over and over again.

Living with a time bomb

Those years were incredibly hard. It was like I was living on top of a time bomb that could explode at any moment. Each new attack followed unexpectedly quickly on the heels of the previous one. The frequency increased to six to seven times a year, and the length of the attacks could be as long as eleven weeks. I was dizzy more than half of every year! Most of the attacks were severe; on several occasions, my doctor had to come out two days in a row to shoot me full of Primperan and Haldol, on the one hand to stop me from puking and on the other hand to reduce the severity and duration of the spinning.

The year 2009 is etched into my memory. I had already had four serious attacks. The last of them, in the autumn, totally turned me upside-down. It was a series of super-heavy attacks, the acute phase of one flowing right into the acute phase of the next.

My neurologist was perplexed. He could not do anything to turn the tide. I had a total of five major attacks in twelve days, followed by seven weeks of recovery, during which anything more than the smallest of movements - even things as simple as sitting up straight, lying down and bending over - would set off a new attack. There was a strange rolling sensation somewhere behind my right ear, inside my head. I had double vision and could not focus my gaze. My doctor dropped by time and time again to see how I was doing, without my even asking him to come. I can't take it any *more*, I screamed. I didn't want to go on living like this. Would my suffering never end?

I could not leave the house on my own, could not go to the drugstore, could not even visit a friend in my own neighborhood. I could not use public transportation, could not ride my bike, did not dare drive a car. Go grocery shopping by myself? No way! I was petrified of having another attack and being hauled off in an ambulance.

At work, they instituted safety precautions in case I had an attack. The corners of tables and desks and drawers were padded. If there wasn't someone in my office with me, I left the door open so I could call for help. I was on perpetual red alert - every slightest disruption in my balance sent me figuratively if not literally staggering. There was only one place I felt safe: on the ground.

A light at the end of the tunnel

So 2009 was the worst of my twenty years of balance disorders. Each attack imprisoned me for up to eleven weeks in an uncertain world. Filled with despair, I sank into a swamp of negative thoughts.

And then the Internet brought me in contact with Tania. She lit a flickering light at the end of the proverbial tunnel. She gave me hope for a literally more stable life. And at the same time she helped me to find a measure of peace. Peace because I had finally met someone who didn't dismiss my experience with a mere 'oh, that's not so bad' or 'you will get better.' She understood what I was going through - not just the physical limitations but also the psychic hell I lived in. My reality was recognized and acknowledged. There were lots of other people like me, I discovered, and each of them knew the same feelings of frustration, of powerlessness, of being marginalized and ridiculed.

Tania's story was almost exactly the same as mine. And for her there turned out to be a solution. On my doctor's and my fellow sufferers' advice, I contacted Tania's doctors and went through a series of tests.

And, yes, my situation was basically the same as hers, with one difference: I was afflicted in both ears. After a series of back-and-forth emails and while I was in a quiet phase, between attacks, I decided to get in touch both with Professor Wuyts and the ENT specialists Tania knew. Several visits and treatments later, my balance disruptions began to decrease, the severe attacks replaced by a smaller number of less serious ones. I wrote up my story for the first edition of her book - and I read the complete book when it came out.

Symptom-free at last!

Several years have gone by since then. In 2017, I celebrate my sixth anniversary of a symptom-free life. I am not exactly sure why the attacks became so much less severe after my *annus horribilis* of 2009 or why the last six years have been so completely stable. My balance disorder was correctly diagnosed when I had my very first attack, back in 1989, and I was treated repeatedly with the Epley or Semont maneuvers. The attacks kept coming back, though, sometimes afflicting one ear, sometimes both. Sometimes mild, sometimes extremely intense. So I can only guess at the reasons.

I see two possible explanations. One is that Professor Wuyts was the first person to apply the maneuvers properly, accompanied by constant vibration at the height of the mastoid bone. The other - which I also consider plausible - is that the attacks stopped when I hit menopause, which altered my hormonal balance, which perhaps in turn changed the composition of the viscous mass in which the crystals are located. That might allow the crystals to settle back in place more quickly, fast enough to prevent the onset of dizziness.

Who knows? For me, the most important thing is that my *world* has settled back into place. But it's also important to see a reference work like *Dizzy Me*, in which every patient can recognize herself and be acknowledged, that offers peace, advice, insight, and a release from fear.

A family affair

My balance disruptions have stopped, but there is clearly something wrong with my genes. I have passed a tendency for balance disorder on to my two daughters - who are thirty-one and thirty-two years old - and through them to my granddaughter ... although in her case the problems are thus far minimal and probably the result of an inner-ear infection. Both of my brothers have also had personal experience with balance issues.

My daughters are afraid they may eventually have to deal with the same physical and emotional problems their mother has lived through: the severe and frequent attacks, the feeling that their world can at any moment be turned upside down, the debilitating uncertainty. The scepticism I used to see in their eyes - Is mama exaggerating? *It can't really be that bad, can it?* - has been washed away by their own experience. Only now do they understand what I went through for all those years....

My brothers also seriously underestimated the impact of my attacks. Now I offer them the support they need and try to calm them down. I have taught them about the various types of attack and the various possible causes. I have explained that there is a really good reference work they can consult, and I have shown them *Dizzy Me*. Each of them wanted to read it, to learn more. So Tania's book has worked its way around my family. It has resonated with them, has given them insight. One of my co-workers has read it, too. Clearly, it's a book that is meeting a need.

Keep on keeping on

It can't stop with this one book, though. Our knowledge must continue to grow. Every day, medical science takes another step forward, a step toward greater insight. New and better treatments must be found and then shared with the world. Because there are thousands of people adrift on this same angry sea, and they need help.

— Viv
Limburg, Belgium

IRIS

Noise puts me on a roller coaster.

On July 5, 2002, I awoke to find the world spinning wildly around me, even when my eyes were closed. I could not sit up straight in bed, kept falling over to one side or the other. Over the phone, my doctor diagnosed me with vestibular neuritis and prescribed a histamine agonist. After this first attack, I soon realized that loud noise was the trigger that sent me off on an endless roller coaster ride. After any exposure to a racket, I needed time to recover.

Over the next few months, I saw several neurologists and ENT specialists, and they all sent me home with a well-intended but scornful 'the problem's *between* your ears, not *with* them'. Eight months after that first terrible attack, an ENT specialist finally told me that my oversensitivity to loud noises had a name: hyperacusis.

I eventually stopped looking for a doctor who could explain the cause of my hypersensitivity. Now, fifteen years later - unable to work because of the hyperacusis and several other chronic conditions - I have adapted, and I am able to enjoy the little things in life. After all these years, I am used to telling people that noise makes me dizzy. I am happy, I accept my limitations - but I would still like to know why I can't manage an evening out with friends, why I can't enjoy listening to music the way I used to. I think it's time for me to see Floris Wuyts....

— Iris
West Flanders, Belgium

DONIA

Mapping Donia's dizziness for a Donia 2.0.

Seasick

Buon giorno, my name is Donia, I am a fifty-five-years-old Italian lady living in Belgium and my story started about eleven years ago. It was a beautiful morning in early spring, March. I woke up with the morning sun and I immediately noticed that strange feeling in my head. I had a bad dream; I got on high sea in the middle of a seastorm. I woke up feeling very seasick. I felt horrible for half a day; I got over it in the afternoon, after a power nap.

Landsick

Only a few months later, I got that strange feeling again, while I was at work. I was very focused on my job, when suddenly I felt a twitch, right in the middle of my forehead. Imagine that feeling of an uncontrolled trembling eye... I got that same feeling on my forehead. Maybe it took only one nanosecond, but that twitch on the forehead made me lose control over my eyes and I ended up dizzy. I started sweating and feeling nauseous, but lucky me it was over in fifteen minutes. Despite that, I felt landsick the rest of the afternoon, feeling strange in my head - what we would call lightheadedness - and unstable on my feet. It worried me, so I went to see my GP that same evening. After a neurological check-up all seemed normal. He thought I was tired, stressed or experienced some hormonal issues.

Fit as a fiddle

'Why don't you do some sports', my doctor suggested me. So I decided to go for a 'start to run' at work. Sports would do me good. But no... The more effort I did, the more I tried, the more dizzy I became. I didn't tell anyone, because I blamed it on my condition. So I did all I could and ran those five kilometers. Well done

Donia! I continued my joggings and on sunday mornings I used to go for a five- to thirteen-kilometer walk. But every time I noticed that strange lightheadedness and pressure in both ears. After consultation of a sports doctor, a cardiologist and a neurologist, I was declared fit as a fiddle.

Being unbalanced

I must confess my parents had to move to a retirement home very unexpectedly; it was a very emotional period in my life. Add a job with a lot of responsability, leading a team of seven.

One year later, it was May 2007, I had a bad dream and woke up bathed in sweat. I wanted to turn on my left side, when suddenly vertigo hit. I had no control over my eyes, could not stand up, the room was spinning that bad, so I had to lay down again.

Second attempt to get up. The vertigo got even worse, with nausea and vomiting as a result. I panicked. My darling husband, who didn't know what to do, called my GP. The doctor told me my vestibular organ was out of balance because of a cold or the flu. Oh yes, probably he was right; for weeks I had been fighting a cold and it didn't get any better. He prescribed Agyrax for the nausea and the vomiting and sent me straight to the physiotherapist. Maybe the physiotherapist could try to free me with a manoeuvre, in case I would have 'some cristals floating around in the semicircular canals of my inner ear'… [note of Dizzy Me: he is suggesting another probable diagnosis: BPPV.] After one week of therapy and rest, I was ready to go back to work.

Calming myself down

Unfortunately, each time I moved, I noticed I got unstable and I experienced that lightheadedness again and again. And that happened to me each time I had to bend over or when I read a book. Going to the supermarket was a challenge... Each time I had to reach out to get something on top of the shop rack, my world started spinning. I got nauseous, I began to feel hot and cold, and very anxious of what would happen next.

I started to calm myself down, and whispered to myself 'come on, this will pass, don't overreact'. It always just turned out I didn't leave my shopping cart, each time I kept undergoing this... I did not dare to share my problem with anyone, because I was convinced I was only making this up, I thought it was all between my ears, this was the result of emotions and stress.

Calling the ambulance

This game went on for weeks with ups and downs, until in June that same year. The day my sister turned fifty and gave a birthday party, it all went completely wrong. I woke up in the morning, and when I turned to the left the room started spinning. I could not stand up; if I tried lying on my back, the spinning sensation got even worse. My eyes went in nystagmus and I lost all control.

Extreme nausea made me vomit, I could not eat, nor drink some water. I spent three days in bed like that, and then I got extreme headaches on top of that. My husband was desperate and called the ambulance. This was my first stay at the hospital. I underwent several tests and scans, but everything seemed to be normal. They told me my vestibular organ was out of balance because of a viral infection of the nose. The neurologist suggested it could be hormonal too, and hyperventilation, nothing to worry about. Three days later I was sent home, cured as they said.

Find excuses

For months I tried to survive with that feeling of unstability; every time I did an effort, I got dizzy, when I took the car, I got carsick, when I went to the cinema, I had to leave early because it made me sick… I can go on giving you examples. I lost weight, lost my *joie de vivre*, I was anxious all the time of what was to come next and scared to change my head position. If I kept reading too long it was hell, if I looked down I got sick. I felt weakened and barely dared to enjoy life. Leaving my house was an ordeal, taking the car, no way. So I was finding excuses all the time so I could stay home and safe. I got sick while watching fast moving images on TV... The next vertigo attack was just waiting around the corner.

Betting on a diagnosis

Two months later. Another vertigo attack. I decided to take the lead in the management of my own health and to consult an ENT specialist. That man prescribed me diuretics; in his opinion the dizziness was the result of a fluid accumulation in the inner ear, caused by a viral nose infection.

The drugs didn't get the vertigo under control. On the contrary, they gave me palpitations. The vestibular tests didn't make us any wiser. Nothing particular to be noticed. So he thought it could be migraine. And he prescribed Sibelium 25 mg. The only result was that I got less nausea attacks. I could eat again and regain some weight. A few consults later I was told he didn't know what could be wrong with me and that he couldn't help me anymore. He sent me to the physiotherapist. Many months and sessions later I got another vertigo attack, this time at the physiotherapist. She called a friend of her, being an ENT specialist. They discussed my case and a few days later I was invited for a consult. Several MRI scans of the brain, cerrebellopontine angle, the inner ear... Everything seemed normal. What a relief! But that didn't solve my health issues. A second vestibular test revealed I had a slight deviation in the inner ear, caused by a viral infection, as the doctor explained. He assumed that was the reason why I developed Ménière's syndrome. He suggested to start the Ménière's therapy immediately: 3 Betaserc 16 mg tablets a day. Finally a name for my disease. A few weeks later I started to feel better. No more heavy vertigo, just the lightheadedness, but I could live with that. I could breathe and live again, and I was relieved it wasn't between my ears as many people suggested. But I noticed stress was a trigger, so I did everything to reduce that stress, and stress management did help me to get a bit better. Even the lightheadedness was dissapearing.

Visual trigger

Another issue... July 2009 the doctor said my bad eyes could be a trigger. Having a diopter of -8.25 L and -9.25 R, he could be right of course. So I went to the ophthalmologist. It was a very nice professor who told me right after the tests there was nothing wrong with my eyes. In his opinion I suffered from migraine. After a laser treatment of my eyes in September 2009 I thought 'all right, another trigger has been solved'.

My fault?

Each time I went for a consult, every 3 months, I heard that same stress, hormones and migraine story. But actually no one was able to help me or give me a decent explanation. As it's almost impossible to live a life without stress, I started to do breathing excercices; I was convinced I developed chronic hyperventilation and blamed it on fear. I did yoga for two years. I handled each possible trigger, tried meditation, went on retreat – that was in February 2011, 1 month after my mother died – and looked for a less stressy job. Despite all my efforts and the medication, I didn't manage to become vertigo-free. Okay, it occured less frequently, and I stopped fighting it; I just underwent it. Fighting this disorder took a lot of my energy. I was so tired! The more I tried to rest, the worse it got. I started taking supplements and those did actually help me to get better.

Mapping my dizziness

I managed to get a clear overview on my dizziness. The vertigo mostly hits when I wake up, very often when I turn to the right after lying on my back. Only occasionally when I turn to the left. When it happens during the day, then it's because of a sudden change of head position, or because I was bending or leaning over. And in most cases I feel that twitch followed by uncontrolled eye movements, with heavy dizziness as a result. And this always happens to me in spring and autumn, after having a bad cold.

Keep on guessing

I always had the idea it wasn't Ménière's. That is the reason why in November 2011, I went to consult Dr. Vincent Van Rompaey, ENT specialist at UZA Antwerp. Another battery of vestibular tests in January 2012, causing nausea for three days. Scans revealed it isn't Ménière's. My new diagnosis is called vestibular migraine.

Now I must avoid CATS: no more aspartame, light products, light drinks, coffee and tea. I changed my diet immediately. After trying two Bètablockers, with horrible side effects and many bad episodes later, I have had it. I got tired again, exhausted, lost all energy.

I lost all hope and concluded for myself I was just one of those many patients where no one could tell what was wrong with us. Even the doctors could only guess, so one day I gave up the search for a better health. I gave up my job in April 2012 because stress was a trigger to me...

January 2014, I still experience about two bad episodes a year. Usually one in spring and one in autumn. I must try not to get a bad cold for a longer period; that is usually when the dizzy monster shows up.

Just because of my rhinosinusitis causing dizziness, my local ENT specialist decided to go for a surgery; in February 2014 I got septoplasty and a sinus rinse. After surgery I was given cortisone, making me more stable on my feet, like I used to be years ago! Of course, it is not a good idea to take cortisone for longer periods, as the ENT specialist warned me... What a pity!!

Dizzy Me shows me the way

Thanks to Tania and her book *Dizzy Me* a new world has opened up to me. I read I am not the only one with this problem. Many patients are dealing with the same issues like a long search for a right diagnosis and a cure or decent treatment. They have mostly tried several treatments before having any result. Thanks to the book I got many answers. And the SO STONED checklist finally made me understand I am not a Ménière's patient. I think I got a mixed or multi-vestibular disorder, but this is way too complex for me. Tania suggested me to go to the UZA for another consult, with the assistance of Prof. dr. Floris Wuyts, who knows… But no way I want to be sent home again with medication to try, and get even worse!

Fear takes away all my freedom

The fear to get worse holds me back to take a new initiative... Fear as a result of the games that dizzy monster is playing with me. Each time I start something, I panick 'what if I get dizzy again?' My liberty to operate gets smaller and smaller. And that is unacceptable!

— Donia
Flemish Brabant, Belgium

Note from Tania

Donia celebrated her fifty-fifth birthday in the summer of 2016 and she was one of the six dizzy Deans & Donna's who finally went for an umptieth opinion on my advise. I joined them all that day, it was August 2016, on the same day I went to the UZA to support Richard.

It's been ten years now since Donia got dizzy, and she already got lots of opinions and diagnoses such as dizziness caused by a viral infection of the nose, BPPV, hyperventilation, something hormonal, Ménière's disease, migraine and vestibular migraine. She even landed in hospital, while having a bad vertigo episode.

New appointment, new hope. 'You are a complicated case', Wuyts said. While the four of those six patients got a quick diagnosis, she needed more tests in September and October, to confirm what is supposed to be her diagnosis, and to rule out other disorders mentioned before. A Donia 2.0... that would be a fabulous birthday gift!

And so she went back several times, to find out she has an extremely sensible right vestibular organ. The treatment? Get rid of the Betaserc and start ball sports. Today Donia plays badminton and even some football with her little grandson. In fact she was doing pretty well and felt a lot better without the medication and she felt a lot stronger while doing sports.

Sometimes it takes more than one appointment to get the exact diagnosis and even Floris can be wrong at first sight. That is normal. But it's the research attitude that makes the difference for a patient like Donia. Keep searching until there is no more doubt… It was January 2017, after three dizzy-free months, when suddenly another vertigo attack hit Donia again. I sent her to Floris Wuyts the next day. This time he could see clearly that Donia suffers from vestibular migraine on top of having a very sensitive vestibular organ. The vertigo also being the result of building down *the – in her case useless - Ménière's Betaserc prescription. Treatment? No new drug prescription, no more Betaserc and continue ball sports. Donia was not amused when she found out her GP had not even read the Dizzy Me book she gave him, not happy that he forced her the day before to start the Betaserc and build up from 3*16 Mg to 3*76 again, telling her she is nothing more than Floris' guinea pig. She will not accept this from a GP who doesn't get updated with the latest knowledge. And you know what? This is exactly what I was being told in 2007: I got misdiagnosis, I got wrong medication (being Betaserc) and I was given the same message that I was doctor shopping and only serving as someone's guinea pig. Well, who got cured? Who was wrong? Well done Donia!*

SONJA

Two decades in search of a proper diagnosis.

I am a sixty-two-year-old widow with two children and three grandchildren. My first attack came around my fortieth birthday. I went out to a restaurant with my family, and, the next morning, I was throwing up and dizzy. I thought it must have been something I ate, but I stayed nauseous and 'floaty' for two days. The only thing that gave me any relief was sitting straight up in bed. It was hard to move my head. My doctor sent me to the hospital. They gave me a stress test on a stationary bicycle for my heart and lungs, and an EEG. No diagnosis. They told me to start taking Betaserc.

Things got a little better - but a few months later I had another attack, worse than the first one. I was out of commission for longer. My doctor sent me to a neurologist, who referred me to an ENT specialist. Diagnosis: Ménière's disease. Treatment: more Betaserc.

It wasn't long before my next attack. Another ENT specialist tested me again… and put a drain in my ear. I had them take it back out. The attacks started coming more often. I finally saw a physiotherapist who specialized in vertigo, and then another physiotherapist who was able to reduce the pressure and tension in my ear with a needle in my neck. Then I started experiencing tinnitus in my right ear. I still have that today. Again, the diagnosis was Ménière's.

Another day, another expert

I know an aunt of Tania's, and she put me in touch with Floris Wuyts. Another battery of tests, the Epley maneuver, the spinning chair, hearing examinations… and now my diagnosis was Ménière's plus BPPV. Floris said that surgery wasn't an option for me. I went on taking the Betaserc.

And I continued looking for help. After CT scans and an MRI, a neurologist said I had BPPV and only that. Another neurologist told me it wasn't BPPV, wasn't

Ménière's, either. 'It's stress, madam. Your neck is completely stiff. Massages might help.' I tried alternative doctors. My spleen and small intestine were not functioning properly. Go on a lactose-free diet, I was told.

Blame it on the neck vertebrae

Eventually I wound up seeing Dr. Bockx in the Orthopedics and Traumatology Department at the Paul Brien Hospital in Schaarbeek. A test that involved poking my fingers and toes with needles showed that they were totally numb. And during or right after an attack I have rapid left-and-right eye movements, a phenomenon called nystagmus. Dr. Bockx explained that my symptoms matched those of Ménière's patients. So, more CT scans and an MRI of my neck. My CD-ROM collection kept growing… if only they were gold records!

In April 2013, Dr. Bockx operated on my neck vertebrae: disc disease at the C5-C6 level, with secondary neuroforaminal narrowing due to osteophyte formation. He replaced the intervertebral disc with an artificial one, held in place with screws. There was also narrowing at the C6-C7 level, and I took Hendronate in the hope of avoiding another surgery.

And then?

Although I felt some improvement, I stopped going to work. I had to spread my household chores out over longer periods of time. If I took the car to do some shopping, I often had to pull over for a while. Walking was also an issue. I could not handle loud parties. I avoided big stores with bright lighting. Vacations were a challenge. Maintaining social contacts and self-confidence - hard! And my family simply didn't understand what I was dealing with.

I had two mild attacks during which I felt a lot of pressure in both ears. I have been to a vestibular physiotherapist several times. When I got nystagmus in my eyes, I needed to sit on the swivel chair and focus my gaze on one point. The therapist then stopped the chair from spinning, and I had to report the moment I could feel that I stopped moving. That could take several seconds. When my pupils were different sizes, I was dizzy and more sensitive to light and sound. After she checked my eyes, she projected a quick series of shapes on the wall - cubes, circles - and I fixed my gaze on one point again. These exercises seemed to be helping, and the attacks were coming less frequently.

Six months after my surgery, my husband passed away. That was a terrible blow. But my self-confidence was growing every day, and I became more independent.

Some time ago I wound up seeing the Orthopedics and Traumatology Department again, because my neck was still blocked. Another MRI, more needles in legs and feet, showing my neural pathways at the leftside under my collarbone were interwoven. So I got another surgery in February 2016. That seemed to give result. When I go out or when I am nervous, sometimes I take Oxazepam (15 mg), but I am glad I can tell you I had no more vertigo attacks since my last surgery.

I don't have the life I want, but I have not given up.

— Sonja
Flemish Brabant, Belgium

VERONY

The Utermöhlen prism spectacles.

These glasses gave me part of my life back. After an awful number of incorrect diagnoses I finally, finally got the help I needed. Except, at the time - the day Dr. Visser measured me for the Utermöhlen spectacles - I didn't know that right away.

It was 1989. I was thirty-two. I had had my first serious attack when I was eighteen, on the last day of a seaside vacation. I was overtired, we thought, I had eaten something that disagreed with me. And so my search for help began.

The Story of Eye

I had a history of eye problems, so we thought the dizziness must have something to do with my eyes. I had already had several surgeries - since I was a child - to correct issues with my eye muscles. Since the last operation, things had gone downhill. I could feel it as soon as I came out of the anesthetic. Something was wrong. My head felt so strange. But that was impossible, they told me. My eyes were fine, and the surgery had been successful.

But the spinning sensation, the constant feeling of being in motion, the seasickness just got worse. I found an excellent doctor, but wound up so sick that something as simple as walking up a flight of stairs would knock me out for the rest of the day. Postpartum depression, they said. I wasn't emotionally capable of handling the responsibility of caring for a baby. But three years later I was still just as sick, and the doctors began to doubt my earlier diagnosis. My husband and I decided to take matters into our own hands, and - under the guidance of my eye doctor at that time - we started researching my condition.

Coincidentally, I stumbled across some information about the Dutch Foundation for Ménière's Patients. I got on the phone, and the woman I talked with told me about a special kind of glasses. I will never forget that conversation: everything she said sounded exactly like she was talking about my case. But my eye doctor read all the information they provided, and he was very sceptical.

Complaints combined

Despite that, I made an appointment with Dr. Visser, an ENT specialist in his late seventies. Actually, he was retired from practice, but he agreed to see me. The minute he began his examination, I realized this was different from what I had grown used to. The man knew *everything*! He looked at each of my symptoms as part of an organic entity. He talked about my eyes *and* my balance and how they influenced eachother, how things went wrong when both systems were sending faulty signals to the brain. He spent two hours with me and measured me for the Utermöhlen spectacles, gave me tests that were totally new to me, some of which had nothing to do with my eyes but instead with my balance and how balance and vision worked together. He told me I would be a new person in six weeks.

People began to notice a difference in me after only *three* weeks. I was walking more confidently, talking faster and more clearly. I noticed that I was sleeping better. After five weeks and four days, I woke up to the strangest sensation. I could not identify it at first. And then it hit me: the world was standing still! Now that nothing in my field of vision was unstable, I realized how much everything *had* been unstable in the past. But now the world around me had stopped spinning at last, even when I moved my head. People started telling me things they had held back from me before. Like, 'You know, you used to walk as if you were drunk.' I was so ashamed. But I got past that. At long last there was peace inside my head.

My eye doctor had to admit that the spectacles were working. He had been following my progress closely, and he saw the changes. It was not easy for him to acknowledge what was going on. If those spectacles really did what they seemed to be doing, he said, then there were fundamental errors in our understanding of the human eye. Ophthalmological knowledge would have to change.

Well, my life certainly changed! I still had certain limitations, but I had regained a part of my life.

'Mr. Gorbachev, tear down those walls!'

Now I am almost fifty-seven. It has only been two years since I got my diagnosis. Unfortunately, it was a rather complicated and not very pretty picture. Eyes, brains and balance: three different specialist fields, unfortunately still separated by thick walls. Every specialist looks at me from the perspective of his/her own area of knowledge. But given my reality, a single viewpoint was not going to be good enough to help me. *Au contraire.* Looking at my situation from a singular point of view - and in fact refusing to acknowledge the importance or even *existence* of other points of view - resulted in poor decisions being made. And that led to irreparable damage. I live with the consequences of those bad decisions every day, and they are not easy to deal with. To survive, I have had to educate myself, to search for answers on my own. I have studied all three fields, and thank God I have come across two wonderful doctors willing to see the full picture. Because of that, my life today is at least bearable.

I still wear my Utermöhlen spectacles. Don't confuse them, by the way, with the prism glasses some eye doctors prescribe - those don't have anything to do with balance, and in some cases they can make things worse, not better. My spectacles - when correctly prescribed - allow me to maintain a measure of balance. Over the last thirty-five years, they have helped many people with problems similar to mine. I try to convince as many people as possible of their value. But the walls that separate the specialist fields still stand. Eye doctors, ENT doctors and neurologists go right on ignoring the potential benefits offered by the Utermöhlen spectacles. It's understandable, I suppose, since none of their fields are broad enough to allow them to see the interconnections with the other two.

Research, sí! Sectarianism, no!

'People with Ménière's disease are victims of the medical world's sectarianism,' a very knowledgable professor said recently. And I know that I have been victimized by exactly that sectarianism. It angers me to see things continue this way. History goes right on repeating itself, and that makes me mad… and impatient. I want to help wake people up. I want to make those different specialists work together for the benefit of their patients. We need to do more research into the effectiveness of the Utermöhlen system, to give it the scholarly underpinnings it needs. People need to take this unconventional treatment seriously. It's not an instantaneous 'magic bullet', but it allows people like me to live more bearable lives.

PS: For thirty-five years, I have been told by orthoptists and ophthalmologists that the Utermöhlen system uses large prisms and causes damage to the eye muscles. But the truth is that the Utermöhlen system uses much *smaller* prisms than the orthoptists and ophthalmologists use themselves, specifically in order to produce a better integration between eyes, balance, and brain. This is the #1 misunderstanding that I would like to help correct.

— Verony Manders
Limburg, The Netherlands

WABIPS (Utermöhlen spectacles)

Hypothesis for understanding the possible beneficial effects of prism therapy
Subtracting the retinal motion signal from an internal reference signal

– by Dr Eric Vente, Utermöhlenstichting

The hypothesis for understanding the possible beneficial effects of prism therapy, arises from knowledge about the mechanism used by the brain to maintain a percept of a stable non-moving world during eye and head movements that cause images of the world to sway across the retinae. In a formal sense thismechanism can be conceptualized as a subtraction of two signals: a retinal signal, encoding the retinal image movement, is subtracted from a reference signal, encoding how the eyes and head move (latency and gain internal code). Only a difference between these two signals, scaled to perceived distance, can generate a perception of motion. Normally, if a retinal image movement is caused by an eye or head movement, the two signals are equal and their difference is zero,[1] so no motion is perceived and the world remains perceptually stable. Conversely, real motion is only perceived when the two signals differ, because that difference corresponds to the extent to which the brain cannot attribute retinal image motion to eye or head movements (see Wertheim[2] for a detailed review of the literature describing this mechanism). The relevant point here is that if there is a vestibular deficit, as in Ménière's disease (MD), the reference signal which encodes the eye and head movements may be incorrect. If so, an unwanted difference with the retinal signal would occur, causing a loss of perceptual stability of the visual environment and a distortion of motion perception when real motion must be perceived. That, in turn, may cause dizziness and balance problems. By affecting the position and motion characteristics of retinal images, prism spectacles might change the retinal signal such that its difference with the incorrect reference signal is reduced. In addition, as mentioned earlier, base-in prism spectacles affect the optical information for distance. Since to obtain perceptual stability, the differences between the two signals are scaled to perceived distance, prismatically induced changes in perceived distance could somehow contribute to making motion perception more veridical. These factors may improve both perceptual stability of the world around us and perception of real motion, concurrent with eye and head movements,

thus reducing the risk of dizziness and balance problems. One attractive aspect of this theory is that it does not relate to presumed eye movement deviations caused by MD, which fits our lack of findings with respect to optometric parameters.[3]
A complicating factor in the application of weak asymmetric base-in prisms (WABIPs) in MD results from the simple observation that ENT doctors generally do not prescribe spectacles, whereas eye doctors generally do not treat MD patients. Moreover, from an ophthalmologic point of view especially the weakness of the prisms can be doubted as well as the phenomenon of habituation to, or 'eating up' prisms.[4] Yet, it should be reckoned that these objections relate to ophthalmologic disorders, while the WABIPs as explained here typically concern a vestibular disorder We conclude that the fact that the treatment itself is relatively simple, non-invasive, low-cost and has a high degree of patient acceptance, and there is support from the literature for a working mechanism as reported , speak in favor of further studies on the effectiveness and working mechanism of WABIPs in MD.

1. http://www.nature.com/nature/journal/v389/n6653/full/389849a0.html
2. Wertheim, AH. Motion perception during self-motion: the direct versus inferential controversy revisited. Behavioral and Brain Sciences 1994;17:293-355.
3. de Wit G, Vente PEM, Bos EJ, Bles W. Het snelle labyrint ten dienste van het trage oog. Ned Tijdschr KNO-Heelk 1999;5:7-10.
4. Campos EC, Catellani T. Further evidence for the fusional nature of the compensation (or 'eating up') of prisms in concomitant strabismus. Int Ophthalmol. 1978;1:57-62.

Notes from Tania

- *Dr. Vente in the Netherlands is specialized in reduction of vertigo symptomatology with chronic use of weak asymmetric base-in prism spectacles (WABIPS) in vestibular migraine patients. Today, WABIPS is the new name of what we used to call Utermöhlen spectacles.*

- *Verony helped many people by explaining the principles of overstimulation of the brain by multiple stimuli. First people have to introduce stimulis-free periods to give the system a chance to rest, recover and reset. Because compromised balance can lead to overstimulation:*

- o *Compromised balance causes incorrect information to be sent to the brain. The brain - and other parts of the body which play a role in balance - constantly have to make corrections and compensations for this inaccurate data. As a result, our brains, ears, eyes and balance system wind up overstimulated, overloaded, and overtired.*

- o *Poor hearing, tinnitus and hyperacusis also cause overstimulation and exhaustion. Another consequence can be sleep issues - and such people generally need extra sleep to rest their overburdened systems.*

- o *In addition to other symptoms, overstimulation of the brain causes exhaustion, reduced ability to concentrate, memory loss, compromised coordination, speech difficulties, and increased sensitivity to stimuli. This happens because the overstimulated, overloaded brain becomes less able to manage cognitive functions and coordination. In some cases - such as instability and exhaustion, for example - extra stimuli cannot be properly processed.*

- o *Introducing stimulus-free periods into your routine gives your brain, eyes, ears and balance system a chance to rest. They can recover and 'reset' themselves.*

- o *Stimuli that can trigger the problems discussed here include sound, light, TV, radio, computer, laptop, tablet, cell phone, reading, talking, physical activity, and stress. This can vary with the individual.*

Please be aware that the purpose of all this is not to become an invalid person laying down all day for the rest of your lives, but to become stable and ready to take the next step: building up again, always taking into account your individual situation.

- *Just like me, Verony has always been there for everyone. Nobody could maintain that pace forever. One-way engagement has been the death knell for many worthy projects. And Verony's thirty-five years of experience are far too valuable to get lost in people's heads. That is why she started a facebook page* 'Eerlijk over Evenwicht' *- which means the truth and nothing but the truth abouth balance - in order to share this information... This change of strategy will give her some peace, and allow her to focus her time and energy on furthering our cause. Curious?* https://www.facebook.com/eerlijk.over.evenwicht/

ROB

Letter of disbelief: IMAGINE...

A while ago I wrote this letter, because I felt the need to shout out my disbelief about the way medicine keeps relying on the knowledge of thirty years ago, when diagnosing and treating dizzies.

Note from Tania

Rob wrote this letter after having been informed by dizzy patients, telling us they attented an information session in the Netherlands, where an expert (ENT) gave a presentation based on very outdated knowledge. The infosession was organized in 2015, by a well-known organization who raises awareness on vestibular disorders. Why outdated? The event was organized to give an update about Ménière's disease. The presentation on Ménière's disease was quite okay, but the organization did make a huge mistake by only covering vestibular disorders having a link with hearing loss. They are not familiar nor up-to-date about the other category of vestibular disorders. I contacted them several times as Dizzy Me, asking them to widen their horizon and start by at least mentioning the list of vestibular disorders where patients don't suffer from hearing loss. This is so important, because spreading only a part of the existing knowledge leads to even more misinformation and misdiagnosis. I offered them free books several times in order to raise awareness. I contacted the organization again as Dizzy Me a few weeks before the event took place, begging them again not to isolate Ménière's disease from other vestibular disorders at the event and to mention at least the list of disorders. I sent them two free-to-use and up-to-date presentations. Hard work, no result. I was very disappointed when I received the slides of the PowerPoints from my dizzy friends; they had not changed since 2009. Although I was happy to find that Dr. Vente did make use of some of my slides in his presentation. But what can we do more to finally wake them up?

Rob continues:

Last week Dizzy Me posted a message about the same way publishers are acting and how they think and select their 'books with potential'. Reading the answer of one of those publishers to her book proposal, I got that same feeling again. Here is my letter:

Imagine…

(Dear Verony, I hope you don't mind I have written this.)

Imagine you were not allowed to use the knowledge and computer/ICT and internet revolution of the past thirty years!!! How would you feel about that, how would the world feel about that…

Imagine if a cardiologist suddenly would have to carry out his surgeries based on the knowledge of thirty years ago... Would his patient survive?

Imagine if your oncologist would tell you 'Oh no, dear patient, I can only treat you based on the knowledge, research methods and medicine of thirty years ago.' Because that knowledge suddenly disappeared or I am not in the mood to use it today. Really? Could that be possible?

How come that so many doctors working in the field of ENT or dizziness are not ashamed they do actually keep operating like that day after day?

When I saw that presentation of that ENT specialist in 2015... This could have been 1990! So I could not stop myself from writing this.

Thirty years ago my wife Verony and I started our own long search to find out the cause of and a cure for her dizziness. What a relief I got her out of that hospital, what a relief we were able to stop the useless and dangerous medication, what a relief we kept searching for ourselves and did not believe the doctor straight away.

We were lucky we found out about Ménière's and very lucky we finally ended up in doctor Visser's office and in the care of doctor Vente. Our life, Verony's, mine, the life of our family, having two little children, became acceptable again step by step.

Of course we were hurt deep inside: especially Verony by those many eye surgeries, disabled for the rest of her life. But we found some peace. This happened thirty years ago.

But today we are 2016! I can't believe my eyes and ears, noticing that eye specialists, ENT specialists, GP's and an organization raising awareness on vestibular disorders still don't put their heads together to bring change, and still not manage to get up-to-date.

I get frustrated when Vente cannot be heard yet with all the expertise he has got. But I keep hoping. I get frustrated when doctors feel too high and mighty to talk to patient/ambassadors and when people tell us we should only respect doctors because they are doctors…

When they carry out needless surgeries, when they prescribe needless or wrong medication, when they say 'Just go for a walk, it's between your ears, get over it,' that is not a diagnosis. That does not make him or her a good doctor.

This is why I admire Tania Stadsbader, Floris Wuyts and my wife Verony of course. Day after day they try to break the silence and become changemakers in medicine by shedding light on balance. If we all help them, people will finally be able to learn about the latest knowledge and misdiagnosis will become some bad memory of the past.

IMAGINE…

— Rob Manders
Limburg, The Netherlands

JOOP

It was a miracle. I could walk again, the way I used to!

My name is Joop. I am seventy years old. In 2001, I contracted a bacterial infection while traveling abroad. I returned to The Netherlands and was admitted to the hospital. I became very sick, with a high fever.

They treated me with a massive dose of antibiotics. Because of that, my vestibular organ was destroyed, and I suffered significant hearing loss. But we only realized that later on. I spent almost eight years going from doctor to doctor. No one could figure out what was wrong with me. They said I was 'weak'. I finally got to see Professor Kingma. I was walking very poorly by then, as if I was drunk, and I had become dependent on my wife and children. It was Professor Kingma who told me about the damage to my vestibular organ. My whole life came to a standstill.

Brace yourself

But the professor had developed an artificial balance brace, and he allowed me to try it. It was a miracle: I could walk again, just the way I used to! When I am not wearing it, I am like a drunkard. But with it, I can drive a car and do things without help. I have my old life back.

— Joop Doornkamp
Limburg, The Netherlands

Note from Tania

Joop and Dr. Herman Kingma were interviewed together on the Dutch television program Good Afternoon, Limburg. During that broadcast, it was mentioned that high doses of antibiotics can in fact damage a patient's hearing and balance system. The way the balance brace works was demonstrated by showing a film of Joop walking both with and without his brace.

At the moment the team of Kingma (Maastricht, the Netherlands) is working on a vestibular implant (next-generation brace, being developed and tested in cooperation with Genève), but it is too soon to speak of any successful outcome. To be continued! And the brace? That is a vibrotactile device giving balance cues to the patient, currently being used in research projects and not commercially available. That's a pity!

LIESBETH

Ping-pong diagnoses.

I am thirty-four and, until recently, I was a lively, enterprising woman. In late July of 2014, I had just begun a new job as editor-in-chief of *Plotsdoof*, a magazine published by the Sudden Deafness and Adult-Onset Deafness Foundation in the Netherlands. Between a pile of other information, I found a book titled *Dizzy Me*. That interested me. I know that dizziness is often reported by people who have problems with their hearing, cochlea, vestibular organ, or ossicles. All those tiny little elements inside our ears.

The usual diagnosis is either Ménière's disease or a virus in the vestibular organ, and most ENT doctors look no further than those two possible causes. My husband once found himself unable to move without throwing up. 'You are either suffering from positional vertigo or an infection of the vestibular organ,' the doctor told him. 'There is really nothing we can do for you.'

But seriously, folks...

Unfortunately, I have been wrestling with my own balance issues and spinning vertigo since April 2014. Since I also have hearing problems, Ménière's disease was immediately suspected. I had the usual examination by an ENT specialist and answered the usual questions about my medical history, and, since I was also experiencing facial pain, I had an MRI to check my auditory nerve and rule out a possible neurinoma. Once that had been excluded, it was decided that hyperventilation was the culprit, and I was referred to a physical therapist. That diagnosis just seemed so *wrong* to me, though. I felt insulted, like my complaints were not being taken even remotely seriously.

I wanted to have a copy of *Dizzy Me* at home. Not that I could read it, since my dizziness made reading impossible. The lines of print blurred into each other, the words danced crazily on the page. In connection with my job, I did a joint interview with Tania Stadsbader and Floris Wuyts. That turned out to be the last bit of work I was able to complete before becoming too ill to continue functioning.

Dizzy Me had an enormous influence on me, and I was inspired by Tania's determination. Thanks to her, I understand how important it is to share our knowledge. After fifteen years of struggle, Tania has happily recovered from her complaint, but she continues to fight to help others receive proper diagnosis and treatment. Together with Floris Wuyts - her 'partner in crime' - she pushes for more research into and awareness of vertigo, of dizziness in all its forms. What gets me is the scope of the problem: we know so much, but there is so much we still *don't* know. And there are so many people who simply cannot function due to these debilitating symptoms.

What exactly is the cause of *my* condition? That remains a riddle for now. Like Verony - whose story precedes mine in this new edition of *Dizzy Me* - I have had several previous eye surgeries. Is that what has compromised my balance? Or could it be MS, a possibility that has the doctors picking petals off a daisy and chanting, 'It's MS, it's not MS'? It's all very confusing. The doctors have prescribed a cocktail of various medications, and all they have done is make things worse.

For two years now, I have been confined to bed. I am so unstable, so subject to attacks of spinning dizziness, that I cannot even walk with my eyes open. If I dare to try, I become horribly nauseous and lose my balance. I can't walk without assistance, and of course I can't ride a bike. I can't read, can't watch television because of the moving images and the bright, flickering lights. I can't work. I guess I am 'lucky' I don't have children to take care of. Because this condition turns your whole world literally upside down. And not just *your* world, but your partner's, and everyone else you are close to.

A normal person in a crazy world

In 2015, I spent more than four months in a Dutch hospital. In the absence of an accurate diagnosis, I found myself someplace where I really didn't belong: first in a geriatric ward, and then in a psychiatric ward. I wasn't crazy, they assured me. The idea was to wean me off my medications and prepare me for an examination by the professor who cured Tania. But I just got sicker there. It was obvious the staff didn't know what to do with me. After talking with Tania, I spent two days in Antwep in Belgium, where a multidisciplinary team re-evaluated my medical records. I underwent testing, and Floris explained to me that, nowadays, the biggest problem is overmedication as a result of misdiagnosis. I returned to the hospital in the Netherlands, and in September 2015 I went back for more ENT and neurological testing in Antwerp. After testing at ENT, Wuyts told me 'vestibular there is nothing wrong. The problem is to be found on a neurological level.' He also told me, if I want to get better, I should get rid of that medication cocktail. But we ended up stuck at neurologist, as we still didn't make progress in getting a diagnosis or in getting a decent follow-up treatment. Eventually, I hope we will get a complete picture and be able to help me get better. But I am still waiting and fighting my symptoms today…

We are family

Meanwhile, *Dizzy Me* has become a 'thing.' Over and above the sharing of valuable information, the Dizzy Me community has become a lifeline for me. When I hear about someone else's experience and find myself thinking, *that sounds so familiar*, or when I have trouble putting what I am going through into words but other members of the community just *get* it, anyway - you have no idea how helpful that is. I get e-mails and letters from people I have never met, but we 'know' each other, thanks to *Dizzy Me*. The support, the sense of connection, is amazing, and it does me a world of good - it's a literal lifeline that gives me a smile and lightens my load.

— Liesbeth Duits – *hearme2.com*
Gelderland, the Netherlands

Note from Tania

We are 2017. Until now no doctor was able to help Liesbeth. She doesn't have a diagnosis, nor treatment which makes her better. She is bed-bound day and night. We can only hope that her story in this book may reach some physician who will be willing and able to help.

RICHARD

A single diagnosis may not be enough.

October 3, 2011. I roll over in bed - and the room suddenly stands upside down. Off to the doctor, who says my symptoms indicate a balance disorder. Everything should be back to normal in a few days or weeks. But the symptoms persist, and I am referred to an ENT specialist. There I am told I have BPPV, and the Epley maneuver will take care of my problems. It doesn't. It's like I am drunk. Add nausea to the mix. Things are worse when I am surrounded by activity.

Back to the ENT for an electronystagmography (ENG) test, which suggests that my left vestibular organ is only working for 35% compared to the one on the right. This partially explains my situation, but not entirely. They draw some blood and do an MRI, but that all comes back normal. The ENT specialist decides I must have Ménière's disease, and he gives me betahistine and Cinnarizine. Avoid crowds and stress, he says.

I go to the University Medical Center in Groningen for a second opinion. No talk of hyperventilation, but definite evidence of Ménière's. Another ENG, and this time my left vestibular organ is 42% off normal. A Duplex scan shows a small problem with the blood flow in my neck.

Off to see the wizard

In 2015, I go to a dizziness clinic. Yet another ENG and, this time, an autonomic function test, which reveals several noteworthy results. The problem with my left vestibular organ has worsened to 54% malfunction. I don't have Ménière's, but I *do* have recurrent vestibulopathy, polyneuropathy (I have been a diabetes patient since 2002) and BPPV. Another Epley maneuver, this time lying on a surgical table. Still, though, no constructive results.

Finally to Floris

It has been more than two years since Tania tried to make me understand she never believed in my diagnosis, nor treatment. In her opinion, something wasn't right. But she also felt my fear for the unknown, my fear for change, so she didn't force me at all to try and find for another opinion. She simply kept telling me, each time when I had another vertigo attack, each time when I came back from the doctor, that if I would be ready one day, she would do an effort to get me to Antwerp as quick as possible. She believed, whithout promising the best outcome, if I could just visit her miracle man, I would get a serious chance to get better.

All little hints together, one day I decided to give it a try. I got my appointment, traveled from the north of the Netherlands to Antwerp and found Tania in the waiting room to support me. That was in August 2016.

Yes, I got a new diagnosis, Vestibular paroxysmia, which is a neurovascular conflict, visible on MRI. Floris sent me home with new hope and antiepileptics: Carbamazepine. He advised me to build up slowly – from 2 x 100 mg to 2 x 400 mg a day) and to come back three months later, to evaluate my progress. Hell yeah what a progress. In November I got my second appointment and ENG: diagnosis confirmed as correct. Since October 5, 2016, I got no more vertigo.

Enjoying my second life

One day in September, Tania came to visit me and my wife in the Netherlands. I wasn't completely dizzy free yet, but she found me riding a bike. I could ride my bike again! We went to a model car swap meet with her kids, we went to the restaurant, things I couldn't do before. Incredible. My wife is very happy: she can go shopping without being worried about leaving me at home, we can go shopping together and we can travel again.

In March 2017 we slowly lowered the drug dose with the intention to stop it completely. Last appointment was in April 2017. The good news: for more than half a year, I had no more vertigo. I often go cycling with my wife; we made many day trips and enjoy this new life. Let's hope my dizzy life is gone forever.

Dizzy Me is a scientific contribution to solving the problem of providing more knowledge about balance disorders to both doctors and patients. The book has brought me into contact with a pleasant group of '*Dizzy Me* Believers,' where fellow sufferers can freely discuss their experiences.

— Richard Brinkman - *evenwichtblog.nl*
Friesland, the Netherlands

CORINNE

Walking a tightrope between hope and acceptance.

I became really sick in 1997. I started having dizzy spells that lasted for days. I still have them. In between the attacks, I also began experiencing other problems that seemed to have an assortment of causes. I consulted several ENT doctors, and also a psychologist, an internist, an eye doctor, and quite a few alternative and semi-alternative care providers.

In 2008, I ran into a brick wall: I could not go on working, the ordinary chores of daily life were too much for me, I was burned out, and once again I began to suffer truly devastating attacks of vertigo. What exactly was wrong with me was unclear, but certainly more than 'just' vertigo: I had so many complaints, so many symptoms… and so few answers. Although the health-care professionals tried to dissuade me, I went on searching for the cause of my misery. The *Dizzy Me* blog - and, later, the book - helped.

A place for everything, and everything in its place

In 2011, a multidisciplinary team finally diagnosed me with vestibular migraine. This was strange, because I had no history of migraines, no headaches at all. And yet the following months showed me that the diagnosis was accurate. Symptoms I had been dealing with throughout my life - a tendency to motion sickness, neck problems, breathing issues, a tendency to excess muscle tone - everything seemed to fall into place.

I probably made things worse by trying to function normally for so many years. Vestibular migraine and chronic fatigue syndrome (CFS) often go hand in hand, and my actions made the CFS worse and led to the development of a chronic form of vestibular migraine. Because of the broad range of symptoms and triggers, I have become very limited in terms of what I can do in my daily life, and dependent on the care of others.

The road to acceptance

It has been hard for me to accept that this is my life now. And the unpredictability of vestibular migraine makes it even harder. I have had to be as flexible as I can and give in to the demands of the disease. Naturally, I still hope for improvement. I live on a mental tightrope between hope and acceptance.

My main concern today is to be as conscious as possible of the energy I have, in an attempt to get my resilience back. Partly because I have developed a chronic condition, my road to recovery is a long one. I continue to appreciate the opportunity to share experiences with my fellow sufferers.

Health-care professionals need to be better informed about this condition. A book like *Dizzy Me* was - and still is - an absolute must!

— Corinne
South Holland, the Netherlands

RENÉE

The artist behind the painting 'Dizzy'.

My name is Renée, I am a sixty-one-years-old lady living in The Hague, the Netherlands. About ten years ago I experienced my first bout of dizziness; after laying down on the bed, or when reaching for something on the top shelf of the kitchen cabinet. It just came out of the blue. No idea or clue what exactly caused my condition. I started googling and immediately had a lucky shot: a stumbled upon a website of a physiotherapist mentioning BPPD or BPPV (which is the same). To me the diagnosis was all clear.

Since that event, I suffer from BPPV in episodes. The first day is always the worst; I feel that horrible I can't do anything but stay at home. Next, symptoms remain for a couple of days, sometimes rather slumbering for several months.

About eight years ago I went to see my GP, who confirmed what I already found out myself. He suggested me to take medication that would only have result after three weeks. To me that wasn't a good plan, because mostly, by that time, I already got rid of the worst symptoms. So I did not follow his advice.

I learnt to live with it, realizing I am only suffering from a mild BPPV, not disabling me to live a normal life besides the occasional vertigo attacks. I continue enjoying sports, hiking, cycling, (except when having vertigo) which certainly has a positive impact on quick recovery. I have my own built-in security tools and tricks: a Nordic walking stick, a guardrail, someone in front of me when I go down the stairs...

I painted 'Dizzy' during a winter stay in Spain, the day after the paving stones started their vertigo dance right under my feet.

— Renée
South Holland, the Netherlands

Note from Tania:

Renée suffers from BPPV, which means taking medication is useless. But doctors prescribing Ménière's medication for BPPV patients is still a very common mistake.

BPPV symptoms (vertigo, nausea, vomiting, nystagmus) are self-limiting. This means these symptoms fade away slowly. Knowing that, you must realize you can get the impression medication helps... but in fact the 'fade-away effect' of your symptoms is just a natural process in case of BPPV, not the result of the medication prescribed. On the contrary, the medication will keep you ill for an even longer period.

Conclusion: in this case it was a very wise decision of Renée not to follow the doctors medication advise. I wasn't that clever as a patient at the time and I took them – luckily my instinct encouraged me to only take them occasionally, but to my doctor's opinion I should take them every day and the rest of my life –, but that was just because I got the wrong Ménière's diagnosis as a BPPV patient for fourteen years...

What Renée does actually need when she will have her next vertigo attack, is a well-performed Epley maneuver. And then continue moving a lot, like she does already.

For severe BPPV cases, there is a canal plugging option, but this is the last option in the care step ladder. It helped me, as a severe case.

JEAN-FRANCOIS & CAMILLA

Uniting parents of dizzy little people

We are a French-English couple living in Switzerland. Our second son Elio was born in the summer of 2015 with a number of health issues including club feet, poor eyesight and severe hypotonia. After weeks of blood tests, genetic screening and MRI, we went along to an ENT appointment. We were not expecting much from this appointment as we didn't have any particular concerns about his hearing, but it quickly revealed that Elio has bilateral vestibular loss without being deaf, which is, apparently, quite rare.

While the doctors still think our son has an underlying neurological problem, this diagnosis was a huge help in giving us a starting point from which we could begin to help him.

After many days spent on internet, we realized that there was not much information regarding this disorder in small children. We set out to try and find out more.

First of all we created a Facebook group to share our experience and try to unite children with the same issue as well as their parents and specialised doctors.

We decided, with the support of our family, friends and local doctors, to create an association for children with vestibular problems. The name is Children's Vestibular Disorder Association and our goal is to share the consequences of this disability with the maximum amount of people we could, to support the research in this domain, to provide guidance to the parents how to help their child, and how to live with it as parents.

We have been delighted by the interest in our Association so far and are gratified to see that we have had so much input from parents and medical professionals alike. We hope to be in a position soon to help raise money for further research and development into possible methods of alleviating some of the challenging effects of this disorder and making life easier for dizzy little people.

— Jean-François and Camilla, Founders Children's Vestibular Disorder Association, *cvdassociation.com*, Geneva, Switzerland

BETH

My Lyme Story

Over the last four years, I have had a total of three surgeries, eight invasive medical procedures, spent over six months in hospital and have had three trips to the USA for medical treatment. I have only just started my very long road to finally getting better...

My health story began when I was just 14 years old when I had suspected appendicitis. I had not long returned from an outdoor camping trip but at the time I didn't see this as being significant. I have always been the outdoor adventurous type. I had my appendix taken out, but I did not recover as expected. I continued to be misdiagnosed over the following 12 years of my life. I was out of school for six months as a result of thyrotoxicosis, asthma and what doctors told me was chronic fatigue syndrome. I eventually got back to school, college and University. I even managed to do some traveling. This did not come without health problems and over the years I have struggled with Hashimoto's disease, IBS, hip tendonitis, frequent infections, asthma attacks and symptoms that the medical profession could just not explain. I was fatigued constantly which I assumed was just a 'normal' way of life when you are a busy student. Little did I know that all of these things could in fact have a root cause. This 'mysterious' root cause continued to damage my body, puzzle the medical profession and made me more and more disabled.

SSCD - the start of the biggest fight of my life

I was on my final ever nursing placement when I started to experience severe vertigo attacks. I had just turned 23 and it was a day that my life changed forever. When I returned home from placement I collapsed as I walked through the front door as I was too dizzy to even stand anymore. The world was spinning and I could not move without throwing up. My GP thought it was just labyrinthitis and encouraged me to get back to University and continue applying for nursing jobs. I got offered two dream jobs as a paediatric nurse and despite the fact I could barely move my head I was over the moon. Little did I know that the following four years were going to be the biggest fight of my life.

After six weeks, I was referred to an ENT doctor but kept being dismissed and told 'I would just get better'. I would love to tell them how wrong they were. After six months of not being able to work I knew that there must be something very wrong. I had balance tests which showed I had lost the balance function in my right ear. I was told it was straightforward to fix with physiotherapy, but this just made me sicker. In March 2014 I got a second opinion and scans revealed I had a rare inner ear condition called superior semicircular canal dehiscence (SSCD)… finally! I was so relieved to have what I thought was the answer to all my problems. If only.

Health hits rock bottom

In September 2014, my health hit rock bottom and I was admitted to my local hospital with dehydration as a result of severe vomiting. This was put down to dizziness and not investigated at all. I spent two months in hospital before having my first surgery to repair my inner ear and what we thought was causing all my debilitating symptoms. I managed to get home a week later, but it soon became obvious that it had not worked. I was, in fact, in a far worse state. I was admitted into hospital again in December before having a second ear operation in February 2015. This did not make me better. I was completely bed bound at this point, too dizzy to even move around the house let alone look after myself properly. I was completely desperate for help.

Assuming that the unfixed SSCD was the cause of my ongoing problems I began researching surgeons abroad who could help me. This is when I came across Dr Daniel Lee at MEEI in Boston. As I was out of options on the NHS, the decision was made that I would travel to Boston to have a third surgery on my ear. This surgery was no walk in the park and would cost over £ 70,000.

Getting Beth Better

My amazing brother, Tom, set up a fundraising campaign 'gettingbethbetter' to help cover the huge costs. I cannot put into words what an incredible time this was, to see my friends, family and complete strangers come together to raise money to help me get better. We raised nearly £ 60,000.

The surgery went as planned and I even noticed some small improvements in my balance after a few weeks. However, things quickly spiralled downhill and in September 2015 I was admitted back to hospital again. Just like before I was suffering with severe dehydration due to constant vomiting. This could no longer be put down to my ear as this had been fixed and I continued to puzzle every single doctor who met me. I lost so much weight that I was put on TPN (nutrition that gets pumped through your veins). I was referred to London for specialist scans which revealed I had severe gastroparesis: delayed stomach emptying. Yet another rare condition. I have had seven PICC lines and now have a port placed in my chest (central line), to continue giving myself IV fluids at home. Two years as a qualified nurse and the only patient I had looked after was myself. Surely there was a cause for all of this?

Following further tests in London I was also diagnosed with a condition called POTs: an autonomic condition where your heart rate shoots up when you are up right. This was making me almost pass out every time I stood up. This then lead to another diagnosis of Ehler Danlos Syndrome: a connective tissue disorder. Then Mast cell activation disease: an immunological condition which causes severe allergic reactions. I also kept getting mysterious infections which would land me in hospital barely able to talk. My immune system was shot to pieces and I was getting weaker by the day. I could not understand why so many things were going wrong. Why was I still dizzy despite a successful surgery? Why all of these rare conditions? I was not prepared to be told that there was no longer a cure. I could not just 'accept the way I was'. Surely there was an answer. I kept fighting for a cure.

Shedding light on Lyme

As conventional medicine options had supposedly ran out, I opted to see a naturopath at the Hale clinic in London. Best decision of my life. She took one look at me and my history and said 'I think you have Lyme disease'. I looked at her completely blankly. Lyme disease?! I didn't even know what this was exactly and not to mention that this could actually be the cause of all of my problems. I left feeling even more puzzled than ever but after two months I finally decided to get tested privately for Lyme disease and co infections.

In the meantime, I had returned to Boston for vestibular therapy as I thought this might be a way to push myself forward to getting better. I didn't think Lyme could really be very significant. After SSCD surgery you lose the function of one of your balance canals so your brain has to learn to compensate. Made sense. Despite vestibular therapy my brain could not compensate. Two weeks into my trip my blood work came back positive for Lyme, Bartonella and Ehrlichia. This is when everything started to make sense…

After doing some research I started to question whether everything I have been through since my camping trip was all down to Lyme disease. Turns out it is. I found a Lyme disease physician in NY state and traveled there for treatment in December 2016. My mind was completely blown by this doctor's deep understanding of my entire health history. To him I wasn't a 'medical mystery' at all, just another patient who had been misdiagnosed time and time again. My health puzzle was complete. I had found the answer I had been looking for for over ten years of my life.

I spent six weeks in the USA having treatment at the Stram Center. A place full of hope. My health needs were understood on a level no one else had ever got. My Lyme disease journey is very much only beginning and I have an incredibly long way to go. Being so ill for so long means there is lots of things to fix. But it is possible and I am putting everything into it! I haven't had any setbacks and continue on my treatment plan in the UK, working alongside Dr Stram. I have the amazing support of people I have met on my journey and greatly appreciate the support of LDUK and their support group. With little help from medical professionals in the UK it really is a lifesaver to have people who truly understand what I'm going through.

This is my story and I hope it can help anyone else out there reach out for help if they think they are suffering with Lyme disease. Please contact me if you have any questions about my history or treatment!

— Beth Rye
Somerset, UK
gettingbethbetter.com

POLLY

Polly's 'Dear whoever' blog post on UK Rare Diseases website

Polly is a MdDS patient, and like many other patients she does not only struggle with 'the disease as such', but also with the impact of having a 'rare' disorder... As if suffering from a neurological condition affecting the vestibular function, or simply a vestibular disorder (there are twelve disorders, but doctors seem to have difficulties in differentiating them all) isn't hard enough...

Anyway... This blog illustrates amazingly the problems almost all 'rare disorder patients' are dealing with.

'Dear Whoever...', she starts, and then she fantasizes about things she would love to write to various clinicians and decision makers.

I especially invite doctors and decision makers to read her imaginary letters.

'Dear Whoever' Letters from a Mal de Débarquement Syndrome (MdDS) patient

On behalf of my MdDS family

I have noticed a trend on social media sites dedicated to conditions such as Ménière's and migraine for people to write letters to these conditions, explaining why they have such a hard time with them – and, sometimes, with their doctors. I have a hard time with Mal de Débarquement Syndrome (MdDS). But my letters would be directly to the various clinicians and other decision-makers involved.

The first would be to the ENT consultant who diagnosed me in 2006, following a classic disembarkation trigger. Amongst other things it would ask 'What was the point of writing "I would probably advise her not to take vestibular sedatives" in a letter I wasn't able to read until I bought my medical record, many years later? You could have just told me at the time.'

To the GP who wrote 'She knows not to take vestibular medication' I would say 'No, I didn't. See above.'

To the one who wrote 'She doesn't have true rotational vertigo.' I'd say 'I know, I told you that. And I also asked why you kept recording MdDS as 'vertigo', to which you replied "We always record balance disorders as vertigo." Great; a pervading systemic error which might be replicated for patients with perilymph fistulas, SSCD, balance symptoms that result from concussion or strokes, gluten ataxia, etcetera, etcetera. Brilliant – not. Especially when doctors in a hurry then try and do the Epley Manoeuvre on me, which can trigger or hike MdDS symptoms.

To the consultant who told me I was lucky not to have Ménière's I'd write 'I agree, it's a terrible condition. But – look at the amount of research that gets done about that, compared to MdDS. Also, the Ménière's researches hang out on facebook. So far, ours don't – although they are very generous when it comes to responding to emails.'

To the consultant who failed to copy me in to a letter saying 'I didn't mention the possibility of MS' I'd say 'Well I wish you had. I have learnt a lot of tricks of the trade from the MS crew, after I spotted the relapse/remission connection and all the overlaps in symptom presentations.'

To all the clinicians who have reported on scans etcetera by writing 'You will be pleased to know we could find no cause that can explain your symptoms', I'd say 'I am delighted, but since those were ruling-out tests, I am not surprised. Could you please get a move on and figure out what does cause them so I can work out which treatment might be appropriate – on the off chance that any of the trialled protocols are ever available on these shores.'

To the GP who wrote 'Her symptoms are medically unexplained' I'd say 'That euphemism has dangerous connotations – apparently Professor Wessely gets death threats when he uses it. If you meant 'It's unfortunate that, although Charles Darwin's Dad wrote about this condition, clinicians have only recently started researching it and the full pathology is still unknown' I would agree with you. Meanwhile, the EDS research should tell you everything you need to know about the problems associated with the term 'medically unexplained' so please stop using it. Thanks. Same goes for 'functional' – having had that label slapped on MdDS by the 'Sleep Clinic' I had to go to London to get re-diagnosed before my former GP would take it seriously. Total waste of NHS resources – and mine. Having lost my job through being 'an uninsurable fall risk' funds are a bit tight and I didn't need that extra expense.'

To the benefits agency I'd write 'Could you please explain why I was eligible for health benefits in 2010 when the condition was still episodic but, now I am in the chronic phase, I am not?'

To the so-called 'health professional' who assessed me for PIP I'd write 'Your notes were almost entirely inaccurate. They were nearly as bad as the ones in my medical record, which are the reason I now call MdDS 'Mal de Débacle Syndrome'. It's par for the course for people with rare conditions to have errors in their medical records but it really didn't help when your inaccuracies were used by a judge to discredit my claim.'

To my beloved Dad, a retired GP who is not in the best of health himself (and pushing ninety) I say, very often, 'Thank you for supporting me financially, Dad. Having a rare condition is notoriously expensive and being able to afford to go to the osteopath helps a lot. Not much left over to go towards fundraising for research but I chip in when I can.'

If she wasn't off sick I would write the following to my fabulous new GP. 'You are a star – and you are winning awards right left and centre on our social media sites. I know you can't cure me but it helps that you are moving heaven and earth to get me the referrals I need to figure out what made me susceptible to MdDS in the first place. The intel from the cardiologist didn't help much, I know, since there are no dysautonomia clinics here. But the report from the neural-ophthalmologist was considerably more useful, given how many of us with MdDS also have convergence insufficiencies. By the way, Dr. Dai, our opto-kinetic researcher e-mailed me to say he wasn't sure of the mechanisms behind vagus nerve stimulation and that it would probably only mask the symptoms (as happens when I use a TENS machine). But, if it will not do me any long-term damage, I would like to give it a go. Under research trial conditions, of course. Meanwhile I am looking forward to meeting the genetics team in the Autumn – bit bizarre that I had to schmooze the local Professor at a public lecture to get there, but needs must when 'the intractable devil' drives, to quote Dr. Dai's definition of MdDS.'

It's far more bizarre that to get to my new GP I had to discriminate against her predecessor on the grounds of his gender. That man had the nerve to tell me not to do any more research. Whereas our researchers – and the rare conditions advocates – say the exact opposite.

If many of these issues were not relevant to others with different rare conditions, I might not bother to say or write any of the above. But they are. In just one example I read about a woman with Wilson's disease who wrote that 'bad advice permeated my notes like a virus' and my heart went out to her in recognition. She also mentioned that clinicians were causing 'havoc' in her medical records (through gross inaccuracies) and this resonated with many of us with MdDS too. At one point this poor lady was told she had a 'conversion disorder' and that the symptoms were that she had seen too many doctors whilst trying to get a rational diagnosis. She finally found doctors who were willing to read the information and advice she had sourced directly from the lead researchers and says she feels very lucky.

I am in the same position now. But I know of far too many rare conditions patients who are not – including those with MdDS.

So the last letter I would write would be to a hearing therapist I met last year. She has MdDS too and told me her GP was 'useless'. It would say, very simply, 'I hear you.'

— Polly Moyer,
United Kingdom

About Polly

Born (1961) and brought up in Yorkshire I moved to Bristol to attend university. I then worked in outplacement before being recruited to the Civil Service. From there I was seconded to The Prince's Trust and later worked for CLIC, co-ordinating their teenage support group. My last job was in student services at a post 16 centre. I took an MA in 2010 and am now a self-employed writer and teacher. I am also a qualified Laughter Yoga Facilitator :) With the support of a mentor supplied by Findacure I run a small campaign group for people with MdDS in the UK and also write a guest blog for Findacure under the banner of 'Treasure the exceptions'.

JOHN

Hearing loss vs. dizziness: if i could choose!

I was about nine when hearing loss in my left ear was first detected. The audiologist explained to me that as a result, I might not be able to hear birds singing as easily, and that I might need to concentrate more to understand words starting with 'sh,' 'k,' or 't.' Sensing my alarm, she tried to reassure me by saying it was unlikely that the hearing loss would affect both ears, and if it did, it would likely not be to the same extent. I compensated in school by simply tilting my right ear toward sound sources.

Over time, my hearing loss became bilateral and progressive, and its cause remains unknown. In graduate school I began using hearing aids and later received a cochlear implant in my left ear. I continue to use a hearing aid in my right ear, and thankfully for the past eight years, my hearing has remained stable, if stably poor.

Hearing loss has sculpted my career path

While I do not consider my hearing loss to be a profound limitation personally or professionally, it has certainly sculpted my career path. After receiving my undergraduate, master's, and doctoral degrees, all in the biological sciences, I settled on a career in auditory neuroscience to better understand hearing loss. I also reasoned that auditory research conferences would likely have assistive listening technology to allow me to participate more fully.

As I entered my forty's, I experienced vertigo for the first time. The clinical data do not fit with a diagnosis of Ménière's disease, and the link between my vertigo and hearing loss is unclear.

When I have an acute attack of dizziness, my visual field scrolls from right to left very quickly so that I must close my eyes to avoid profound motion sickness and vomiting. I must lie down until the dizziness subsides, which is usually twelve to sixteen hours. I honestly cannot do anything - I can only hope to fall asleep quickly.

Vertigo is a profound limitation for me. With no disrespect or insensitivity intended toward the hearing-impaired community - of which I am a passionate member - I would take hearing loss over vertigo in a heartbeat. Dizziness incapacitates me, and I cannot be an effective researcher, educator, husband, or father. Some people perceive an aura before their dizziness occurs, but I do not get any advance warning. Unlike hearing loss, I cannot manage my dizziness - it takes hold and lets go when it wants to.

I recall one episode especially vividly. I was invited to give a seminar at the National Institute on Deafness and Other Disorders and experienced a severe attack just hours before my flight. Vertigo forced me to reschedule my visit, which was tremendously frustrating. That night, I slept in the bathroom (my best solution when vertigo hits). Vestibular (balance) dysfunction is quite simply a game changer.

Looking for tailored therapies

A satisfying part of my research involves trying to define treatments for hearing loss and dizziness. Usher syndrome is a condition combining hearing, balance, and vision disorders. In Usher syndrome type 1, infants are born deaf and have severe vestibular problems; vision abnormalities appear by around age ten. In working with a group of dedicated colleagues at various institutions, we have evidence that fetal administration of a drug in mice with Usher syndrome type 1 can prevent balance abnormalities.

As part of HHF's Hearing Restoration Project (HRP) consortium, I have been working on testing gene candidates in mice for their ability to trigger hair cell regeneration. This research is exciting as it is leading the HRP into phase 2 of its strategic plan, with phase 3 involving further testing for drug therapies. The probability is that manipulating a single gene will not provide lasting hearing restoration, and that we will need to figure out how to manipulate multiple genes in concert to achieve the best therapeutic outcomes.

It is an exciting time to be a neuroscientist interested in trying to find ways to help patients with hearing loss and balance issues. I am hopeful that we will make progress in defining new ways to treat and even prevent vertigo in the near future as well as determine effective therapies tailored to address the unique causes of hearing loss and tinnitus.

— John V. Brigande, PhD
Portland, USA

Note from Tania:

Hearing Restoration Project consortium member John V. Brigande, PhD, is a developmental neurobiologist at the Oregon Hearing Research Center. He also teaches in the Neuroscience Graduate Program and in the Program in Molecular and Cellular Biology at the Oregon Health & Science University.

KIM

Trek to balance.

I am Kim, fifty-seven years old. So you can better appreciate my story, let me share with you who I am as a person, professional, wife, mother, and friend.

Adventure girl!

I was a Seattle Mountaineer in my teens, a natural pastime for one who was called a 'mountain goat' as a young girl by my dad. I have hiked, biked and climbed my whole life. My serenity is the outdoors, fresh air and natural beauty.

My life has been filled with outdoor adventure with my family and friends. I was also fortunate to find and marry my adventure partner in life, my husband Larry. Together, Larry and I have climbed mountains and built a life exploring the beauty of the Northwest and the world.

We have lived in the same community for over thirty years and have a vast network of friends, family, music groups, beer groups, adventure groups, book groups and stitch groups. We are surrounded by support.

Professional career

My lifetime career in the health profession was where I belonged. It was a career choice that allowed me to validate patients, give compassion, and heal with caring. I have worked in an environment of trauma, drama, adrenalized events, stress, loss and teamwork. In this field, I was able to multitask, use critical thinking and gear down in the face of crisis to implement care and healing.

I set the stage of our lives, because my course of health has rocked our boat, has challenged us on every level, has redefined us, and has confronted me with the question, 'Who am I now?' My story is probably not unique, but I believe that my healing process has been. I hope it is inspirational to you.

March 6, 2014

I leaned over to kiss my husband goodnight, and the room began to spin. My initial thought was that I just needed to get some rest.

The following morning, I tried to stand and fell into the wall, several times. Finally I held on to the furniture and, despite some mild vertigo and imbalance, I was able to get ready for work and drive the two miles to the hospital to my nurse navigator role in an office. I did not speak of my symptoms - 'Mind over Matter' has always been my motto - and tried to work.

It quickly became apparent that, not only was I having difficulty on the computer and with thinking, but I was unable to stand without the room spinning. I was ineffective. It was suggested to me that I pop on over to the emergency department for an evaluation. Of course, as an emergency department nurse, I am a minimizer of my own symptoms. 'If you all could just drive me home,' I said, 'I am sure this will resolve with some rest and over-the-counter medication.'

But I did not improve. My condition continued to worsen, and by the time I ended up in the ED for a stroke workup three days later, my symptoms were consuming. I had a headache, vertigo, nausea, visual changes, left-side motor changes, difficulty walking and inability to think straight. The workup I received was comprehensive. A stroke was ruled out, and I was diagnosed with BPPV and advised to follow up with an ENT specialist and consider the Epley maneuver.

My daughter Becky and I attempted the Epley maneuver as described on YouTube, but my symptoms only got worse. Within a week, my ability to walk without assistance was greatly compromized, and I needed assistance with my daily living.

Roller coaster of testing

Larry and I entered the fast track with the ENT follow-up. The differential diagnosis was Cerebellar CVA vs Vestibular Neuritis. We were both thankful that my ataxia (an odd way of walking), motor and perceptual changes were being validated. We set off on a roller coaster of testing and emotions: Balance and Hearing lab, VNG workup, vestibular therapy, neurovestibular specialist, neurologist, neuro-ophthalmologist, functional optometrist, a neuropsychiatrist for cognitive testing…

Was this a central or a peripheral problem, we wanted to know. Was MS ruled out? Was my condition progressive? Would I recover?

I underwent repeated MRIs and ultrasounds.

My primary diagnosis: vestibular migraine disorder. Six months later, I got a second opinion: left vestibulopathy.

Living with loss

I cried every day, experienced loss every day, doubted my resiliency, strength and stamina every day. I was spiraling downward.

Healing started the day I met Julie Groves, a vestibular therapist. Julie not only validated my symptoms, she gave me hope, encouragement, tools to accommodate my symptoms and, most of all, she joined me on a journey to health. She addressed all aspects of a vestibular syndrome: the physical, cognitive, emotional, and functional impacts that the disorder includes. She saw me as a whole person. My symptoms were predictable, she said, and she was able to anticipate them. I had hope!

Julie recommended that I get an evaluation by an optometrist who specialized in the functional, neurological aspect of vision. Larry and I were so grateful for this recommendation. The evaluation validated my visual changes that involved tracking, depth perception and the fact that my eyes were not working well together. Therapy was recommended.

Breaking through a bubble of despair

Multiple practitioners steered me to the Vestibular Disorders Association (VEDA). Their website explained my condition and my challenges in plain terms.

I began to look outside my bubble of despair. I started letting my friends and family in. I tried to stop focusing on the diagnosis and instead work with the symptoms I had, to let go of what I had lost and see opportunity, instead. This was the hardest job of my life.

Balance

Vertical balance is a physiological process. Life balance is who I am. Who am I now? What will I do next? How do I focus on healing while I am being evaluated for disability? What do I contribute to life if I am not working? How do I deal with variable symptoms on a daily basis? How do I handle my inability to process or think clearly as I am interpreting my environment?

I am stuck like glue to my guide

Maeghan Culver of the Bastyr Center for Natural Health, the teaching clinic of Bastyr University in Seattle, has given me direction and guidance in rebuilding my day-to-day life. In her words - which I love - I am 'on a sabbatical for health'. This involves my feelings of self worth, fueling my body for success, and a viewpoint that is kind, caring and loving of self. I found her through an article she wrote for the VEDA website, 'Staying Grounded in an Unstable World: A Meditative Approach to Coping with Chronic Dizziness & Imbalance.'

Rewiring my brain

The one thing I know for sure is that, no matter where I go, there I am! I take my disability with me, everywhere I go. I am not driving. I am not working.

I am living life. I am rewiring my brain. Playing the bass in a band, sitting down, camping and hiking with Larry and friends, hiking and spending time with my adult children, enjoying my kitties, my garden, my birds. Getting together with my girlfriends. Planning adventures that hopefully will be possible in the future. Allowing myself to dream again.

I am in transition. I recognize that every day is different. Some days I have increased difficulty with balance or vision or cognition. Other days are better.

I hope that, by sharing my story and my adventures with you, I can give you hope. I truly feel this is a daily choice to trek towards balance. I am so thankful to my husband Larry for becoming my #1 supporter in spite of all the ways this has impacted him. He validates me. Thank you to my children and family for their tolerance, listening ears, assistance with so many things… and for loving me and believing in me. Thank you to my dear friends who have been my chauffeurs, my walking partners, who share a laugh and a great beer with me, who love me for who I am. I have such gratitude for you all.

— Kim Kutz Striber, VEDA Ambassador
Kirkland, Washington, USA
trektobalance.com

DAVID

Stroke survivor with misdiagnosis.

I am one of Tania's American VEDA colleagues. I am fifty-three years old. I went to my local ER on August 5, 2013, with sudden onset of dizziness. The on-call doctor told me I had vertigo and sent me home to rest. Two days later, I was feeling much worse and could not walk. I was transported by ambulance to my local ER, now showing all signs of stroke. That diagnosis was confirmed per MRI.

I have had a fairly slow recovery, and I still have ongoing vertigo. Exactly one month after I had my first stroke, my brother - a year older than me - was rushed to a different ER with sudden onset of dizziness. The doctors were about to send him home with a diagnosis of vertigo when our sister intervened and asked the ER doctor to do an MRI. The doctor was reluctant to do this test; she thought it was a waste of time and money. But she did the MRI, and it came back as a left brain stem stroke… same as mine.

They gave my brother appropriate medication. He was discharged from the hospital within a week and back to work after missing just a month. He has no ongoing physical disabilities. I, on the other hand, am currently disabled, unable to drive or work, with ongoing vertigo that seems to have stabilized with the help of medication at six months post stroke.

Bitterness

After this six-month period I was left feeling very bitter. Someone from my job - which I had started nine months previous to my stroke - came to my home after my stroke. I was told to take my time and recover. 'We will be there for you,' he said. He collected my company car and iPad - and I never saw him again. The following week, just six weeks after my stroke, the company called my wife while I was in rehab therapy and told her they were terminating my employment. That also meant I lost my health insurance.

I was so angry that I cried and lashed out in anger. How could any company do such a thing, while I was busting my ass to get better so I could return to work? I actually did a little work from my hospital bed, just a couple of days post-stroke, to try to tie up some loose ends. But six weeks after a stroke, they let me go. I thought, *You have got to be kidding me!* I mean, they give mothers *eight* weeks after having a baby.

Turning anger into passion

I was feeling a lot of anger and grief, but then something changed. Jay, a friend of my sister's, took me into his physical therapy practice and did therapy on me for very little money. Jay helped me more than the previous two or three therapists I had seen in the hospital. You see, I wasn't like most stroke victims. I was left with severe vertigo and balance issues. So it wasn't about making my muscles stronger. It was about what would help me regain some of my balance.

Jay was the only one I saw who *got* me and what I was talking about; I needed balance to regain some of my life. He worked tirelessly over a period of months, encouraging me and scolding me if I wasn't working hard enough. This was just what I needed, and soon I was on a path of recovery. Although I didn't regain all I had lost, I did gain enough to live a life that's a lot better than most stroke survivors. For that, I am very grateful to Jay.

It is from this point that my life changed. If I could turn all of my anger into passion to help others in similar need, I thought, what a way to pay it forward. So that's where my new journey began.

I started researching causes of strokes and came across a neurologist at Johns Hopkins Hospital who was working on a project to help differentiate between common vertigo and stroke. I was interested, because two members of my family had experienced sudden onset of dizziness, and we both were initially diagnosed with vertigo. To my surprise, the busy doctor called me back within the week, and we had about an hour of conversation regarding what role I would like to play in helping develop his new device.

Out of the ashes....

He told me to contact the Vestibular Disorders Association (VEDA), a group that helps people who are experiencing balance and dizziness issues. VEDA helped me to understand why I was dizzy and to find ways to cope with my disorder.
I quickly became involved in a lot of conversation with this group and realized that there are millions of people all over the world who suffer daily from this invisible and disabling illness. I now wanted to be a part of the solution, to help as many people as possible to better understand and cope with their disorder.

I started a local support group in my area of Maine in May 2014, and I have since become the chairperson of a group of VEDA Ambassadors. Our goal is to create a grassroots campaign to spread the word about this often-misunderstood condition. I also do volunteer work for a group called the Society to Improve Diagnosis in Medicine. We partner with doctors and patients to help find better ways to decrease misdiagnosis. And I also work with the American Stroke Association, advocating for rights for stoke victims.

I never thought that my life would take this path. But now that it has, it gives me great pleasure to turn a negative experience into something positive. As the saying goes, 'out of the ashes rises a phoenix.'

– David Morrill, VEDA Ambassador
Dedham, Maine, USA

Just as the 'SO STONED' method helps doctors diagnose vestibular disorders, the 'BEE FAST' method helps diagnose stroke. David raises awareness for lifesaving stroke care.

All of the signs and symptoms listed below are acknowledged by neurologists and stroke specialists. Keep in mind that it's possible to have only several or even only one of these symptoms and still be having a stroke!

B – **B**alance: sudden loss of balance or coordination

E – **E**yes: sudden change in vision

E – **E**xtreme headache that comes on suddenly

F – **F**ace: sudden weakness of the face

A – **A**rms: sudden weakness of arm or leg

S – **S**peech: sudden difficulty speaking

T – **T**ime to call 911!

KATHY

A hat & sunglasses to stay grounded

My name is Kathy, I am fifty-eight and Canadian. I began having dizzy spells approximately seven years ago. They would occur once or twice a year and last a very short time, usually over a weekend and then I was fine to go to work on Monday morning!

Positional?

The last couple of years the spells were occurring more frequently. I went to physio to learn what exercises I should do to help with what they described as a crystal lodged in my ear (positional vertigo – *note from Dizzy Me: what they call BPPV*). I made many trips to my physio until eventually it went away.

Left vestibular hypo function

Christmas time 2014, the vertigo was very intense and I ended up going to the hospital by ambulance. The vertigo came out of nowhere and my symptoms were the worst I have ever experienced. Intense spinning, vomiting, that lasted hours. To make a a long story short, I ended up seeing an ENT specialist who referred me to the University Hospital where they did caloric testing. I was told I would experience intense dizziness or possibly vomiting during this test. To my surprise I experienced none of this. They repeated the ice water test on my left ear and found that there was no response. I was diagnosed with left vestibular hypo function.

Develop new pathways

I was off work for over a month where I was referred to physio to a therapist who was a vestibular specialist here in our small city of St. Thomas Ontario (Corinne Roos physical therapist – The Dizziness & Balance Program centric/ Lifemark Health, she is listed on the VEDA site). I was not optimistic this would work but it was explained to me that my brain needs to develop new pathways to compensate for the complete balance loss of my left ear (*note from Dizzy Me: what they call neuroplasticity*). Needless to say I was devastated, angry, and I cried a lot, feeling my life was over.

I got over that and thought 'Well I was able to beat one disability (I have had severe back issues), so I can beat this.' I dried up my tears, scoured the internet looking for support and came across the site *vestibular.org* and read through it getting lots of advice on how to kick this invisible disability. I purchased a cane, hat, wrap around glasses and worked hard at the exercises.

Strategies

I experience vertigo in places like shopping malls, hiking in the woods, but have learned to manage by using strategies like focusing on an object in front of me rather than everything around me. I get frustrated, but I am refusing to let this control me. I am on no medication for this. Initially when they thought it was crystals in my ears, I was on Serc but the specialist said it will not help me (*note from Dizzy Me: indeed Serc is prescribed to treat Ménière's but does not help if you got the crystals related – BPPV – disorder*).

My fear in all this is 'when will my next severe bout occur and what are the chances of losing all the balance in my right ear.'

Since Christmas 2014, I continue to experience slight vertigo many times throughout the day. It's hard to explain how my brain feels during these small episodes. I feel pressure on my head that waves in and out and causes dizziness. These occur frequently during any given day. At times I experience a loss of balance and a wave of nausea which only lasts a few brief moments.

A hat & sunglasses to stay grounded

My hat and sunglasses are my best friend these days in helping me to stay more grounded. There are times where I become teary out of sheer frustration, but remind myself I can continue to be strong and fight this.

I made it through 2017 without any further hospital visits and am thankful for that. I try and stay positive and am thankful to have found the support of vestibular.org and Dizziness and Associated Illness support group. I continue to seek out information from *vestibular.org* but have not read any articles on vestibular hypo function!

— Kathy
Canada

MARGARET

When a therapist needs therapy.

My name is Margaret, and I just turned sixty. I live in Texas. In a time not so long ago, I was a happy, vivacious, respected COTA (Certified Occupational Therapy Assistant). Working with children was a perfect match for my childlike spirit. I was the kind of person who didn't think twice about donning a ballet tutu over my clothes, if that's what it took to get the children to participate in therapy, I did it! I guess I should explain what Occupational Therapy (OT) encompasses. This is the official AOTA definition:

Occupational therapy is the only profession that helps people across the lifespan to do the things they want and need to do through the therapeutic use of daily activities (occupations). Occupational therapy practitioners enable people of all ages to live life to its fullest by helping them promote health, and prevent – or live better with – injury, illness, or disability.

Sneezed into dizziness

During a treatment session, I was sneezed on, so unexpected, it hit me square in my face and MOUTH! Yes, sneezed into my mouth! My professionalism flew out the window. I jumped up, ran to the sink, washed my mouth with antibacterial foam soap, spit, wash, repeat! I quickly dashed out. Spit! More spit! By the end of my work day, I was feeling like I had the Flu! It certainly wasn't the first time I got sick from the children, actually it happened fairly often, but this was different. After a week off, I knew I had to go to the doctor.

Scary night

That night I woke up to go to the bathroom, but when I turned over to get up, *Vertigo* hit. I had never experienced that before and it was a disturbing sensation. I laid there for a few minutes, then got up. I might have taken ten steps before it hit again and I was flat on the floor… in the dark… my husband snoring so loudly

he didn't hear me at first. 'Mike! I have fallen and I can't get up!'
I screamed. '*Where* are you Margaret?' 'Mike, I am on the floor and everything is spinning, I need you right now!' He turned on a light, jumped out of bed to find me attempting to 'hang on' to the floor. 'My eyes are doing something weird, I don't know what's going on…' I whined. Then the nausea and vomiting hit! Mike helped me to the bathroom, then put me in bed. This was officially a scary mess now.

No help & breaking bones

A visit to the ER the next morning was a joke! A virus was going around, so that was my diagnosis. They ignored my complaints about how my eyes felt, like a slot machine was my description, but all I got was a shot for the nausea.
I would remain in a constant state of nausea/vomiting for the next 1+ years! An appointment with an ENT specialist was scheduled, but it was not for months. Back at work, I quickly realized I needed to be touching the walls as I walked for stability. I had to look at my feet and the floor when I walked. If I became too dizzy, I put my back against the wall and slid down to sit. Professional? No, practical! My driving to schools stopped the day I turned my head to check traffic and the next thing I know, I'd gone up a curb. Now I worked in the facility only. I was putting everything on the ENT to save me, which proved a huge mistake.

All usual Vestibular tests (from the 1950's!) turned out normal. *No way*! My eyes were still going nuts, I was still throwing up daily and I'd fallen breaking my tailbone. Using Scopolamine Patches (usually for sea sickness) for one year and a half until becoming allergic to the adhesive! I went to part-time work, but still had more falls breaking more bones! My co-workers set my ankle more than once, more than once I used a wheelchair to get around. Back and forth to the ENT for over one year before a *major* meltdown in his office that could have gotten me arrested, all to get a referral to a neuro-otolaryngologist in Dallas.

Chronic labrynthitis & vestibular neuritis

It took over one year of me fighting for my right to a correct and accurate diagnosis, but I finally received one after tests in Dallas. It was also my birthday ironically, December. I endured a six-hour battery of tests. I was throwing up before, during and after the tests. I carried a 'Christmas' bag lined with plastic bags, for the just in case. One woman said, 'I see you have been shopping'... Lady if you only knew!

This doctor knew his stuff! I was diagnosed with chronic labrynthitis and a vestibular neuritis on the VIII cranial nerve (our *balance* nerve). He assured me there were 'newer and more current medicines to help me' (remember my 1950's ENT?) and he wanted me to do VRT – vestibular rehabilitation therapy – with his chosen physical therapist (PT). I did therapy for over one year. In total, I broke seven bones during my journey.

Early retirement

I did everything I was told to do, but unfortunately I never got back to the person I used to be. Being 'off balance' and working with people does not go together. The day I took a very early retirement, was the day a big piece of me died, and I mourned my loss. I have stubbornly kept my COTA License even though I no longer practice.

New purpose has been found as an Ambassador for VEDA (Vestibular Disorders Association), I am the only one from Texas! I blog about my experience if you want to read a more extensive 'telling' of my story: visit my sneezemedizzy blog!

— Margaret
Texas, USA
sneezemedizzy.com

JEFFREY

That bastard of a disease in my head.

It was a normal day in 1994. I was working in my office going over routings and schedules trying to find some one-offs that might work for specific venues for an artist or two when sudden a roaring noise entered my left ear. I looked to the window to make sure a truck wasn't about to crash into the building. That sudden movement sent the whole room into a fast back and forth flicking fast movement unlike any dizziness I'd ever experienced and then the nausea, vomiting, and my head smacked the top of my desk and I literally could not pick my head up again.

My assistant heard me throwing up and came in concerned that I had suddenly developed the flu or something worse. I could not talk to her, I could not raise my head, I could not move. Everyone then thought I had experienced a stroke and called 911. The EMT's arrived and my pulse was racing, my heart pounding, still throwing up, still could not move…they transported me to hospital.

Twenty-four hours later I was released with a diagnosis of a major migraine. That was the beginning of a three-year long battle of going through the same 'attacks' over and over and over again with no notice until finally I found a doctor willing to do the tests, make the call, tell me the hard truth… Ménière's disease. It fell on me like an anvil. What I had suspected, read about, feared… an incurable, almost untreatable, bastard of a disease was now in my head.

Deal with it

I learned to deal with it adjusting diets, taking pills, all the usual things for twenty-some years. It was left-side oriented. Then in 2001 the disease became more and more devastating to the point that it was a weekly event. I had a shunt placed in my skull to help drain the fluid. That seemed to help for a few months, then the attacks came back with a rage on a daily basis so the decision was made in 2002 to have a vestibular section. My left balance nerve was cut. No more vertigo. Relief, but I still had the pressure, the tinnitus, and now I could not walk a straight line if my life depended on it. But just to have the vertigo gone made life livable.

Things were going along fine until the summer of 2013. My hearing had begun to dissipate on the left side until it was gone completely. I was half deaf then, and one hot summer night I woke up in a full-blown Ménière's attack! I was convulsing, throwing up, and major vertigo just like that first attack so many years ago… but how? I didn't have a balance nerve on the left side anymore! Another call to 911 and another trip to hospital. I was released the next morning with another diagnosis of migraine.

Hearing 'off'

I went to my neurologist who said it could have been a mini-stroke, I had had one in the past, and my ENT said he wanted to do some tests. My hearing suddenly became noticeably 'off' on the right side about the same time. The tests came back positive… bilateral Ménière's disease. The disease had played enough in my left ear and decided to take up residence in my right ear now.

Learning sign language

Since then, I have had many more attacks, my hearing is down to only about thirty percent on the right side and depending on the weather I have weeks at a time with one hundred percent deafness. My doctor says it is only a matter of time when I will not come out of one of the attacks with any hearing at all. So, I am back in ASL class re-learning sign language. The attacks are currently in remission. The tinnitus is predominately left-sided, but sometimes roars into the right side just for fun. And I deal with it…

That's all I can do. We all deal with it in our own ways. There is no cure right now. Perhaps through this book and the associated science there might come some encouragement to find a cure? I certainly hope so.

Thank you Tania and your partner... Keep up the good work so we don't have to... deal with it.

— Jeffrey Bowen
CEO Starbooker Presents

Note from Tania:

Jeffrey announced his retirement recently because of his disease. But finally he picked up work again.

CHRIS

The cruise of a lifetime.

Imagine, if you will, a once-in-a-lifetime cruise. Mine took place on the Rhine River in Germany, in December 2012. It is still with me now as I rock and sway. I was based in Nuremberg, visiting my dearest and oldest friend Sarah. We grew up together in Melbourne, Australia. She married a German and decided to live there. Hence the reason for my many visits. This time, Sarah had to work for the first week of my stay, so I booked my cruise… to visit the Christmas Markets.

It was a fabulous journey, fitting in well with the rest of my travel plans. Since I work as a travel consultant, I was able to secure my cabin at agents' rates, a mere $ 400 for a French balcony cabin.

What a price to pay.

My name is Chris, and as a result of that once-in-a-lifetime cruise, I now suffer from Mal de Débarquement syndrome.

When I returned to Nuremberg, I experienced rocking sensations, like being back on the boat. I was so tired in the afternoons. When I lay down, I felt like my head was being tilted backwards. My holiday was ruined. I still had two weeks to go. And it was Christmas. I truly do not know how I managed Christmas Day. I guess it was the love of those around me.

I always take a half empty suitcase with me when I travel. As Sarah's husband says, I help the German economy, because I love to shop. But even shopping became an effort and unpleasurable. Dealing with crowds, noise and bright lights. As I know now, all typical of MdDS symptoms. I managed to make it through the holiday season, and my return to Australia marked the end of one journey and the beginning of another.

I was home, on solid ground. But my body told me otherwise. My return to work was not fabulous. I was unable to sit for any length of time at my desk in front of the computer. I was even clumsy at making a cup of tea. My doctor diagnosed BPPV. He attempted the Epley maneuver, and I was given a series of exercises to do at home. To no avail.

Deal with it

A second visit to my doctor resulted in a diagnosis of labyrinthitis and a referral to an ENT specialist. It was she who diagnosed me with MdDS. She recommended a month off work with complete rest. In the interim, my CT scan and MRI came back normal. The ENT also referred me to a neurologist - which made sense, since MdDS is a neurological condition. I paid $ 230 for the privilege of being told: 'Go home and deal with it. If you had a broken leg, you would deal with the pain and get on with your life.' (MdDS is a chronic condition, by the way - unlike a broken leg, which is acute.)

After four weeks of 'resting' the best I could, I had a meeting with my employer. He suggested that perhaps I should find another, less stressful job. I knew I was going to have to resign. What really upset me was that, before I did so, my company was already advertising for a new travel consultant.

I resigned. I endeavoured to find support and joined the American Yahoo Support Group. I posted in the hope of finding other Australians suffering the same fate. Lo and behold: four other ladies, all within a one-hour drive. MdDS Australia was born.

From self-diagnosis to raising awareness

MdDS Australia, albeit only just over three years young, has grown to over one hundred and forty members, many of whom have a story to tell - from misdiagnosis to treatment not fitting their condition. I feel very blessed to have these people in my life. Some of them have become very good friends. Soul mates, in fact.

A survey was put out to the MdDS Australian Community in December 2014. Interestingly enough, it showed that almost fifty percent of the group was self-diagnosed. The rate of diagnosis by a neurologist was but nineteen percent. A follow-up survey in December 2015 demonstrated a significant change. Selfdiagnosis rate was down to thirteen percent and that by neurologists up to forty-six percent. MdDS Australia has certainly come a long way in raising awareness.

Once I gave up work, I applied to the Department of Human Services in Australia, seeking a disability allowance. It was rejected on two occasions. I was informed that my condition was not fully treated. Excuse me, but MdDS has no effective treatment nor cure. After nine months, my second appeal saw MdDS recognized as a disability, allowing other Australians with MdDS to make a claim.

We have also been fortunate to have a neuroscientist in Melbourne take an interest in research. Alan Pearce (Associate Professor at Swinburne University Melbourne) has done some fabulous work with Repetitive Trans Magnetic Stimulation (rTMS). His results to date have been promising and were published in January 2015 in the *Journal of Neuropsychology*. Unfortunately, I don't meet the criteria for his treatment due to other (non-MdDS-related) medication I am taking. In addition to which, MdDS Australia has an established Medical Advisory Board comprising of a neuroscientist (Alan Pearce – Associate Professor), two neurologists (based in Sydney and Melbourne), a leading vestibular physiotherapist in Adelaide (Dr Margie Sharpe) and an Assistant Professor in Neurology at MT Sinai in New York.

Onward and upward!

I have a chronic neurological balance disorder, which is with me 24/7. Some days are better than others. I have a list of over twenty exacerbating factors - including low weather pressure, hormonal changes (I am premenopausal), fatigue, stress, anxiety, confined spaces, bright lights, to name but a few.

I am a believer that there is a purpose to our lives. Mine is to help raise awareness about MdDS and to assist in research efforts. I trust that this account of my journey will be of benefit to those who read it.

I would like to thank my partner, Alan. We only met three months before my onset of MdDS. This wonderful man has been at my side ever since and supports both myself and MdDS Australia. Plus, to my children, Peter and Timothy. They didn't understand in the beginning. My Mum (in-law), who loves to cruise, my sister Sue Muller, together with all my dear friends. Not forgetting Alan Pearce. His support in raising awareness has been invaluable. And, of course my GP at Point Clare Medical Surgery.

– Chris Daws, Founder of MdDS Australia, VEDA Ambassador
Central Coast, NSW, Australia

CHERYL

I never got my land legs back.

My name is Cheryl, and I was first diagnosed around 1998. My initial onset was from a plane trip: I went on holiday to an island, and from the time I returned I was never the same. I could not stand up straight and had the feeling that a pendulum was going backwards and forwards, constantly on the go. I went to the local GP, and he said that sometimes after a trip it can take a little while for some people to get their land legs back. He advised bed rest and told me that, if I didn't feel better within two weeks, I should come see him again. Two weeks later, I went back, and he got me in to see a neurologist that very same day.

After about two months of tests, I was still feeling terrible and unable to work. I was referred to another neurologist, who ran further tests and diagnosed me with MdDS. But he left me feeling that it was all in my head, and told me there was nothing to be done to remedy my problem. I was still unable to work, and I kept on looking for more information on the Internet. I found the MdDS website in America, and at least it showed me that I wasn't alone.

Façade.

Despite the rocking, I was eventually able to go back to work. I was strong, and I maintained a façade, but people had trouble looking at me: I was making them feel sick with my rocking. I went on raising my family and ignoring how I felt, mostly because of that second neurologist, who had made me feel like I had created all these symptoms myself, and they were all in my head. Every day I would get out of bed feeling the motion, and I would persevere through the day, ignoring everything. Finally, after about a year of this, I woke up one morning and realized that it was gone. *Hip hip hooray*, I thought. *It's over!*

But you know what they say about counting your chickens...

Ignorance isn't bliss

Second onset. It was summer, and my family spent a lot of time near and on the water, but I would always stay ashore. On this particular day, the weather was beautiful, the water was very calm, and I let myself be talked into going with them on the boat.

Well, the next two weeks I once again had to have off work. When my body and brain got used to how I was feeling, I again ignored everything, kept it all to myself, and returned to my job.

I remember playing with my nephew, running after him as we were playing chase and catch. We were on a hill. I ran after him and caught him, but I kept going to the ground as gravity weighed me down. I grabbed my nephew and toppled onto him, which must have been very painful for the poor boy. He was crying, and blood was everywhere. I felt so bad!

From then on, I vowed I would not even pick him up, as my balance was clearly unstable. I kept making excuses so I didn't have to explain my situation, as I felt that for some reason my brain was making this all up.

After a few years, I divorced. I eventually started to date, but I would not tell anyone I began seeing that I could not go on plane trips or boat trips. I just kept defending Australia, insisting it was better to see our country by road.

Brain fog

When I met the man who was to become my new husband, I explained my condition to him. Most of the time, my rocking was under control - although my brain fog often interfered with my everyday life. I noticed that, the older I got, the more often the brain fog came. There were times when I could not even talk properly. I kept saying that I wasn't feeling well or was getting older and could not cook and run the everyday chores the way I used to… menopause, old age, getting slower at doing things, excuses, excuses. As the years passed, I would sometimes take a day off work, go to the doctor's and advise him that my work was very stressful. He would give me a couple of days off, not letting my employers know the real reason I was staying home.

A rare disorder

At long last, I saw something on a current-affairs program about people with seasickness - and, lo and behold, I learned about MdDS. Finally, after fifteen years, I could admit that I have a rare disorder. It's not in my head. I didn't make it up.

I have now started to see a neurologist again. He is trying me on medication, and hopefully I will get some vestibular therapy down the road. I also found the Australian support group for MdDS - and suddenly I was not alone any more. I was over the moon.

Unfortunately, the older I get, the more the MdDS is prevalent. I rock, I sway, I go to bed in a waterbed, I am taking more and more time off work.

Hard times

You see, I am a customer-service operator, and I work constantly with computers and phone calls. Sometimes when I answer phones, I can't even get my name out. It's now getting to the point where I am incapable of leaving my house, especially when the weather is bad. The only thing I can do is lie down with my head against a pillow and try to stop my body from rocking. I rock so much I can't even cook. I can't contribute to paying the household bills. I feel I am letting everyone down. I can't go out the door: people look at me as if I am a drunk, my head rocks backward and forward, I feel sick.

I used to play the piano, but now I get all the notes around the wrong way. The notes say to play one thing, but I end up playing something completely else. It's like I am dyslexic. When I type, I get some of the words backwards, too. I can't remember how to spell things, and I sometimes can't remember even the simplest of tasks or conversations.

Feeling helpless

Who knows what is around the corner for me? As I said: the older I get, the worse this becomes. There is no information on this rare disorder to advise on the outcome for people like me. Will I eventually be so completely housebound that I cannot even make a cup of tea, because I can't get the water in the cup? If I had a broken leg, people would provide support and sympathy. With MdDS, people look at me like I am a freak - and when they do, I feel so hopeless and helpless.

I am not dying, I know that. I don't have a fatal disease. But MdDS is very demoralizing.

— Cheryl,
Sydney, Australia

DONNA

Nurse becoming a patient.

My name is Donna, ex-nurse with Mal de Débarquement Syndrome (MdDS). Up until five years ago I was a very healthy and happy single parent of two teenagers; I worked full time selling caravans and my hobby and coping mechanism was dance.

In 2010, my then new partner and I decided we would take a trip. One I had dreamt of since my childhood... EGYPT. Until then I had never travelled by air any further than Vanuatu, which I had done on six occasions.

Hell, that was supposed to be my Dream trip!

October 2010 we left for our wonderful trip to Egypt, flying business class all the way to Cairo via Singapore and Dubai, in total luxury with flatbed sleeping available for our twenty-three-hour flight.

On arriving in Cairo, I was very wobbly on my legs and was feeling rather nauseous. I put it down to the pollution and the amount of hours we had travelled.

Over the next few days nothing seemed to change and I was having the strangest experience. Every time I walked out on balcony I felt like it was on slope, which gave me the sensation I was going to fall over the edge. Having a shower was the worst feeling of spinning and felt like I was going to fall over. Walking into the pyramids was terrifying! The ceiling of the tunnel is only about 1.3 m high and downhill roughly 100 m. I had that falling feeling the entire way down and it was so hot. When I got to the burial chamber I could hardly stand up because of the crazy rocking sensation. I started to realize I had problems with my balance as soon as I bent over or looked up at anything. It made visiting the temples very difficult and the constant nauseous feeling was wearing me out each day.

Labyrinthitis?

We were in Egypt for twenty long and hard days. The return trip was a non-eventful except for the overwhelming wrung-out feeling. Melbourne at last, fresh air and no pollution! No, I was still rocking and feeling ill. Two days later I ended up in hospital and the doctors were totally at a loss. After a week I got discharged, medicated with Serc and diagnosed with labyrinthitis, and being told it would be gone in six weeks.

Sent to se(a)e an ENT

Six months later, still rocking and sent to see an ENT specialist; after many tests, his wonderful idea was for him to put grommets in my ear, 'You will be fine then'. My old nursing brain said 'NO'. I agreed to be put on Moduretic to help keep my ears dry. After reading up on the internet I started to think I could have MdDS. I went to see another ENT specialist and got diagnosed with 'It's all in your head with your attitude – you will learn to live with it, and get on with your life.'

My world crashed down

I could not be a proper mum for my kids, or dance, and was only working part time by then. I was not coping on the inside but all looked good, yet wobbly, on the outside. The ex-nurse in me losing all confidence in the medical profession and myself, the permanent fake smile – the teenage kids not believing me anymore.

More of the same

Another ENT specialist. All becoming more expensive each time, as I climb the ladder. This one says Ménière's. After three MRIs and twelve hours of testing over the year I say 'No way', I have no hearing loss. I have this big inbuilt magnet inside me that pulls me to the right, constantly rocking, fatigue, Brain Fade, affected by weather change and can't go near a shopping center on my own, this is MdDS, I am sure.

Drug game

Next stop is a neurologist who diagnoses me with vestibular migraine and we start the drug game, three months on this, two months on that. I just go with the flow, he is one of the best, he must know what he is talking about. I am also told I must be medicated or I will get worse. I have trouble functioning, can't think for myself. My partner says, we are getting married and you are moving in with me. The kids can stay at your house, which is just around the corner and they are now in their early twenties. My partner is also my boss, and has known me for twenty years. I give in and say yes.

Floor contact

The week before our wedding I have my first bad fall, broken thumb and legs black and blue and one beautiful black eye. We all, including kids, laugh about it and move on. That was the first of three bad falls; I also fell out of an off-road caravan and tore my rotator cuff.

Tai Chi, yeah right!

April 2015, I go and visit my drug happy neurologist who still thinks I have vestibular migraine and I inform him I have been off the brain-numbing Topamax for two months and feel fine, but still rocking and fatigued but that is normal for me after four years. He is not happy when I suggest, could it be MdDS. His answer is no, because I still have the rocking motion when I lay down and MdDS does not last this long, I would be well and truly over it by now. His new suggestion: 'Maybe you should go and do some Tai Chi to relax.' Can you just image doing Tai Chi with no balance!

Making contact with the neuroscientist

I decide it is time to take my health in my own hands and look around for a doctor who does know about MdDS.

One week later I see a write up in the Melbourne Paper about a neuroscientist Dr Alan Pearce and he describes MdDS and a new treatment trial using TMS he is working on. I send him an e-mail that day, describing my symptoms and he makes contact suggest joining the facebook group of MdDS Australia.

What a breath of fresh air!

MdDS Australia, finally people the same as me! Instantly I lost my feeling of being alone and someone to talk to. The suggestion was to find a new doctor, one who understood my condition. My wonderful new GP supported me on my self-diagnoses. I found the brilliant Dr Luke Chen (neurologist) who agreed, most definitely MdDS. At the moment there is not a lot that can be done, but at least I have not gone mad and I have support.

Five years since my onset of MdDS, I am still rocking, have a frozen shoulder from my falls, and my body has decided it needs to stay on Moduretic or my feet and legs swell, but oh well, that is life when you have the Rare Disease called Mal de Débarquement Syndrome not many doctors know about it or seem to want to know.

Tunnel-vision specialists

Most of my nursing years were spent in a Theatre Suite so I have an understanding of how most specialist think; they have tunnel vision and don't like being questioned about a diagnosis and can be very closed minded when it comes to something rare.

All in all, I consider myself pretty lucky, MdDS cannot kill me but just rather debilitating. I have a wonderful new husband, two very happy and loving adult kids, four fabulous stepchildren, four beautiful grandsons and now I can just put on the music and close my eyes and dance in my head. Life is good. Now I have two doctors that support me and not put me down.

– Donna
Melbourne, Australia

Note from Tania

MdDS is still very unknown by doctors and needs more awareness and education quite urgently. I hope this story can help us all to accomplish a breakthrough.

IGNACIO

Dizzy boy in Chili becomes devoted kinesiologist.

My name is Ignacio, I am twenty-six years old and I live in Chili, South America. I was only ten when I experienced my first vertigo crisis. I was playing with my brother when suddenly my world started spinning. Since that day my life has changed for good.

Doctors reported I had a – bilateral – congenital malformation in the inner ear. I have moderate hearing loss and I am using hearing aids. I suffer non-stop from dizziness and I am pretty sure more people must be suffering like I do. I decided to devote my life to studying and rehabilitating vestibular patients.

From illness to devotion

Sixteen years have passed. Today I am a kinesiologist specialized in vestibular rehabilitation. I hope that this area will become more known in our country, so that patients do not have to live in the shadow and they can enjoy life just like every normal person.

I am regularly attending courses in South America to get updated on knowledge.

I always tell my patients: 'Each one has what he can endure, being out of balance modifies the way you think, feel and relate to people.' They are my patients, they feel like me.

I am a professional member of the Vestibular Disorders Association (VEDA) and raise awareness on social media. Check my facebook page 'Rehabilitación Vestibular V región'.

— Ignacio Novoa Cornejo, Chili,
South America

RIRI

In Indonesia, the Internet is the best doctor.

I am Riri, an Indonesian thirty-two-year-old female. In my country, we have lots of alternative approaches to health care, such as Traditional Chinese Medicine (TCM), acupuncture, etc. I work fulltime as a government employee in the IT sector. This job requires me to use a computer on a daily basis. I have already been diagnosed with tinnitus in both ears, but somehow both of my ears make sounds like an airplane engine the day before I have a vertigo attack.

Early one morning in March 2014, out of nowhere I felt a little bit wobbly. My hands were sweating, and I felt like I was walking on a boat. A couple of minutes later, I noticed that everything around me was either jumping or shaking. My friends took me to the nearest clinic. The room was spinning, and I puked a lot. I was not able to move my head. My heartbeat was very fast. After all that calmed down, I started to poo a lot. Miraculously, after that I was able to walk again. My GP told me that it could be Ménière's disease or just vertigo. She prescribed a betahistine and nausea medication.

The Internet is my best doctor!

After that, I have been to a TCM doctor, an acupuncturist, an ENT specialist, and a traditional massage therapist, but no one could tell me what type of vertigo I suffered from. You may laugh out loud, but it's true! Most doctors only said, 'You have vertigo' and nothing more. But vertigo is a symptom, not a disease. So I diagnosed myself, using Google and visiting various online support groups. I learned what to do and what not to do. I requested specific medications and blood tests, based on my research on the Internet.

Limiting my social life

Vertigo does limit my social life. I never have the confidence to go outside and meet people without having my family or friends nearby. This really bothers me, since I am a single traveler who enjoys exploring new places. I always bring my medicine everywhere I go and tell people around me that I can get an attack out of nowhere. I am very curious to read the book Dizzy Me. I am sure this will help me and a lot of patients like me! All I can say is I will survive!

— Riri
Jakarta, Indonesia

TANIA - SILLY ME

Silly Me...

Hi there. It's me again, Dizzy Me. Being cured from my vestibular disorder since 2008, at the end of 2015 I got a nose surgery due to severe malformation causing bilateral pan sinusitis infections with fever. Blah...

Nose issues

On 26 November I got a septum correction and cystectomy. Fine, hoping for the better to come. But it didn't turn out better that easy. In fact, the wounds after surgery were healing well, but it was the start of a very difficult recovery process. Blah again...

Tough recovery

First I didn't respond very well to anesthesia. But allright, that happens to many of us. Right?

To keep my new septum straight, I got internal nasal splints for five days, splints made of silicone. That caused my second disappointment, because my nose kind of rejected them; I didn't stop sneezing, which was actually a 'not done' issue after surgery, and that sneezing caused a lot of blood issues and was definitely exhausting me.

Then I got two more weeks of intensive nose and sinus care (non-stop rinsing with salt water and follow-up treatments in hospital) and plenty of bad nights. I ended up exhausted, caught a cold from my kids and wrestled with severe headaches and persistent feeling of sinusitis.

So I googled desperately what could help me to get rid of my persistent headaches

– especially focusing on the eye and sinus zone – and I went to the pharmacy to get myself a wonder treatment for head colds and stuffed nose, not subject to medical prescription, and containing those ingredients I wanted: kalium bichromicum, cinnabaris and silicea. After some advice I got some chewing tablets containing an extra ingredient which would relieve my severe pain: belladonna.

That cruel belladonna

I came home and told it to a fellow patient – one of my dizzy me believers, Verony – who warned me I should be very careful with belladonna, as this could trigger the vestibular system; she got too many of that in eye drops for eye tests and in anesthesia products, causing severe damage to her system. But, giving the fact that she is a 'severe case', I judged for myself this product would not harm me, as my vestibular system is doing just fine since I had my canal plugging surgery for BPPV in October 2008. I started to take two pills three times. That same day I had to take my car to get my medical papers in order, and felt severe eye focus problems. But didn't make the link yet.

I must mention also, since a few days before taking those pills, I already experienced a slight dizzy sensation when moving my head in bed. Not that bad, but present. Perhaps caused by the sinusitis effect, I thought. But it awakened old BPPV memories and fears, for sure.

The day after. First severe dizzy incident. I reached for my medical dossier on a chair, bending over with my head. Immediately I felt the world shifting. I felt I would fall over. Surprised by the event, I got myself through the kitchen door, searching for the walls with my hands, but then the world around me started moving again. I could not do anything else than prevent worse by letting myself fall gently on the cold kitchen floor and sit down there, until I was able to stand up again. Incident closed. And wanting so much to forget it. In the afternoon I noticed my ears started ringing. Didn't make the link... yet.

At night I had my second dizziness attack. It started with slight dizzy feelings in bed, getting worse each time I moved, lasting for hours. I got so bad, recognized all the symptoms, just like when I was suffering from my old BPPV troubles, with that one big difference: it wasn't the vertigo like I had before, it was more a feeling of 'the world shifting', and being extremely drunk.

At the end I got that sick I had to go to the bathroom with the help of my husband. All the experience and knowledge on dizziness I gathered during the last twenty-two years didn't stop me from panicking. I tried my dizzy-me tricks to stimulate blood flow in my neck, without result. I became very anxious and felt horrible. Sweating, panting, breathing vigorously, starting to hyperventilate (even when I was counting to breathe out three times as long to get it under control), needing to go to the loo, my arms both sleeping (side effect of the hyperventilation, caused by the dizziness and not vice versa!), and almost fainting, trembling, crying. Got on the floor with a bucket; the nausea made me vomit. Blah. Blah. Disgusting!

After that we managed to get upstairs and I decided to spend the rest of the night under a blanket on the sofa, keeping my head upright. Too anxious.

'WhatsApp?', Floris said

My kids found me the next morning, horrified by what happened to me after all those nice dizzy-free years. My oldest son asked me if I didn't need to call my GP. No way, I said. Not because I don't trust my GP, but this was too complicated to get a right diagnosis. I would have to hear that I had an inconvenient but harmless dizziness attack. 'No one would be able to help me', I said, 'besides my co-author Floris'. And as five years of being co-authors resulted in my deep respect for the expertise of Floris and a nice friendship, I *WhatsApped* him my horrible story and cry for help that night.

The next morning I was invited by him to come in for some tests to sort out as quickly as possible what was happening to me. My husband went working early, so my son Matthias, who experienced and remembers my dizzy life the most – since his birth till he got eight or nine years old – managed to get me to the bathroom to get dressed and ordered me a taxi from my neighbor to the hospital.

Same story passing again

In hospital I had an audiogram – the last one was in 2009, my hearing now was okay – and a Dizziness Handicap Inventory questionnaire to answer. Next, Floris and his ENT colleague went through my whole post-sinus operation and medication history and the dizzy events of the last days. Then they did the video nystagmography test and they went through my old brain MRI images taken for my canal plugging surgery in 2008.

They found out what had happened to me and discussed this in my presence, which was really nice for me, it enabled me to understand perfectly what was going on. This wasn't BPPV. The canal plugging is still okay – I did Paris-Roubaix, which contains more than fifty kilometers on cobbles, I would have noticed then if there was a problem with that...

A different devil

One issue they could see on my old MRI is the blood vessel and the vestibular nerve 'making contact'. This happens to many people, and it could cause vestibular paroxysmia, or not. It never occured to me before. So what did happen to cause it now?

First, anesthesia can trigger the vestibular system and especially that VP (blood vessel widening drugs, but I don't know what anesthesia products they gave me). It even doesn't mean you feel the impact immediately.

Second, the belladonna. Stupid me... belladonna is an atropine – and often anesthesia products just act the same. So I got a temporary VP triggered just by taking that.

Detox Tania

I stopped taking the medication, and soon started to feel the difference. My system was eliminating the last bits of belladonna. Probably I will not have to feel this horrible VP again. In case it would appear again, he wrote me a prescription of anti-eplieptica to eliminate the symptoms, but lucky me I didn't need that!

Belladonna. Look it up. Wikipedia tells a lot. They give it to soldiers after a gas attack, or when doing reanimation on heart patients. It stimulates the nervous system and can be toxic. Be careful when you have a sensitive vestibular system and when you buy products containing this ingredient.

Don't become like Silly Me.

— Tania (Dizzy Me)
Belgium

MARC CUBAN

Virtual reality gave me my brain back

No, this is not a joke. It isn't a set-up for a routine or comedy. It is a real title for a very real and nerve-wracking experience I had.

On May 20th, 2015 I was in New York City. Like I love to do on a nice day, I took a long walk through the city. When I say long, I mean long. From Columbus Circle down to the Alphabet Streets and back. My step count was through the roof. I got back to my apartment, showered and soon after I had a headache. I rarely get headaches, so I thought maybe it was dirt and grime and whatever that had accumulated on my contacts. Took them out. I was tired. So I went to bed. Expecting to feel better in the morning after a good night's sleep.

May 21st, 2015. I woke up dizzy. My initial reaction was that I had a form of vertigo. I had experienced vertigo multiple times before. Once when I was staying in Manhattan Beach, I woke up with vertigo, thought we were in the middle of an earth quake and rushed to alert my neighbors. All of whom made it clear that there was no earthquake. There had not been an earthquake. And maybe I had too much to drink the night before.

My most recent vertigo experience was a good ten years ago and with a trip to the doctor I was given a few pages with a series of head movement exercises. By the next day I was fine. It was as if nothing had happened. So on May 21st, 2015 my expectation was that all would be fine shortly. I did my exercises. Unfortunately, they did not work. At the end of the day I was still what is easiest to describe as being dizzy, but it was far more than that. My brain was in a fog, I felt hungover. I felt some nausea, without having had a drink. My face and ears felt full. I can't fully describe it or give justice to just how off I felt. My balance was fine. My body below the neck was fine. I never felt better. But inside my head something was definitely wrong. I headed back to Dallas still believing it was vertigo related and I was just missing something.

I visited my doctor who suggested I get more electrolytes and see if that helped. It did a tiny bit, but not much. After which I started 'the rounds'. He sent me for an MRI of my head - nothing. My neck. Nothing. An MRA. Nothing. All of which was obviously good news at the highest level. It did not appear to be anything life-threatening. Then I made the rounds to ear, nose and throat (ENT) doctors. Nothing. I was in tip top shape. Then my doctor suggested I visit a neurologist. She immediately concluded that it was not physical and completely stress related and that I should see a psychiatrist, but first here is some Klonopin for you to take to help you. That made me even worse. I would take dizzy and nauseas over how the klonopin made me feel any day and I knew it wasn't a psychological issue. So I got off of those meds quickly.

Then I found another physician who had more experience in treating dizziness and related issues. To his credit, he pushed me to do the full battery of tests that are normal for these types of issues, but unfortunately it was now the second week of June and I had to head to LA to start shooting Shark Tank in a couple days. I don't remember how we got to it, but he suggested valium.

Boom. It worked. Mostly.

I was no longer dizzy. I actually felt alright. When I took nine milligrams of valium. The problem of course is that I wanted to lay down and take a nap all the time. But it got me through the first shooting pod of Season 7 of Shark Tank. So when you are watching, if you notice I look really, really relaxed and maybe a little tired or sleepy, now you know why. While the valium certainly helped, it became obvious to me that taking nine milligrams of valium a day was no way to go through life. So I began trying to reduce my dosage. I got it so that within a couple weeks I could take half a milligram in the morning and half in the afternoon and get to an acceptable state. I also found that the busier I kept myself, the less I thought about it and the better I felt. Of course the doctors were sure at that point that if valium worked (as did drinking. Drunk felt like every drunk night before it), that it must be stress. It was not.

I would be lying if I didn't say that I was concerned as my family headed off to Southern California for a vacation. I didn't want to drive with my family in the car. Every terrible possibility I could conjure in my head as a problem, I did. I read everything and anything that I could about dizziness. Unfortunately, dizziness is a symptom for almost everything. I found nothing. I was miserable. Valium was not a solution. Not a way I wanted to go through life.

Dizzyland

Then I stumbled onto a website dizziland.com. It claimed to cure 95% of patients who come in with dizziness. I was desperate. It was a thirty-minute drive from where we were vacationing, so I made an appointment. It was for first week of August.

Dr. Mango and his crew put me through about five hours of tests. From what I understand they were traditional, for the most part. I got spun, turned, twisted, ballooned and then they put me in a dark room, strapped me in to a chair and asked me to use a joy stick to demonstrate that I could align a red line absolutely vertical, and absolutely horizontal. My vertical was no problem. Horizontal? I was convinced I was laying the line down so it was absolutely flat. As it turns out I wasn't close. I was off 38%. That was good.

The audiologist, Dr. Pearce, told me that was the information they needed. She was confident she could get me back to normal. When I asked what caused the problem, there was no answer. It could be an inner ear infection or something else. But she was fairly certain that an otolith in my vestibular system had been damaged. The way she explained it, and I am paraphrasing, I was dizzy because my eyes, the otolith in my vestibular system and brain were out of whack. My damaged otolith was telling my brain I was falling or off balance, but my eyes were saying everything was normal. So my brain was confused and working overtime, resulting in all the problems I was experiencing. Obviously I was thrilled. But getting back to normal wasn't a quick process. In my original blog post you will find a video I asked to do for Dizziland to tell people who were experiencing what I was experiencing that there was hope. What you cannot really see is that I am in front of what is called an Epley Chair.

If you watch the video, you will see the spinning chair. For my case, the chair was in a dark enclosure. Dr. Mango had created the special enclosure for the chair, but more importantly, he created a protocol of videos that would be projected against the walls. While I watched the videos there were cameras looking at my eyes, measuring the response of my eyes. It was a solution that he had integrated and it was working. In the dark room, the protocol would sometimes show star like objects projected against the walls of the room. Sometimes I would be still. Sometimes I would be moving. Sometimes they would be slow, sometimes they would be faster. All in all I would be in the chair about an hour. Every day.

I was making progress. But my time in Southern California was coming to an end. I had to get back to Dallas. Which was a problem because my brain really benefited from daily treatment. There were no chairs available to me in Dallas. There were only twenty in the entire country. Almost all in Veteran's Hospitals where they were used to treat servicemen and women who had suffered various types of head trauma resulting in dizziness. The closest to me was in San Antonio and it did not run the protocol Dr. Mango had created.

Desperate

I literally was desperate. I was making progress. I was getting closer and closer. So I looked into buying my own chair and enclosure and hiring one of Dr. Mango's audiologists to move to Dallas to start a Dizziland branded office in Dallas. It would help not only me, but also others who could benefit from the same therapy. It was September going into October at this point and I was at what I would call about 60%. But unless I could just go back out to Southern California and stay until I was fixed, I was going to have to wait several months to put all this together. To try to mitigate the problem and buy time, the doctors gave me videos to watch on a laptop screen in the dark. It did not help. I was not getting better and on some days it was much worse.

Then it hit me. Why not put the videos on my phone and look at them in the Samsung VR set I had bought just to try to learn more about VR. Bingo. I started using Dr. Mango's protocol in the Samsung VR Glasses every morning and every night and started making progress nearly every day. Day after day, night after night I was in my bedroom or a hotel room with my Goggles on watching white boxes on a black background scroll past my eyes. My doctors had me standing sometimes. Laying down sometimes. Standing on a pillow in the morning, rolling side to side while watching at night.

By November I was 75%, by December 90%. By the end of January and into February I had days where I felt completely normal. I was able to reduce my use of the googles to every third day. Then every week. Today, I use them for maintenance every couple of weeks just to play it safe, but I am back to normal and happy. Virtual reality along with Dr. Mango, his protocol and some amazing audiologists, Dr. Pearce and Dr. Nava, gave me my brain back. I cannot thank them enough. VR worked so well, Dr. Mango and I are now patenting the entire protocol and program and he is already testing it with great results with some of his other patients. Hopefully it can have the same impact on others that it had on me.

Mark Cuban - July 16, 2016

American businessman, investor, author, television personality & philanthropist
Owner of the NBA's Dallas Mavericks
Co-owner of 2929 Entertainment and chairman of the AXS TV
Known from the ABC reality television series, Shark Tank

ALEXANDER HANDY

Dizzy in a virtual world

Much has been written about VR's undeniable potential. Unfortunately, conversation about the risks remains muted or trivialized. 'Everyone is cautious about new technology' is a common retort. Yet, the stories and science of motion sickness is real and must be addressed. If not, VR will at best remain a niche, and at worst keep making people ill.

So what happened to me?

Last year I was trying out a demo experience that a developer friend of mine from California had built. The experience put the two of us in a virtual world at the same time. We could interact with objects, talk and move around at full-room scale in real-time. But there was one feature which, quite literally, threw me into a spin.

This virtual world could be made to rotate and replicate the sensation of walking side by side with a friend. This sounded interesting so I was keen to give it a go. Problem was, as we were walking and talking, I wasn't walking, I was standing still.

I had been in the experience for over half an hour by this point so didn't really notice the change. We continued for another fifteen to twenty minutes and then said our goodbyes. I removed the headset and initially felt fine. Fifteen minutes later I had a severe headache and dizziness. I wasn't hugely surprised by this. Having reflected on the unusual sensation that my brain had just been put through (thinking it's moving when my body is not) I expected some backlash.

What surprised me, was that my dizziness and sporadic headaches had not gone three days later despite taking anti-vertigo medication. It would take almost six weeks, a trip to Accident & Emergency, three scans and vestibular physio for my symptoms to fully disappear.

Unfortunately, your average consumer may have no idea that things could go awry. Given VR is being used by millions and millions more people, it's important for the community to be mindful that we have an incredibly powerful tool in our hands.

This can do amazing things, but also cause harm.

Alexander Handy
VR and AR freelance consultant
Founder VsportR
United Kingdom

EMPOWERED PATIENTS FOR CHANGE

Letter to WHO (petition addressed to World Health Organization)

– The story behind a DreamTeam Empowering for Change

Imagine a world where dizzies received a fast diagnosis, appropriate treatment and even a cure. If this were a contract for life, wouldn't you sign immediately?

Reality shows us a very different picture; doctors report they are often poorly trained in vestibular conditions. Young doctors choosing to become ENT specialist want to perform surgery. They receive important training for this, but not enough regarding balance issues. While treating dizzy patients with success implies a multidisciplinary approach, with knowledge in ENT, neurology, neuro-ophthalmology. Today this is rather an exception. Misdiagnosis is a very common phenomenon. Worldwide.

It is obvious, when you read the threads in many Facebook groups: vestibular patients all agree 'we need change'. But change will not come if we wait for some other person or some other time. We are the ones we have been waiting for. We are the change that we seek. Change is 'waiting for us'. We can make a difference, if we take action, bottom-up, to awaken the world.

This is why I convinced a group of eleven empowered patients to initiate that famous petition to the World Health Organization calling for better awareness of vestibular disorders among medical professionals.

Our goal? Give vestibular patients a better chance for accurate diagnosis, a cure or appropriate treatment. Asking for a worldwide agreement on education of medical students, further training for existing specialists. And asking for the establishment of medical guidelines regarding vestibular disorders.

Who are we? Verony, David, Chris, Tamar, Kim, Polly, Margaret, Richard, Beth, Liesbeth and Tania. Eleven e-patients from the USA, Australia, the UK, the Netherlands and Belgium (most of them have their stories published in this book).

Okay, it was a huge effort to get this started. Skype seemed too difficult to talk with one another when some of us live in Belgium, the Netherlands or the UK while the USA and Australia are asleep... But even different time zones and scrolling issues – you know, dizzies can't handle that! – could not stop us from working together. Using Messenger groups with several themes: one for brainstorming, one for gathering petition material, one for listing people to contact. As simple as that!

After a few drafts, we quickly agreed on our petition text. Although it isn't the easiest text to read, and this 'level of communication' can discourage some people. Dizzies having difficulties in reading it all. We ask that you do read and sign it. Arguments are key, if you want to make a difference when knocking on the door of a World organization like WHO.

We decided to make use of the beautiful artwork of my daughter, to catch people's attention and visualize the idea of multidisciplinarity. With many variants from different dialogues, used during Balance Awareness Week (#BAW).

The results? Well, first of all, the idea of taking bottom-up action, showing the world that patients are getting empowered, raising their voices in a positive way, has not shocked but rather charmed many doctors. Some of them even signed and commented. Hurray! And reading the comments of vestibular patients shows us that this petition was the best thing ever we initiated as a team. We even received some success stories as a result of the petition; doctors using SoStoned and patients who finally got a correct diagnosis and better treatment.

In four months time, we have gathered almost 2500 signatures. Working together to achieve this was the most wonderful thing to do, with lots of happy, funny, even emotional moments, and some new friendships too!

Please join and support this wonderful action. We hope we will get many more signatures before we can address this to WHO and get the change dizzies are asking for. Will you join us?

https://www.change.org/p/world-health-organization-who-vestibular-patients-for-smarter-doctors-and-better-patient-care

Thank you so much,
Your Dizzy Dream Team

Petition Text: Vestibular patients for smarter doctors & better patient care

Goal

We aim to give vestibular / neurovestibular patients a better chance for swift and accurate diagnosis, a cure or appropriate treatment. We ask for a worldwide agreement on education of medical students, further training for existing specialists and the establishment of medical guidelines regarding vestibular conditions / disorders.

The problem/situation today

'More than 1 in 20 US children between the ages of 3 and 17 have dizziness and balance problems.' [Sciencedaily]

'A variety of balance disorders affects up to 30-40% of the population before they reach the age of 60. About a quarter of those affected will have to take time off work, with a large socioeconomic cost when untreated. However, because of complexity of the balance control mechanisms, patients with balance disorders may have to see several doctors / consultants at primary and secondary care level before a correct diagnosis is made. Therefore vestibular / neurovestibular patients may remain without a correct diagnosis and without appropriate care for very long periods of time.' [EMBalance]

'The presence of dizziness in the elderly is a strong predictor of falls, which is the leading cause of accidental death in people older than 65 years.' [Frontiers in Neurology]

Doctors report that they are often poorly trained in vestibular and neuro-vestibular conditions. 'Misdiagnosis rates in the Emergency Department for peripheral vestibular disorders are estimated in the range of 74 to 81%.' [Neurologic Clinics]

Additionally, because there is a lack of understanding of these disorders, GPs may prescribe vestibular suppresent medications as a 'treat all' which can cause further damage as these are only suitable for certain conditions and can be harmful for others.

Likewise they may want to treat using the Epley manouver on the basis of symptom descriptions rather than appropriate testing. Whilst this can help with BPPV it can be harmful for people with other vestibular / neurovestibular conditions. So the guidance here needs to be for GPs not to treat the symptoms until an accurate diagnosis has been made.

Likewise they prescribe Betahistine; it works for Ménière's, but can keep a patient with another disorder ill for even a longer period.

How to make the changes doctors and patients need

Misdiagnosis / mistreatment being a worldwide problem, we endeavour to empower doctors to help more people regain their lives.

We ask:

1) These basics:

For a greater understanding amongst the entire medical profession of the following principle: that our balance is not only a matter of our vestibular system (and thus coming under the specialism of ENT) but **rather a coming together of 4 sensory systems:** the vestibular system, the visual system, the proproceptive system and central brain processing systems (cerebellum etc).

That **vestibular disorders should not be the expertise of ENT only**. Doctors working in the field of ENT, neurology, ophthalmology / eye doctors, audiology and physiotherapy (physical therapy) – and, crucially, geriatrics for the elderly - should work together in multi disciplinary teams to give their patients a better chance for a cure or appropriate treatment. We also ask them to **share the latest knowledge and new research outcomes across disciplines and with patients.**

That balance and vestibular conditions / disorders become a **mandatory, full and substanciated part of all general medical studies** due to the percentage of the population who present with these conditions.

That **retraining in General Practice should include balance / vestibular disorders training as a matter of priority**. As a result of this, all GPs should know how to make appropriate referrals for testing and treatment. We want them to be aware of these basics: a peripheral vestibular disorder is a dysfunction of the balance organs of the inner ear. A central vestibular disorder is a dysfunction of one or more parts of the central nervous system that processes balance and spatial information. And **each disorder needs a different approach** - *Vestibular Neuritis, Labyrinthitis, Benign Paroxysmal Position Vertigo, Ménière's Disease, Vestibular Migraine, Vestibular Paroxismia, Superior Semicircular Canal Dehiscence syndrome, Mal de debarquement syndrome, Perilymph Fistula, Autoimmune Inner Ear Disease, Persistent Positional Perceptive Dizziness or Triple PD and Bilateral Vestibulopathy, Childhood Dizziness... and even more to be discovered by research...*

2) For diagnosing:

The **'SO STONED' diagnostic mneumonic to be adopted worldwide** to guide the clinician to an accurate diagnosis. Key factors that allow a first approximation of diagnosis identification are based on the time profile, symptom profile, and trigger profile of the disorder. 'SO STONED' comprises eight different dimensions that characterize the vertigo-related complaints of the patient and guide the clinician in his or her decision scheme.

That all doctors **pay attention to these life threathening diseases:**

A **brain tumor** to be ruled out
The **BEE FAST** method to be used to rule out **stroke** when a clinician sees a dizzy patient [World Stroke Campaign] : [Balance – Eyes – Face – Arms – Speech – Time – Call 911 for immediate medical attention].

That all doctors remember to '**Think Zebra**'. Within the category of vestibular / neurovestibular conditions there are two rare disorders: SCCD (peripheral) and MdDS (central). But there are also many other rare conditions which have symptoms that overlap with more common balance conditons, including IIH and the less common forms of ataxia.

3) Certification

That professionals who adopt this approach and develop this expertise be **granted appropriate certification / accreditation** and listings in relevant registries.

4) Medicine to benefit from empowered patients:

That **patients are involved** in this process as much as possible, for example via health conferences that have patients on stage and in the program. Patients also have a valuable role to play in providing training and with the design of research.

Outcomes

As well as revolutionising health care for patients with primary vestibular / neurovestibular conditions this approach will add to the cadre of doctors who are able to support patients with a wide variety of conditions that can have an impact on balance, including Vision Disorders, Parkinson's, Multiple Sclerosis, Cerebral Palsy, Hyperventilation, Neurofibromatosis...

These are my fellow campaigners:

* **Verony Manders (the Netherlands)** is striving for a multi-disciplinary approach for 35 years, based on the principle that our balance is a coming together of the four sensory systems explained in this petition. For 35 years she was misdiagnosed and mistreated and she pays a high price for this; so she is highly motivated to do everything she can to ensure this doesn't happen to anyone else. Now she asks ENT, neurology and ophthalmology to work together. She raises awareness with her page Eerlijk over Evenwicht.

* **David Morrill (USA)** is a stroke survivor and works with a team of Healthcare professionals led by John Hopkins University to help facilitate the difference between acute vertigo and stroke and the propensity to be a diagnostic error in the Emergency Room setting. He is also a VEDA Ambassador.

* **Chris Daws (Australia)** focuses on patients with MdDS, a very under-represented group of neuro-vestibular patients. Mal de Débarquement Syndrome has been with Chris since December 2012, after disembarking from a river cruise in Germany. After two misdiagnoses and being told to go home and deal with it, she now leads a support group for those with *MdDS in Australia*. The aim of MdDS Australia is to raise awareness of this condition. Chris is also a VEDA ambassador.

* **Tamar Schwarz (USA)** is blogging under the name *Visible Person, Invisible Problem* on 'the invisible factor' of vestibular and vision disorders. Vision plays a key role in the entire system of balance. She is also a VEDA Ambassador.

* **Kim Striber (USA)** was once a nurse, caring for patients. Today she is a patient needing expert care. Her life had been filled with outdoor adventure before she got her Central Vestibular Disorder diagnosis. She now runs a page *TrekToBalance*. She is also a VEDA ambassador.

* **Polly Moyer (UK)** campaigns for people with rare conditions and for the organizations set up to support and empower 'zebra' patients. She has blogged for several of these organizations and gives presentations about rare conditions to medical students. In May 2016 the BMJ – formerly the British Medical Journal – published her article '*Healthy approaches to rare conditions*'. Polly is also the co-founder of Action for MdDS UK.

* **Margaret Byrne (USA)** was a Certified Occupational Therapy Assistant (COTA), working with children with Neurological, Sensory, and Developmental Issues. She was misdiagnosed for one year and now has a chronic Vestibular Disorder and blogs about living with one. She blogs under the name *Sneezemedizzy* and she is also a VEDA Ambassador.

* **Richard Brinkman (the Netherlands)** runs a page *Evenwichtblog.nl* sharing his search for a right diagnosis and cure. He recently got the vestibular paroxysmia diagnosis and finally received a successful treatment. He is dizzyfree for almost a year now.

* **Beth Rye (UK)** is a young woman who has been suffering from an extremely rare inner-ear condition called superior semicircular canal dehiscence (SSCD)

since June 2013. Beth's symptoms started at the age of twenty-three, as she was just completing her nursing degree. After eighteen months of trying to get a diagnosis, fourteen weeks in hospital and two failed operations, she was left with very few options in the UK. Her brother started the *Getting Beth Better* crowdfunding campaign to raise money needed for Beth to travel to Boston to be treated for her condition. Beth had surgery in July 2015 and is receiving treatment for Lyme disease nowadays.

* **Liesbeth Duits (the Netherlands)** is a very young woman suffering from an extreme vestibular condition. Her illness started in 2011, but even today no doctor has been able to find the cause nor treatment to get her better. She has a blog *Hearme2* which means 'hear me out' and tells us about her endless search for appropriate diagnosis/treatment. 'Most frustrating is that a patient is no longer a person, but just a number. The struggle against rigid systems and doctors who don't analyze my illness as a team. Not looking at me as a person. And when they don't, I am left with no options for a treatment.'

More info on VEDA: *vestibular.org*

PS I want to thank my lovely daughter Charlotte for making this nice 'balanced' painting (in fact she just painted me and her dad); we will use her artist work with pride to defeat dizziness!

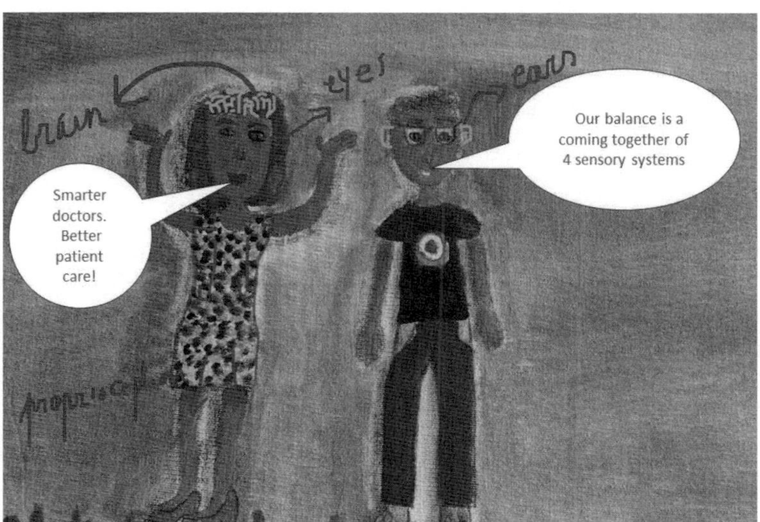
brain
eyes
ears
Our balance is a coming together of 4 sensory systems
Smarter doctors. Better patient care!

Acknowledgements

More than 250 people contributed to the English edition, which makes them all PART of an international book, with voices from all over the world.

Supporter, Fan, Friend, Believer, Contributor, Ambassador, Super Sponsor, Magic Investor, Dizzy Me Fellow or Pioneering Changemaker; our Ulule crowdfunding campaign suggested different formulas, giving everybody the opportunity to find his/her best match gift and be part of this English publication. This was your choice:

- For € 5 or more: 23 funders
- Dizy Me Supporters For € 10 or more: 80 funders
- Dizzy Me Fans For € 25 or more: 85 funders
- Dizzy Me Friends For € 55 or more: 50 funders
- Dizzy Me Believers For € 105 or more: 11 funders
- Dizzy Me Contributors For € 155 or more: 7 funders
- Dizzy Me Ambassadors For € 255 or more: 2 funders
- Dizzy Me Super Sponsor For € 500 or more: 1 funders
- Dizzy Me Magic Investors For € 1,000 or more: 2 funders

Dizzy Me's Super Sponsor

The Belgian company **Stadsbader** became our Super Sponsor by funding € 500 for translation of 2500 words.
Thank you to my family, thank you Désiré, to be part of history!

Dizzy Me's Magic Investors

Miep Hermans – Van Helden of the Netherlands was our first Magic Investor; she donated € 1100 to get 5500 words translated.
Menno and Ineke De Vries of the Netherlands donated € 1200 to get 6000 words of dizzy me translated.
A very special thank you to both Magic Investors.

Thank you to these Belgian, Dutch, American and Australian Dizzy Me funders, and thank you to my family and friends who are not dizzy but who believe in this project:

Gerrit Achterland, Alena Aga, Guy Annunziata, Monique Aschman – Bliekendaal, Albert Atkins, Kris Baert, Ann Baetens, Gridje Bauwens, Wim Blaton, Eric Boers, Johan Bombois, Andrea Boogaard – Rutjes, Richard en Grietje Brinkman, Hilde Bruyndonckx, Dirk Bultereyst, Fernand en Monique Buysse, William Buyst, Catherine Callens, Brenda Casteleyn, Nancy Celis, Ineke Ceuterick, Toef Clement, Justin Coenders, Inge Cornillie, Agnes Coron, Boris Cossement, Arn Cowan, Isabelle Cruypelinck, Family Cup, Danielle Dahler, Chris Daws, Carmen De Backer, Bram De Cocq, Esther de Cocq – Piepenbroek, Suzanne De Cort, Eric De Greef, Stephanie De Jaeger, Ann De Jaeger, Meike De Jongh, David De Keukeleire, Wendy De Keyser, Ingrid De Kinder, Joeri De Knop, Etienne De Pauw, G. De Rot, Ann De Valck, Bart De Visser, Kim De Witte, Maarten De Wolf, Esther Decocq, Mike Decocqies, Siglinde Deconinck, Dari Decoster, Rob Dedel, Johan en Kristien Demuydt, Rian Den Boer, Mieke Denys, Katleen Dereu, J.G.W. Derks, Sofie Deruyttere – Martens, Peter Devalez, Draisineken Ladies, Françoise Druguet, Liesbeth Duits, Annick Dumoulin, Sabrina Durieux, Family Eikenaar, Steph Feremans, N. Franke, Ann Gaeremynck, Bert Geens, Monique Geeroms, Pieter Ghijssels, Gemma Hagens, Christel Hanssens, Dieter Hautman, Christel Hemelinckx, Linda Hendrickx, Bas Hendrikse, Armand Hermans, Christa Hermans, Lulu Hermans, Maartje Hermans, Remi Hermans, Silke Hermans, Allan Hodgden, William Horlait, Bets en Fritz Huys, R. Icks, George Ide, Peter Jacobs, Toine Janssen, Peter Janssens, Harry Jaspers – Focks, Wilma Jenniskens – Spreeuwenberg, T.G.W. Jeurissen, Tina Joos and Kris Poelaert, Gerlinde Juurlinck, Brenda Keirsebilck, Ingrid Kempen, Petra Keppel, Peggy Kirsch, Carla Koopman, Jimmy Koroli, Guus Krähe, Anita Langeveld, Mark Langohr, Ann Lanneer, Jenny Lauwereys, Ria Lauwers, Cecile Lems, Els Leunens, Marianne Levering, François Lhermite, Katrin Liegeois, Dirk Lindemans, Jos Litjens, Geert Lories, R.T. Louw, ATC Maessen – Schutte, Miguel Major, Sanne Manders, Verony Manders, Josiane Massage, Liliane Massagé, Marc Mertens, Family Mertens – Stas, Ria Middel, Guy Minnebach, Sarah Moens, Family Moens – Praet, Christiane Moonen, Mariana Moreira, David Morill, Dorien Mot, Polly Moyer, Anne Nechelput, Corinne Niemuis, Inne Nollet, Jerinde Odinck – Talen, Jenny Oosterlinck, Nancy Paternoster, D. Piepenbroek – Staniford, Janneke Piepenbroek – Heijstek, Vladimir Pletser, Lenny Reijnierse, Bert Reyniers, Familie Rijnbende, Willemijn Roeland – De Vries, Luc Roossens, Greet Rozeboom, Jan Rutjes, Annet Scheek, Richard Scholten, Michael Schoukens, Jean – Pierre Schoukens, Tamar Schwarz, Muriel Segers, Leen Seynaeve, Richard Simoens, Noël Sissau, Isolde Sleeckx, Mario Sluijter, Junior Smith, Veerle Snoeck, Luc Somers, Patrick Somers, Jeanne – Marie Speleers, Julien Stadsbader and Anna Abeloos, Helena Stadsbader, Marian Stadsbader, Tania Stadsbader, Fabian Stalpaert, Jaqueline Stogall, Kimberly Striber, Kim Striber, Dimitri Stuer, Thor Talpe, Tina Teulingkx, Christina Thorngreen, Linda Timmermans, Franky Timmermans, WTG Timmermans, Andre tJonke – Devos, Annick Van Bellinghen, Monique Van Boeckel, Betty Van Brussel, Stefaan Van Damme, Karel Van de Keybus, Mieke Van de Wiele, Familie Van den Bogaard, Arthur Van den Hoof, Charlotte Van den Hoof , Matthias Van den Hoof, Thomas Van den Hoof, Patrick Van Eesbeek, Ivan Van Hassel, Fien Van Hove, Brigitte Van Hulle, Greta Van Malderen, Ines Van Obbergen, Joelle Van Oers, Jet Van Os, Stefaan Van Oudenhove, Family Van Rens, Martin Van Schaik, Annemie Van Winckel, Patrick Vanbellinghen, Hilde Vandenbosch, Christine Vandenneucker, Dirk Vanderlinden, Gui Vanderlinden, Elke Vanderperre, Leen Vandeweghe, Geert Vanvaerenbergh, Caroline Vanwynsberghe, Alexa Veller, Johan Venema, Rosiane Verheyden, Patti Verhoeven, Kristien Vermeiren, Frans

Verraest, Iris Verraest, Wim Verreecken, Sanne Verschuren – Van Helden, Barbara Vos, Ingrid Walraevens, Lonne Westhof, Thijs Wiener – Hermans, Rita Wijns and Peter Wilms

No Tania, no Dizzy Me books. That is simple. I would like to thank her for pushing me and supporting me in this huge endeavor and adventure. Priceless is her patience and pressure.

I also absolutely want to thank all the people who supported the crowdfunding, so that Tania's part of the Flemish (Dutch) version of the book could be translated in English. My part took much longer than expected to reach the finish, since I wanted to update the previous version of Dizzy Me. But, given the fast evolutions in this domain, I could hardly catch up with the new findings in the scientific literature. This newest English version however makes me very happy - for now.

I want to thank also all patients for participating in this book or for their support. It means a lot to me.

I want to thank Pieter Rombaut and Luc Sanspoux for their figures and Leen Vandeweghe for her superb pictures, as well as my friend and colleague Pierre – Francois Migeotte.

I want to thank my collaborators, family and friends for their support.

In particular my children Charlotte and Maxim, also for their help in some figures as well as my wife.

— Floris

I must once again start by thanking Dr. Paul Van de Heyning and Professor Floris Wuyts for curing me of my illness. Thank you to my family, my friends and all who've followed my recovery on my blog and my Facebook page. I also thank those of my fellow sufferers, e-patients and VEDA ambassadors who've allowed their voices to be heard in the pages of this book. Thank you Kugler Publications – and our original Belgian publisher ASP Editions – for believing in us and allowing us the opportunity to bring this book to fruition.

Special thanks go to Shana, my Ulule crowd funding coach and also to Dr. Eric Vente from the Netherlands, for promoting the Ulule campaign towards his patients. And how would we have achieved all this without those 250 people who made the crowdfunding campaign for translation a success? Their support made the English publication dream come true.

A standing ovation to Geert Van Hoof, for his support and amazingly professional layout skills. I'm grateful for the lovely front and back cover photos by Leen Van de Weghe. Thanks to photographers Wendy, Floris, Dian, Manly and Matthias. The medical illustrations were drawn by Luc Sanspoux and Pieter Rombaut.

The most challenging job? Finding a translator with experience in medical issues and the writer's gift for fiction style texts and having the talent to write for two different target groups: medical professionals and patients. I found Josh Pachter, equipped with both. He was my perfect match to make this English edition a success! I was surprised how he took the lead in our creative process and how he immediately got into the skin of the real life person behind Dizzy Me. He did the maximum to get to know every personage of my book. With passion for what he does, extreme professionalism, eye for detail & English-language market, and the talent to handle my jokes, tone of voice and rhythm. He feels the author's words. His translations capture so many subtle nuances of tone and the prose seems so natural that the reader can hardly believe the words didn't come directly from my original author's pen. Almost scary for me to read!

Floris, you are a driven researcher, a true professional, and the best co-author I can possibly imagine! Thanks for your invaluable scientific contributions, your unconditional support, your faith in Dizzy Me, your friendship, and your pride in our collaborative work. Can you just imagine, this is our 4th book we made together!

Thomas, your understanding and patience have been endless! Thank you for standing by me throughout this project, and for giving me the time and space to become today's Tania. In return, you get a younger, healthier wife! Still busy being Dizzy Me, and even Wobbly Wilma soon, I guess that is not really what you've had been hoping for…

Matthias, Arthur and Charlotte, I am so glad that, for you, all this history is nothing more than a story, told in the pages of this book. A book with, thank goodness, a happy ending.

— Tania
Dizzyme.eu

Index

NOTES

NOTES

NOTES

NOTES

NOTES

NOTES

NOTES

NOTES

NOTES

NOTES

NOTES

NOTES

NOTES

NOTES